Copyright 1897, by GEORGE WAHR
Copyright 1911, by GEORGE WAHR

ERRATA.

Page 155.—Thickness of gall-bladder wall 1-2 mm. instead of 1-2 cm.
Page 240.—Langhans' for Langhan's.
Page 264.—v. Kossa instead of Kossa.
Page 295.—v. Kölliker instead of Kölliker.

HERRN PROFESSOR ALEXANDER KOLISKO

Zur Erinnerung

an die ertragreichen, im Sektions-saale des

Wiener allgemeinen Krankenhauses

zugebrachten Sommertage

der Jahre

1893, 1894, 1895

gewidmet.

PREFACE TO THE SECOND EDITION.

The first edition of this book, in spite of numerous typographic errors beyond the control of the writer, was very soon exhausted. An apology is due the many, to whom, during the last ten years, a new edition has been repeatedly promised. The writer's only excuse for the failure to fulfill these promises has been the pressure of other work that has prevented such fulfillment. In the final accomplishment of these promises the book has been practically rewritten and more than doubled in size.

The autopsy method given in the main text is a composite one, made up from the Rokitansky, Virchow, Chiari and Nauwerck methods, according to the judgment of the writer as to what was the best in these, and put together with modifications and additions arising out of his own experience. The aim has been to offer a method by which an autopsy can be performed with the greatest speed and ease, and at the same time with the greatest completeness, the various steps of the operation following in logical order in such a way that nothing can be lost or destroyed, and thereby revealing a complete picture of the pathologic conditions present. A choice of methods is offered whenever the aims of the examination may be so varied as to make variations in method advantageous. The general order of the autopsy is the same as that given in the Protocol Blank-book, the present book being designed as a guide and reference-book for that. The points to be noted in the examination of each region are given in connection with the method of examination of that region, and represent the condensed special pathology of the latter. This should be of great service to the beginner in autopsy work, as affording a concise but complete guide to the most important conditions of each region. A text-book on Special Pathology should be used as a reference book in connection with these condensed statements of special pathology.

The technical methods for microscopic examination given in Part II have been brought up to date, and all recent methods of value included. Original methods have been given in preference to modifications; the latter, when of value, are also mentioned. As a rule that method has been chosen which in the light of the writer's laboratory experience has yielded uniformly the best results. An effort has been made to reduce the number of methods to the lowest number as representing the best and most indispensable ones. During the fourteen years of laboratory experience since the publication of the first edition there has been plenty of time for changes in points-of-view concerning laboratory methods. Then an ardent exponent of celloidin-imbedding as a routine method, the writer has now practically discarded it in favor of paraffin-imbedding and the celloidin-sheet made by the dextrin-sugar or molasses method. This combination method is so superior in every way to ordinary celloidin-imbedding that the latter becomes obsolete except for a limited number of conditions. A number of personal modifications of various methods will also be found in this part of the book; indeed, it is intended to be an expression of individual opinion concerning laboratory methods.

The writer's views concerning the value of teaching by *unknowns*,—that is, giving the student preparations or case-material for his own analysis and independent working-out to a diagnosis—are stronger now than they were when the preface to the first edition was written. Experiments with other methods of teaching have always brought me back to this as yielding by far the best results. It accomplishes two things—it not only teaches a knowledge of pathology, but it develops objectivity and the faculties of diagnosis, and accomplishes these with more marked success than any other method of teaching pathology.

ALDRED SCOTT WARTHIN, Ph.D., M.D.

ANN ARBOR, MICHIGAN, May, 1911.

PREFACE TO THE FIRST EDITION.

Pathologic Histology deals with departures from the normal in the various tissues of the body, which, occurring as the sequelæ of disease-processes, or standing in the closest causal relationship to the clinical symptoms and physical signs, constitute the foundation of all diagnostic conclusions, and of all rational therapeutic treatment. Without a definite knowledge of these abnormal changes, of their various forms, of the manner in which they arise and progress, no physician can deal intelligently with disease. The knowledge of the *natural history* of disease, based upon a knowledge of the normal body, makes the wise and successful practitioner; and to such, the autopsy, the microtome and the microscope must ever stand as constant aids in the satisfying of his intellectual curiosity.

It is, therefore, essential that the student in his undergraduate work should be so trained that, in addition to a broad conception of General Pathology, he may acquire also such a technical knowledge as to fit him to carry on his investigations after leaving the laboratory. Not only in everyday practice in certain lines is a knowledge of this technique necessary for diagnostic purposes, but the true physician should so hold himself toward every problem of diagnosis which presents itself to him, that with every opportunity, he will, through excision, curettage or autopsy, make use of his technical skill to further his knowledge of disease, and to aid his science toward a solution of its great problems.

It is for these reasons, that in my laboratory courses in pathologic histology, I wish to give each student a practical working knowledge of the technique of pathologic investigations. That the student become an expert as the result of such undergraduate courses is neither possible nor desirable; it is only hoped that he may be placed in a position to cope intelligently with the questions awaiting him in the field of practice.

For the guidance of the student toward this end, I have compiled this little book of laboratory methods, endeavoring to make it as practical as possible, but yet thorough and complete. The methods given are taken from the original papers, or from the compilations of Friedländer and von Kahlden, but are modified in many instances according to the writer's own experience. The autopsy methods are, in the main, those used by Kolisko of Vienna; but methods of Virchow, Chiari, Nauwerck, and others, are also given.

It is from the study of the material itself, and not from the textbook alone, that the student can obtain a proper knowledge of pathologic changes. The most comprehensive textbook can give no adequate idea of the infinite variety of these changes; there is no absolute *type,* but an endless variety of appearances more or less closely related. Only from a contemplation of this variety is it possible for the student to build up a point-of-view, and to arrive at an independent and unbiased conclusion.

The student who seeks in a preparation only the appearances described in a textbook is not studying in a scientific way. He will constantly accept the author, instead of using his own impressions for the basis of deductions, guided by the experience of others. With an unbiased mind the student should take each specimen for that alone, which it, itself, presents; and upon this he should build his conclusions. He should seek in the textbook the things he *finds* in the material; not *seek* in the latter the things he *reads* in the former. Thus may he escape superficiality, avoid errors and hasty judgments, and build up for himself a sure foundation of knowledge. For these reasons the students in my laboratory course, having been thoroughly prepared for such work by the study of normal tissues in the histologic laboratory, are given the pathologic material as *unknowns,* which under careful guidance, they are enabled to work out for themselves to a satisfactory conclusion.

The student is further aided in the fixing of his impressions, and in their expression, by means of the drawings and written descriptions which he is required to make of the preparations. In this way the faculties of observation and expression receive a training that is not otherwise possible. It is true that such a course of instruction is difficult for the student whose previous training has been deficient in the cultivation of these most important faculties; for this reason it is the more necessary that he should now apply himself to work in the scientific method.

That this method of teaching takes much more of the instructor's time is true; that it takes too much time cannot be granted when measured according to the results obtained. The frequent objection of the student that he cannot draw only emphasizes the necessity of that student's receiving the necessary training to enable him to reproduce his visual impressions.

A greater difficulty lies with the teacher. Not only must he select his preparations with wisdom, so that in the necessarily limited time of the course, the student may receive the greatest benefit; but he must be tactful and patient in leading the student to work for himself. It is easy to give a demonstration and then tell the student to work; it is very much more difficult and nerve-consuming to make the student *see* and *demonstrate* for himself. The relation of the microscopic preparation to the gross anatomy must be shown, and, when possible, demonstrated by macroscopic preparations; further, the relation to the clinical symptoms and physical signs must be made clear, so that the student receive not a narrow conception of pathologic histology as something in itself separate and complete, but as a foundation-stone to the broadest conception of diagnosis, whereby the real unity of his studies will be revealed. Moreover, the teacher must be fully awake to individual differences and needs, and carefully shape his teaching influence upon each student accordingly. The problem of the individual equation becomes especially difficult in a course of this kind.

The laboratory course in histologic pathology, in the University of Michigan, follows the general order given in the second part of this book, beginning with the diseases of the blood and the circulation, and finishing with the special pathology of the most important organs. A preparatory training in general technique is first given. About one hundred and seventy-five prepared specimens, each illustrating some especial pathologic point, are given to the class as unknowns for diagnosis. In addition each student is required to prepare about fifty slides from fresh material, performing for himself all of the necessary technical manipulations, according to the methods given in this manual. To further the work in this course, and to meet the needs of advanced students and of practitioners, this book is primarily intended.

ALDRED S. WARTHIN, Ph.D., M.D.

ANN ARBOR, January, 1897.

CONTENTS

PART I.

THE SOURCES OF PATHOLOGIC MATERIAL AND THE METHODS OF OBTAINING IT FOR EXAMINATION.

Chapter		Page
	Introduction	1
I.	The Autopsy: General Considerations	3
II.	The Order of the Autopsy	24
III.	The Protocol	33
IV.	The External Examination	41
V.	The Examination of the Spinal Cord	53
VI.	The Examination of the Head	63
VII.	The Main Incision: Thorax and Abdomen	96
VIII.	The Examination of the Thorax	106
IX.	The Examination of the Mouth and Neck	131
X.	The Examination of the Abdomen	140
XI.	The Examination of the Pelvic Organs	160
XII.	Special Regional Examination	173
XIII.	The Autopsy of the New-born	177
XIV.	The Medicolegal Autopsy	187
XV.	The Restoration of the Body	193
XVI.	Other Sources of Pathologic Material	196

PART II.
THE TREATMENT OF THE MATERIAL.

	Introduction	199
XVII.	The Laboratory Outfit	201
XVIII.	The Examination of Fresh Material	208
XIX.	The Preservation of Macroscopic Preparations	222
XX.	The Fixation and Hardening of Tissues	225
XXI.	Decalcification	232
XXII.	Imbedding	234
XXIII.	Section-cutting	238
XXIV.	The Preparation of Mounted Sections	243
XXV.	Staining and Staining Methods.—Nuclear and Protoplasmic Stains	253
XXVI.	Special Staining Methods for the Demonstration of Pathologic Conditions in Cells or Tissues	262
XXVII.	The Staining of Pathogenic Micro-organisms in Tissues	277
XXVIII.	The Staining of Special Organs and Tissues	288
XXIX.	Microscopic Examinations for Medicolegal Purposes	305
XXX.	The Study of Mounted Preparations	309

LIST OF ILLUSTRATIONS

Figure		Page
1.	Large section, or cartilage knives	10
2.	Scalpels	10
3.	Long section knife	11
4.	Myelotome	11
5.	Autopsy scissors of various types	12
6.	Enterotome	13
7.	Costotome	13
8.	Large autopsy saw	13
9.	Small autopsy saw	14
10.	Hey's saw	14
11.	Luer's rhachiotome	14
12.	T-chisel or skull-opener	14
13.	Hatchet chisel	14
14.	Straight bone chisel	14
15.	Brunetti chisels	15
16.	Steel hammer	15
17.	Wooden mallet	15
18.	Forceps	15
19.	Bone-forceps	16
20.	Bone-nippers	16
21.	Probe	16
22.	Blow-pipe	16
23.	Hand bone-drill	17
24.	Needles	18
25.	Brass measuring-stick	18
26.	Author's method of removing skull-cap	65
27.	Skull-cap after removal, showing interlocking joint	67
28.	Method of examination of brain (after Nauwerck)	71
29.	Section of brain. Ventricles opened (after Nauwerck)	72
30.	Method of Pitres	75
31.	Base of cranium after removal of brain (after Nauwerck)	79
32.	Incisions for examination of orbit, ear and nose	80
33.	Tympanic cavity after removal of tegmen (after Politzer)	81
34.	Sagittal section through left middle ear, outer half (after Politzer)	84

ILLUSTRATIONS.

35. Sagittal section through left middle ear, inner half (after Politzer) 84
36. The main incision completed (after Nauwerck).......... 97
37. Method of disarticulating sternoclavicular articulation (after Nauwerck) 101
38. Section of left ventricle and auricle (after Nauwerck).... 108
39. Removal of heart (after Nauwerck).................... 112
40. Section of right auricle and ventricle, Nauwerck method.. 114
41. Incision for opening of aortic ring (after Nauwerck)...... 115
42. Section of left lung (after Nauwerck).................. 118
43. Section of right lung (after Nauwerck)................. 119
44. Removal of neck organs (after Nauwerck).............. 132
45. Section of male pelvic organs (after Nauwerck)......... 162
46. Section of female pelvic organs (after Nauwerck)........ 164
47. Method of opening abdomen of new-born (after Nauwerck) 178
48. Section of pulmonary artery in new-born (after Nauwerck) 179
49. Method of demonstrating Béclard center (after Nauwerck) 180
50. A satisfactory microscope for the working laboratory.... 202
51. A good practical microtome 206
52. Cathcart freezing microtome 212
53. Carbonic-acid freezing microtome, Becker model........ 213
54. Bardeen freezing microtome 214
55. Knife for Bardeen freezing microtome................. 215

PART I.

SOURCES OF PATHOLOGIC MATERIAL AND METHODS OF OBTAINING IT FOR EXAMINATION.

INTRODUCTION.

The chief sources of pathologic material are the autopsy, surgical operation, diagnostic excision and curetting, the spontaneous discharge of diseased tissue, and the experimental production of pathologic conditions in animals. To these sources may be added the blood and other body-fluids, as well as pathologic fluids, exudates, effusions, cyst-contents, etc., particularly the cellular elements found in the sediment of such fluids.

That an accurate pathologic diagnosis be secured, the material must first be properly obtained, its gross characteristics carefully noted, the portion to be examined microscopically chosen with discrimination, and, finally, the microscopic examination itself carried out along the various lines indicated. All of these procedures require the knowledge of a certain amount of technique, and the general principles of such technique should be familiar to every student of medicine. While it is not possible that every medical graduate can enter into the active practice of his profession as an expert pathologist, yet the possession of the technical knowledge necessary to perform an autopsy properly and to select with discrimination the tissue for microscopic examination gives to a physician a distinct practical advantage. This advantage becomes the greater if to the possession of this knowledge there be added also a practical working knowledge of the technique necessary for the microscopic examination and diagnosis. Not that this knowledge should be so extensive as to cover the great field of special methods; all that is really essential is a knowledge of the general principles of laboratory examinations; and a very large proportion of practical work can be successfully carried out if the physician possesses this foundation knowledge. In the first days of practice a young physician so equipped often finds that his laboratory training comes to be his chief source of income and opens the way to a successful professional career. It constitutes a professional asset which the older practitioner usually does not possess.

CHAPTER I.

THE AUTOPSY: GENERAL CONSIDERATIONS.

1. **AUTOPSY** (Postmortem examination, necropsy, necroscopy, obduction, mortopsy, section; Latin, sectio cadaveris, sectio anatomica, autopsia cadaverica, sectio, obductio; French, autopsie cadaverique, nécropsie; German, **Leichenschau, Section, Obduction**) is the term preferably applied to the examination of the dead body, conducted for the purpose of ascertaining the cause of death, for the study of the pathologic conditions present with reference to their nature and cause, or for the obtaining of anthropologic, anatomic or surgical data. When carried out primarily with the view of obtaining evidence of legal importance, as in the case of a suspected crime, accidental death, the identification of a body, in damage suits for injuries received, malpractice, insurance, etc., the autopsy is usually styled **medico-legal**, or the German term **obduction** is not infrequently applied. The terms **prosector** and **obducent**, although used originally in a medicolegal sense, are now generally applied to the person performing the autopsy whether medicolegal or not.

2. **IMPORTANCE OF THE AUTOPSY.** The opportunity of performing an autopsy should be regarded by the physician and student as a very great privilege. Even to the prosector with an experience of several thousand autopsies to his credit, each new examination of a dead body becomes a new revelation and extends still farther his intellectual horizon. To the student and physician in practice each autopsy may, if performed in the proper spirit, become in itself an educational factor of the greatest value. In no other scientific procedure is there such a demand made upon the faculties of observation, judgment and interpretation, and in no other is there such intimate correlation between methods of technique and the higher intellectual processes. It is unnecessary to add that the ability to perform an autopsy in the proper manner presupposes a foundation of accurate anatomic and pathologic knowledge as well as a capacity for careful work.

Primarily, the aim of the autopsy is to ascertain the cause of death and to acquire knowledge of the changes produced in the tissues and organs by the disease-process. If for no other purpose than that of extending our knowledge of disease, the autopsy becomes the most valuable factor in furthering the development of medical science. We have but entered into the broad, rich fields of pathology; at any time new facts may be discovered or observations of the most far-reaching nature made. From year to year the statistics of the most common diseases must be revised in the light of new conceptions of disease. Through the autopsy there lies within the reach of every practitioner the opportunity of contributing something worth while to the general sum of medical knowledge. There is not a pathologic condition in the medical category that does not call out for illumination upon some point or other. The phenomena of malignant tumors, the earliest stages of the so-called chronic affections, as well as the majority of the infectious diseases, require further autopsy observations for their elucidation. The autopsy establishment of the diagnosis is also of the greatest importance in giving value to vital statistics. Until we have a more universal confirmation of the clinical diagnosis by the pathologic our vital statistics must of necessity be imperfect.

To the practitioner the autopsy offers further a most valuable control of subjectivity and a guide to methods of diagnosis and treatment. Without such a control no one is so likely to get into a dangerous rut as the practicing physician. The disclosures of the autopsy will enable him to correct faulty methods, and should effectually check any tendency to superficial diagnosis. Particularly is this the case with regard to such diagnostic methods as palpation, percussion and auscultation. Postmortem percussion offers a most valuable means of acquiring precision in this important branch of physical diagnosis. The percussion boundaries may be marked upon the body by pencil, or long pins may be inserted, so that when the body is opened the exact relation of the percussion area to the organ in question may be noted. In the case of palpable tumors the results of palpation before the body is opened should be carefully controlled by the findings when the actual conditions are exposed. Even when the cause of death seems obvious it is worth while to perform an autopsy at every opportunity offered, both for the sake of controlling technical methods and for the pictures of disease revealed. More accurate knowledge of the nature of the processes of disease can be obtained through one autopsy than through months of textbook reading. To the surgeon the opportunity of examining cases dying after surgical operation should be a source of great satisfaction. The review of anatomic relationships offered by the autopsy is in itself worth while, and in the case of healthy individuals killed by accident the survey of the normal appearances of the organs and tissues offers an opportunity for study too valuable to be neglected. Further, it is justifiable to practice upon the cadaver any surgical operation that does not disfigure it. Removal of the spleen, transplantation of thyroid tissue into the spleen, decapsulation of the kidney, transplantation of ovarian tissue, gastric and intestinal operations, anastomosis of bloodvessels, operations upon the uterus and cervix, prostate, vas deferens, thyroid, nose, ear, etc., and many other surgical procedures may be practiced with profit upon a cadaver during the course of an autopsy. The feasibility of a new operative method or the improvement of an old one may thus be demonstrated.

In the case of medico-legal autopsies the ends of justice as well as the life, liberty or reputation of some individual may depend upon the results of the postmortem examination. In all cases to which there is any suspicion attached, or in which the cause or manner of death is doubtful an autopsy should be legally required, but unfortunately this is not yet done in this country. Physicians individually should endeavor to create in the public mind a more healthy attitude toward the autopsy and an appreciation of its usefulness. As to his own share in the advantages derived from it, it is safe to say that no physician can perform an autopsy properly without having his experience widened, his knowledge of disease increased, his diagnostic faculties sharpened and his tendency to subjectivity controlled. Last, but far from being the least, should be his gain in honesty and humility.

3. **LEGAL ASPECTS OF THE AUTOPSY.** The individual cannot dispose of his dead body without the consent of his nearest heirs, except in those States (New York) providing by statute that a person may direct the disposition of his cadaver. The legal rights to the corpse are vested first in the husband or wife of the deceased; if none, then first in the father, then in the mother; after the parents, in the brothers or sisters; after them in the next of kin, according to the course of common law; and then to the remotest degree according to the law of descent of personal property. An autopsy performed with the consent of the relative having the body in custody cannot be questioned, if it is properly performed. In the case of members of societies requiring autopsies the membership cards or certificates should be endorsed by the nearest heir.

A physician who performs an autopsy without the consent of the person having the custody of the deceased does so at his own risk, except in those cases in which the autopsy is in accordance with legal statutes. In the majority of the States there are statutes providing that the Coroner or Board of Health shall order an autopsy whenever a person is found dead and the cause of his death is not apparent, and cannot be ascertained from the evidence given, or from a superficial examination of the body. In such cases no permit from the relatives is necessary, and an autopsy performed under the direction of law is never subject to legal punishment, if it has been performed according to approved methods. Nevertheless, even in these cases it is a better policy to secure the consent of the custodian of the body, when this is possible.

When consent to an autopsy is withheld and the physician feels that such an examination is necessary, he should turn the case over to the Coroner or Board of Health, and act under such direction. Conflicting decisions, however, have been made in different States. The Supreme Court of Indiana (1909) held that a Coroner cannot order an autopsy unless there was a reasonable supposition that death had occurred from violence or casualty. A suit brought by an Indiana physician to recover fee for an autopsy held on the order and under the direction of a Coroner was set aside on the ground that there was not the slightest suspicion of death from casualty or violence. Such a decision is too narrow and not framed in accordance with the actual needs of the times in so far as the protection or enlightenment of the community is concerned. Under such a decision a Coroner or Board of Health could not in safety order an autopsy in the case of a death in which the diagnosis had not been established clinically, when no suspicion of violence or casualty exists, although the establishment of the diagnosis through an autopsy might be of the greatest importance to the family or community.

On the other hand the Court of Appeals in Kentucky (1906) affirmed judgment for the defendant in a suit for damages brought against a physician for performing an unauthorized autopsy to secure a burial permit, the court holding that, if the autopsy was made in good faith for the purpose of ascertaining the cause of death in order that a burial certificate might be granted, and if the autopsy was made decently with due regard to the sex of the deceased and without unnecessary incisions or mutilations, there could be no grounds for damages. This is a reasonable and just decision and laws framed upon it should be passed in all the States. Autopsies performed under such conditions, however, should always be conducted in the presence of several witnesses competent to testify as to the methods used.

In several States legal authority is given to the Board of Health to order an autopsy whenever the health-interests of the people demand such an investigation. Autopsies performed under such orders against the desire of the relatives should always be carried out with extreme care and in the presence of proper witnesses.

State and charitable hospitals cannot be made liable for autopsy performed by Coroner or Board of Health, when the consent of the relatives is withheld. It is high time that all charitable institutions in this country should require an autopsy from all patients dying within their walls. The cards of admission should contain a clause to this effect, and such cards should be counter-signed by the nearest relatives.

Inasmuch as some life-insurance policies contain clauses requiring the presence of a representative of the company at the autopsy or a forfeiture of the claims, it is best to ascertain if such policies exist in any given case, and to notify the company. The Supreme Court of Missouri has decided that an autopsy made in ignorance of such an insurance clause is no bar to recovery if the company be notified in time for a re-examination of the body.

Supreme Court decisions also hold that consent for an autopsy implies removal of organs and tissues for microscopic study, when such is necessary to fulfill the object of the autopsy.

One of the great needs of this country is a uniform autopsy law and the establishment of a proper medicolegal autopsy code, as in Germany. As conditions exist at the present, crimes may be easily concealed, the safety of the community endangered by failures in diagnosis of communicable affections, and our morbidity and mortality statistics become a shame and reproach to the nation. The majority of our medicolegal autopsies are made by ignorant and imperfectly trained coroners and coroners' physicians, mostly political appointees of inferior material. We need in our medical schools a greater amount of attention paid to the teaching of autopsy-technique and gross pathology. The community must also be educated to a realization of the value of autopsies. It is the duty of every physician and layman to work diligently for the improvement of existing conditions. Had the ideas of a former Governor of the State of Michigan been realized there would have been compulsory autopsies upon the bodies of every person dying within the State, and far-reaching results would have been attained. The economic importance of tuberculosis and the venereal diseases would have been made clear, the profession and laity alike educated, and the progress of preventive medicine tremendously aided.

4. **PERMISSION FOR AUTOPSY.** It is a desirable and certainly a wise precaution to obtain a written permit for the autopsy from the next of kin or from the legal representative of the body, in case the examination has not been ordered by law. Some of the legal decisions quoted above offer sufficient grounds for this precaution. The following form is in use in the University of Michigan Hospital.

No.......   Ann Arbor, Michigan................., 19..

Professor of Pathology.......................
    University of Michigan.

    Permission has been given by........................, who bears the relationship of.................to........................, to hold a postmortem upon the remains of..........................., with the understanding that the object of such postmortem is to ascertain the cause of death, and that you are to use such means as you deem best to make a thorough examination for the proper attainment of the object desired, excepting that...

..............................Superintendent.

There can be no doubt that the public in general is beginning to appreciate the usefulness of autopsies, as it is much easier to obtain them now than it was ten years ago. The proper display of tact and a reasonable exposition of the object of the examination will practically always meet the objections urged on sentimental grounds. Aside from these the chief objection usually met with is the fear of mutilation of the body. Emphatic assurance may be given in this respect, not only as to the entire absence of any disfigurement resulting from the examination, but also as to the marked improvement in the general appearance and condition of the cadaver as the result of the autopsy.

While it is obviously difficult to give any specific rules as to the method to be pursued in seeking permission for an autopsy, there are certain arguments that can be used to advantage. Natural curiosity, the general good to humanity, the control of diagnostic and therapeutic methods, new knowledge to be gained, the question of inherited or infectious conditions, the strengthening of insurance claims, etc., are some of the lines that may be followed in working for an autopsy. Satisfaction is always expressed when definite light is thrown upon the hereditary or infectious nature of the condition.

Religious scruples may often be overcome by an appeal to the pastor or priest.

In a certain number of cases the matter is hopeless from the beginning, but in the majority the autopsy may be secured by the exercise of proper tact and patience. The laity should be educated to ask for the autopsy; and even at the present time laymen often show a greater willingness in this direction than some members of the profession. That physicians and undertakers who discourage or oppose autopsies should be avoided is a principle that should be instilled into the minds of the public at large. Undertakers soon come to recognize the aid given them by the autopsy in the matter of embalming and preserving the body, and the prosecutor should always show his readiness to allow the undertaker to profit by his operations, and to render him such definite help as may be within his power.

As a last resort the offer of a small amount of financial aid in the burial expenses will secure sometimes a permission otherwise refused. In extreme cases the physician may decline to sign the death certificate, or the Coroner may be called in, or the case turned over to the Board of Health. Under suspicious circumstances such procedures are necessary, but threats to resort to these expedients should not be made without good reasons.

With the request for the autopsy should be included the right to take such portions of organs or tissues as is necessary for a microscopic examination and for the complete diagnosis. It is, of course, never necessary and certainly unwise in the majority of cases to make any definite statements as to what or how much shall be taken away or left. No specimens should be taken if this is absolutely forbidden; and, while a half autopsy is better than none, the importance of the microscopic examination should be urged, if necessary, as strongly as the performance of the autopsy. The use of a written permission, such as is given above, obviates the necessity of making a special request for material and avoids the complications that such a request often brings about. Moreover, the legal decision above quoted grants the right to microscopic examination as included in the permit for the autopsy when such an examination is necessary to complete the aims of the autopsy.

5. **AUTOPSY INSTRUMENTS.** An autopsy can be properly performed with very few instruments; indeed, a knife and a saw, with a needle to close up the body, would suffice for the majority of cases. But there are very great advantages in the use of certain instruments adapted especially to autopsy needs, and these the

physician should gradually acquire for his work. It is not advisable to purchase the so-called "postmortem sets" sold by the dealers, but far better to start with two or three of the most necessary instruments and gradually add to these. Surgical instruments as they become discarded can often be made to do good service in the autopsy outfit. In private practice the fewer instruments one can get along with the better, as there is much less trouble in carrying them about and in taking care of them, and it is better to make the performance of the autopsy as inconspicuous as possible. In teaching institutions and in hospitals the number and variety of instruments that can be utilized in autopsy work are limited only by the financial means at disposal, but even under the most favorable conditions in this respect it is better to simplify as much as possible. The list given below will meet all requirements.

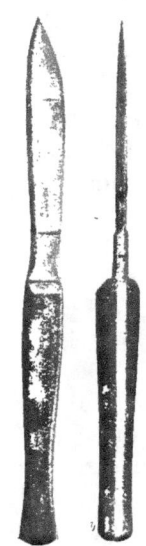

FIG. 1—Large Section, or Cartilage Knives

Knives. The *large section-* or *cartilage-knife* is the most important cutting instrument used in autopsy work. It is a strong, heavy knife 20-22 cms. long, with handle and blade of about equal length. The blade has a heavy back, a bluntly rounded rather than a sharp point (more blunt than appears in the illustration), and bellies at its anterior third, narrowing toward the handle. In its widest part the blade should measure about 1¾ cms. The handle is heavy, 1½ cms. broad, and a little over 1 cm. in thickness toward the blade, gradually diminishing to about ¾ cm. at the posterior third, then increasing to 1 cm. toward the end. This variation in thickness gives a gentle curve to the handle that is of great importance in adapting the latter to the form of the closed hand, so that the knife becomes practically a cutting extension of the fore-arm. With this knife all the chief incisions are made, and it is rarely out of the hands of the operator during the autopsy. The handle or blade may be made shorter or longer according to preference, but the other features of the instrument are most important.

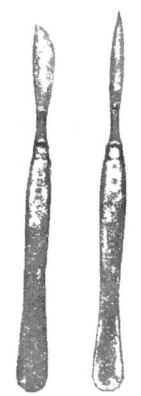

FIG. 2—Scalpels

AUTOPSY INSTRUMENTS.

Scalpel. (See Fig. 2.) A number of *dissecting scalpels* of varying sizes are needed for finer dissections. They should have a metal handle, and are preferably of one-piece construction.

Long Section- or Brain-Knife. In place of the broad thin brain-knife usually advised, an *amputation-knife* can be used to much better advantage in the section of the brain and in making the chief incisions in the large organs. It should have a sharp point rather than a blunt one.

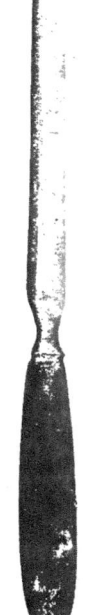

Fig. 3—Long Section Knife

Myelotome. This is used only for the purpose of cutting the spinal cord squarely across in the removal of the brain. It has a slender steel stalk with wooden handle, and a short, thin, narrow blade set obliquely at the end of the stalk. This instrument is not absolutely necessary, as the cord may be satisfactorily cut with the point of the long section knife.

Scissors. (See Fig. 5.) A number of these are of service: one large and strong pair with long handles and short stout blades, another large pair curved or bent with the longer blade blunt- or probe-pointed, a small pair with a narrow, probe-pointed blade for opening small vessels or ducts.

Enterotome. (See Fig. 6.) For opening the intestine the enterotome or intestinal scissors are used. These consist of one long probe-pointed blade bluntly rounded at its end, and a shorter blade with straight end fitting into the longer blade. Neither blade should be sharp-pointed.

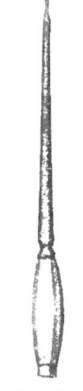

Fig. 4 Myelotome

Costotome. (See Fig. 7.) The cartilage-shears have two short, thick blades, the upper one with a broad belly, the lower one curved. Between the strong handles a spring is placed, and the construction should be such that when the blades are closed the ends of the handles do not touch. The form in which the handles meet and are secured with a catch is a dangerous autopsy instrument because of the severe pinching that the operator's hand is sure sooner or later to receive.

Saws. (See Figs. 8, 9, 10.) A *small hand-saw* (*bone-saw*) is necessary for opening the skull, and the same saw may be used to open the spinal canal. It is sometimes made with a rounded point (*"fox-tail" saw*). For sawing vertically through the base of the skull when exposing the nasal tract a larger *butcher's saw* with a high frame may be used. For sawing the angles of the skull-cap *Hey's saw* may be of service but is not essential. A *metacarpal saw* may be used for opening small bones or the long bones of an infant. *Band saws* are sometimes used in opening up the nasal tract.

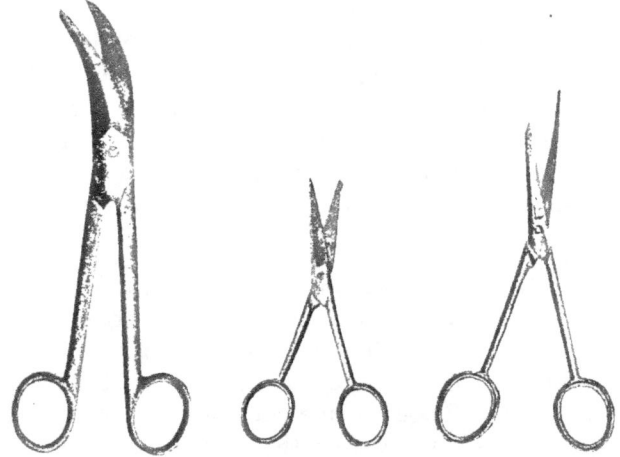

FIG. 5—Autopsy Scissors of Various Types

Rhachiotome. (See Fig. 11.) This instrument consists of two curved saw blades placed parallel to each other in such a way that the distance between them can be regulated by screws. There are two handles, a horizontal one for the right hand, and an upright one for the left hand attached to the fixed saw blade. It is used in opening the spinal canal.

Chisels. (See Figs. 12, 13, 14.) A very convenient autopsy instrument is the *T-chisel* or *skull-opener*, used for springing off the skull-cap and in detaching the periosteum. *Side-* and *guarded-chisels* may be used for the same purpose. The *hatchet-chisel* may also be used on the skull or spinal column. *Straight* and *curved bone-chisels* are also necessary for the examination of the bones and bone-marrow.

Brunetti Chisels. (See Fig. 15.) These are of great service in opening the spinal canal, but require some practice for their proper use. When used with skill they are preferable to the rhachiotome. The chisels are rights and lefts, and have a long, heavy,

AUTOPSY INSTRUMENTS.

curved blade, broadening toward the cutting end, which has on its right or left side a small blunt projection that is introduced into the spinal canal after the removal of a portion of one of the vertebræ. This projection serves as a director and lever, while the cutting edge of the chisel is driven through the lateral portions of the bony covering of the canal by means of blows from a wooden mallet received upon the heavy handles.

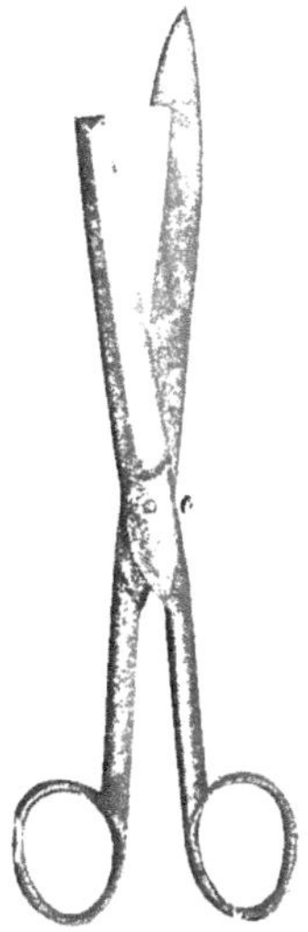

Hammer. (See Fig. 16.) The steel hammer of the amputation- or bone-sets is often of great service in autopsy work. The hook at the end of the handle may be used to lift up the skull-cap after the sawing is completed.

Mallet. (See Fig. 17.) A wooden mallet is necessary for the use of the Brunetti chisels. It may be loaded with lead or the end may be covered with felt to deaden the sound of the blows.

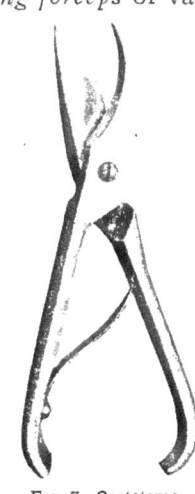

FIG. 6—Enterotome

Forceps. (See Figs. 18, 19, 20.) *Dissecting forceps* of various types are useful in the finer dissections. *Cover-glass forceps* should be at hand for use in the taking of smears. A pair of strong *bone-forceps* may be of occasional service in cutting ribs or small bones. When the spinal canal is opened by means of the Brunetti chisels or rhachiotome the loosened fragments of the vertebræ should be jerked off by means of lion-forceps, or a strong pair of ordinary nippers may be used for the same purpose.

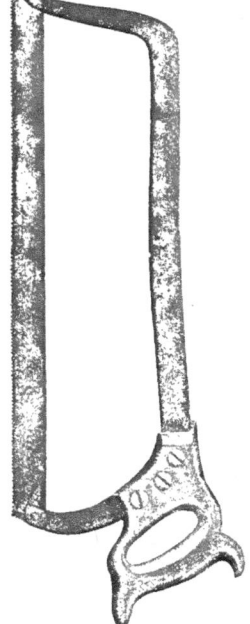

FIG. 8—Large Autopsy Saw

FIG. 7—Costotome

Miscellaneous Instruments. (See Figs. 21, 22, 23, 24, 25.) Probes of various sizes, grooved and curved directors, retractors, catheters, both metal and flexible, injection-syringe, blow-pipe with valve, trocar, canulas, hand-drill for wiring bones, an iron-vise, etc., all find a place of usefulness in autopsy technique. In institution work motor band-saws, trephining or dental engines, drills, etc., may greatly facilitate the progress of autopsies when the daily number of these is great and when special examinations of the ear or nose are required. The needles for sewing up the incisions should be large, strong and slightly curved. A strong linen thread should be used for stitching and for ligatures.

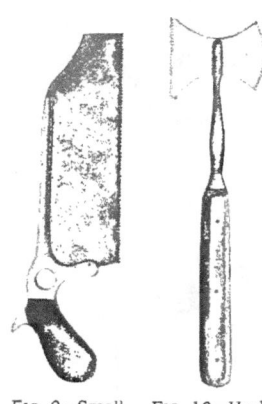

FIG. 9 - Small Autopsy Saw FIG. 10—Hey's Saw

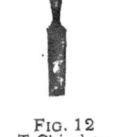

FIG. 12 T-Chisel or Skull-Opener

FIG. 13 Hatchet-Chisel

Besides the instruments mentioned above there should be brass or nickel measuring sticks, one 10 cms. long and one 30 cms. long, a flexible metal measuring tape, graduated glass vessels for measuring fluids, graduated glass cones for orifices, etc. Suitable scales should also be provided. Rounded or triangular wooden blocks are needed to elevate portions of the body. For the display of gross specimens as they are removed from the body, agate dishes or wooden trays that have been infiltrated with paraffin should be at hand. The necessary outfit for the taking of material for bacteriologic examinations should always be present. Likewise cover-glasses and slides for smears, and reagents for the examination and preservation of tissue should be at hand. Sponges, pails, towels, tow or excelsior for filling up the body-cavities, disinfectants, etc., must be supplied.

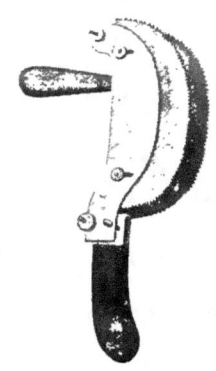

FIG. 11—Luer's Rhachiotome

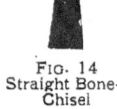

FIG. 14 Straight Bone-Chisel

The autopsy outfit may be extended indefinitely to suit the requirements of the conditions or the ideas of the pathologist. In actual practice, however, the physician may confine his requirements to the limits of a cartilage knife, dissecting scalpel, forceps, one small probe-pointed pair of scissors, enterotome, saw, T-chisel, needles, thread, sponge and specimen bottles. Five or six dollars would cover the initial expense, and the set may be gradually increased. It would seem unnecessary to decry the use of surgical instruments for the autopsy. Once an instrument is used in an autopsy it should be left in the autopsy set.

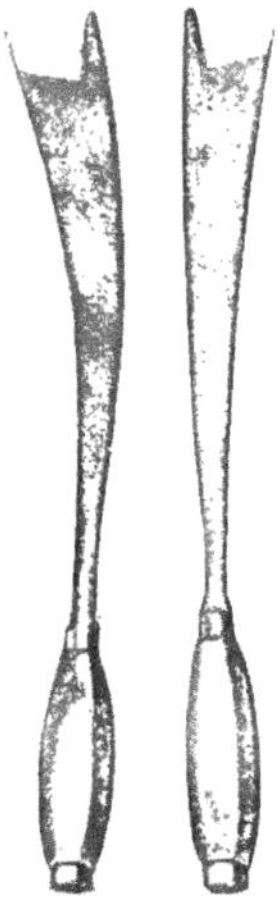

CARE OF INSTRUMENTS. The cutting instruments should always be kept sharp and bright. Care should be taken that when the knives are sharpened the blunt points and rounded bellies are not ground off. After use the knives should be cleaned, disinfected and wiped dry. A tight galvanized iron box containing wire trays and a bottom pan for holding formalin is very practical in institution work. In private practice the knives after cleaning and disinfection may be kept in a holder made of Canton flannel or chamois skin having pockets fitted to the instruments; the whole may be rolled up into a small and compact bundle.

FIG. 15—Brunetti Chisels

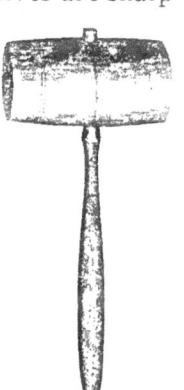

FIG. 17—Wooden Mallet

6. **PREPARATION FOR THE AUTOPSY.** Permission having been obtained, the autopsy should be performed without delay. It is very important that the examination should be carried out before the body has become cold, if any thorough microscopic study of the tissues is to be made. Changes in the finer structure of cells and nuclei quickly take place, and certain tissues, such as parts of the nervous system, the medullary portion of the adrenals, the pancreas, mucosa of gastro-intestinal tract, etc., within an hour or so after death are usually no longer fit for microscopic study. In all cases, therefore, it is best to make the autopsy as soon as possible after death, that is, as soon as positive signs of death appear. In the majority of cases this takes place within an hour, and the most favorable time for the performance of the autopsy falls within one to three hours after death.

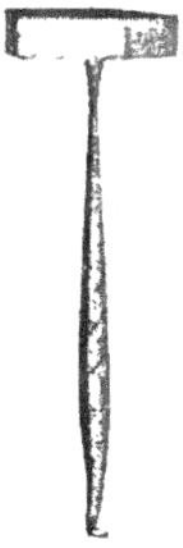

FIG. 16—Steel Hammer

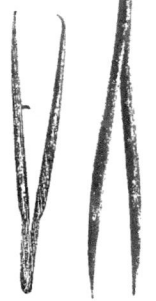

FIG. 18—Forceps

Under certain circumstances it may be necessary to make the examination sooner, but for various reasons the operation is very repugnant when performed within the first half-hour after death. For ordinary purposes an autopsy performed within twelve to twenty-four hours is usually satisfactory. Occasionally it becomes necessary for medicolegal purposes to examine a body some days, weeks, or even months after death and burial.

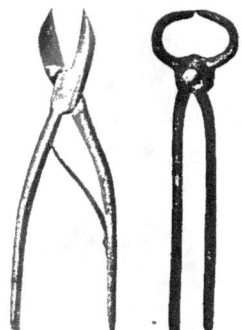

FIG. 19 Bone-Forceps FIG. 20 Bone-Nippers

The body should not be frozen if microscopic studies are to be made. When the autopsy is delayed cold storage just above the freezing point produces less change in the gross pathologic picture, as well as in the finer structure. No embalming fluids, injections, punctures, etc., should be allowed, and undertakers should be instructed not to do these things until after the question of autopsy has been decided and the operation completed. If the use of an embalming fluid becomes necessary, formalin, not stronger than a ten per cent solution, should be advised, as it does not damage the tissues and hinders but little the operations of the autopsy. Strong solutions, as found in the usual embalming fluids, render the tissues stiff and hard and cause color changes, while the strong vapors are very unpleasant to the obducent. The use of arsenical embalming fluids or preparations should be wholly discountenanced. When it is desired to study the mucosa of the stomach or intestine, it may be fixed soon after death by the introduction of a fixing fluid into the stomach or intestine by means of a tube and pump. Finally, instructions should be given that the body shall not be dressed for burial until after the autopsy.

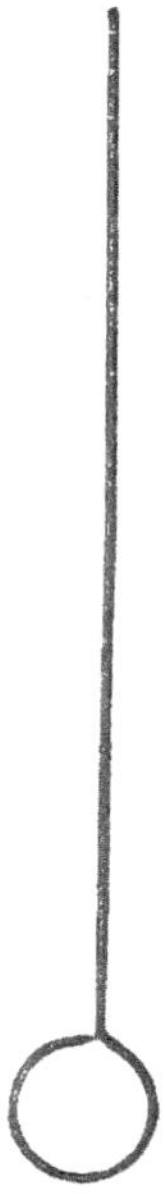

FIG. 21 Probe

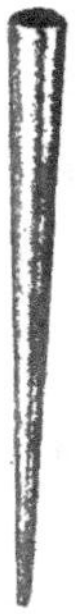

FIG. 22 Blow-Pipe

The necessity of making special preparations for an autopsy depends upon its performance in a regularly appointed autopsy room or under the conditions of private practice. In the former case the autopsy room should be constructed to meet the demands of the work. In teaching hospitals it should be a large, well-lighted and properly-ventilated room with proper facilities for teaching-staff and students, and should be so

PREPARATION FOR THE AUTOPSY.

connected with the hospital wards that the conveyal of bodies may be protected from observation. In the same building there should be the pathological laboratory, library and museum, a waiting-room, and under some conditions a chapel for funeral services. The autopsy room itself should have a grooved concrete floor sloping to a central drain, the furniture should be of simple construction, and so built that the entire room may be washed with a hose. The seats should be arranged in an amphitheatre facing the northern side of the building, which should be constructed practically wholly of glass, the lower sashes containing ground glass or prisms. The northern half of the roof should likewise be of glass.

In the pit, in the field of strongest illumination, should be placed the autopsy table. This should be strongly built, of marble, slate, soapstone, artificial stone, copper, zinc, etc., about seven feet long, thirty inches wide, and thirty to thirty-six inches high. A high table is much preferable to a low one. It should have a top with grooves slanting toward a central perforated plate fixed in the central hollow standard in such a way that the top may be freely revolved. In the standard there should be a drain and ventilating shaft connected with a fan revolving outward. The drain from the table as well as the others from the laboratory should empty into a large catch-basin where the contents may be sterilized before passing into the main sewer. Above the table a combination gas and electric light with hot and cold water-pipes should be arranged. A sheet of blue glass of the proper tint may be used in connection with the illuminating apparatus to give day-light effects.

Extra tables, weighing and measuring apparatus, sinks, lavatories, bacteriologic outfit, sterilizer, instrument-case, etc., may be supplied as needed. In the case of delayed permission, or when the law requires that the bodies be kept a certain length of time before the autopsy, it becomes necessary to provide a proper cold-storage

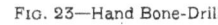
FIG. 23—Hand Bone-Drill

18   THE AUTOPSY: GENERAL CONSIDERATIONS.

apparatus. The local conditions will suggest the most convenient and appropriate construction. In routine autopsy service well-trained assistants and attendants become a necessary factor in the satisfactory performance of the work.

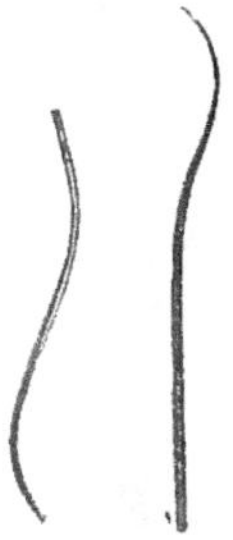

In private practice the autopsy is usually made in a private dwelling or, more rarely, in an undertaker's shop. Under such conditions much depends upon the ability of the operator to make the best of things. In place of a proper table, the cadaver must be examined upon the bed, undertaker's body-rest or shutter, in or upon the coffin, on the coffin lid, box, door, shutter, table or board. It is always advisable to move the body from the bed when anything else can be found upon which it can be placed. The support should be put in front of the window giving the best light and the cadaver placed upon this with its left side toward the window. Care should, of course, be always taken that the operation cannot be witnessed from without. A piece of oil-cloth or several layers of newspapers should be placed upon the floor beneath and around the support. When it is necessary to make the autopsy on the bed or in the coffin an abundant supply of old newspapers tucked under and around the cadaver will usually prevent the escape of blood or fluids.

FIG. 24
Autopsy Needles

An abundance of cold water should be provided, also a slop-pail, several basins, towels, old cloths, sponges, etc. Before the operation is begun the instruments and utensils, specimen bottles, needle and thread, etc., should be arranged. A stick of wood may serve as a head-rest. Material for filling up the body and restoring its form should be secured, according to the need for such. Hay, bran, tow, excelsior, old cloths, paper, etc., may be used for this purpose.

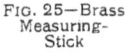
FIG. 25—Brass Measuring-Stick

When all is ready for the operation members of the family or of the laity should be tactfully gotten out of the room. It is always well to ask members of the family if they desire to be present, but this invitation should be given in the expectation that it will not be accepted. The effect of an autopsy upon the minds of the laity is not always a pleasant one, and harm is sometimes done through the misinterpretation of necessary procedures and the resulting gossip. In private practice it is worth while, as a matter of courtesy, to invite several of one's colleagues to witness or take part in the autopsy. An ideal way would be to have one of these perform the operation in expectation of future reciprocation. In the interests of objective observation a clinician should never perform the autopsies of his own cases, but should turn them over to a trained pathologist or to a colleague. The operator is usually in a better position to know what to do than the onlookers, and while the suggestions of the latter are usually futile they may be endured for the occasional great help derived from them.

As far as the obducent himself is concerned he may prepare himself simply by removing his coat and rolling up his sleeves, or he may wear an autopsy coat or apron. While an autopsy can without doubt be best performed with hands bared, the danger to the operator is sufficiently great to lead him to sacrifice the undoubtedly greater technical skill thus gained, to his own safety, by the use of some protective. Rubber gloves of a medium weight, reaching half way to the elbows, are a great protection when carefully cleaned, sterilized and cared for. The sleeves of the coat may overlap the gloves and be fastened to these by an elastic band. When gloves are not used the hands may be covered with carbolized vaseline, or a six per cent solution of guttapercha in benzin. Cuts, abrasions, hang-nails, etc., must be protected by surgeon's-plaster, collodion, finger-cots, etc. When these are used it may be necessary to remove them during the course of the autopsy, as they are easily torn or become loose. Frequent washing in flowing water lessens the danger of infection. Blood and other fluids from the body should never be allowed to dry upon the skin or upon anything used in connection with the autopsy.

Gloves should be thoroughly washed and scrubbed; and, when clean, washed in four per cent formaldehyde and dried before they are removed from the hands. They should be then dusted inside and out with talcum powder and put away dry. When they are again used they should be tested for holes by filling them with water. After having been used several times they easily tear. If the autopsy has been performed with unprotected hands, thorough disinfection of these, particularly of the finger-nails, should be carried out. Unpleasant odors may be removed from the hands by the use of mustard, dilute tincture of benzoin, turpentine, etc., and then washing with tincture of green soap. Rubbing with cornmeal is very effective in removing discolorations of the skin, particularly the blood-stains fixed by formaldehyde that occur so often in the course of autopsies on bodies injected by the undertaker.

Postmortem infections should receive prompt surgical attention, as the smallest one is dangerous and may develop in a few hours to such an extent as to cause the most alarming constitutional symptoms. In a way all autopsy work, like surgical operations, offers a risk to the operator. This is particularly great in all cases of pyogenic infection, tuberculosis, blastomycosis, syphilis and the acute specific infectious diseases. Any of these infections may be received through the unbroken skin by way of a hair-follicle; but previous cuts, abrasions, hang-nails, etc., form a frequent avenue of entrance for the infecting agent, as well as punctures, scratches and cuts received during the autopsy from instruments, spicules of bone, needles, etc. It is particularly dangerous to allow blood, pus or exudates from the peritoneal or thoracic cavity to enter a glove through a hole. A finger or hand so bathed is very likely to develop hair-follicle infections. All wounds received during the autopsy should be allowed to bleed freely, and then should be thoroughly washed in sterile water, alcohol and ether and an antiseptic.

Tuberculous warts are very common on the hands of prosectors having a large autopsy service and not using gloves. A generalized tuberculosis may follow. These warts are easily removed by repeated painting with fuming nitric acid, just sufficient to keep the skin yellow. If this treatment fails such warts should be excised. Syphilis has been reported only a few times as due to postmortem infection; but observations tend to show that the spirochætes may remain virulent for several hours (7-24) after death.

7. **AUTOPSY TECHNIQUE.** *The object of the autopsy is to examine thoroughly, in as short a time as possible, and in the easiest and most convenient method, all of the organs and tissues of the body, with reference to the occurrence of disease-changes, in such a way that nothing will be overlooked or obscured.* The preservation of relationships becomes, therefore, a very important matter; and nothing should be done to disturb these until a complete pathologic picture has been obtained. All unnecessary handling and cutting must be avoided. No hasty or ill-advised cuts should be made. Careful deliberation is often necessary as to the proper course to be pursued in order to obtain the proper result. Each autopsy is a law unto itself in this regard. New complications constantly arise and must be studied before the right way of revealing the solution of the pathologic problem is found. *Above all things nothing should be destroyed until its relationships have been fully*

determined. False steps taken in an autopsy cannot be retraced, and the complete investigation and the successful attainment of a diagnosis may be made impossible by improper methods of technique. As in all other technical matters there is a *best* way of carrying out the different steps of the autopsy; and as this best way must be altered to suit the conditions as they arise, it follows that there is both a *science* and *art* of autopsy-making. Some general rules can be laid down that apply consistently to all autopsies, but strict adherence to one method is impossible in all cases. As in everything else the prosector should be master of his technique and not let it master him.

When everything is ready for the autopsy the operator should take his place at the right side of the cadaver, unless he happens to be left-handed, when it may be more convenient for him to stand at the cadaver's left. This position at the cadaver's side he does not leave, except when opening the cranium, when he stands behind the head. When the spinal cord is removed posteriorly he still remains on the same side of the table, although the cadaver, having been turned over, presents its left side toward him. The instruments arranged in proper order should be on a tray close at his right hand, either on a neighboring table or placed on the autopsy table. As they are used they should be washed and returned to their proper place and not allowed to lie on the body or table.

The cutting technique employed in the autopsy is, as a rule, quite different from that employed in surgical operations or in dissection. For the large incisions the cartilage-knife is used. It should be held in the palm of the hand so that when the arm is extended the knife-blade becomes an extension of the axis of the arm, and used with a free arm-movement, fingers and hand being firmly fixed to the knife-handle. Long, sweeping cuts, adequate in pressure, and giving smooth and even incisions, are made by moving chiefly from the shoulder, with secondary movement from the elbow. The knife-blade should not be pressed or pushed into the tissues, but should be *drawn* through them rather quickly, cutting as it is drawn. The greater the force used, the more swift the drawing-motion should be. All cuts should be clean; if made in the wrong place they will do less damage than ragged, uneven incisions. The toe of the cartilage knife is used for the beginning and end of long incisions and for cutting in hollow or depressed surfaces. For flat surfaces the belly of the knife is employed. The heel of the blade can be used for cutting cartilages. The incisions made in the body should be directed away from the operator, especial care being taken to avoid injuring his left hand or the hands or arms of anyone assisting in the operation. When the knife is held as directed there is not much danger of a slip except at the end of the incision when, the resistance being overcome, the knife goes through with a rush. To avoid this, pressure should always be slackened toward the end of the incision. The main incisions in the organs should be made with the brain-knife or short amputation knife, by a long, sweeping cut made from heel to toe of the knife-blade and beginning at the part of the organ farthest from the operator, drawing the blade through the organ toward the operator. For finer dissections the smaller scalpels are to be employed, and in such cases the dissection-technique of fixed arm and free finger movement must be used. In many places within the body the cutting-edge of the knife should be directed outward rather than inward so that underlying structures may not be injured. Often the fingers of the left hand are used in such cases to take the place of a grooved director. The application of these and other points of technique will be elucidated in the chapters following, whenever it is of advantage to use some especial method. In general nothing should be done to disturb relationships until these have been noted, and cuts should be made into organs in such a way that they may be reconstructed in their original shape and condition.

Order and cleanliness should characterize the autopsy. Abundance of water should be at hand, and after every incision the knife should be dipped into a vessel of water standing on the autopsy table. Practically all cuts should be made with a *clean wet* knife; only in the case of the chief-incisions of the large organs is it of advantage to cut with a *clean dry* knife, when it is desirable to obtain a judgment of the moistness or dryness of the cut surface. Never cut with a dirty knife, as the cut-surface may be obscured. A gentle scraping with the knife-blade often gives a more distinct picture of the cut surface. The water-stream should not be used too freely upon cut surfaces; it should be employed only when there is so much blood or fluid that the surfaces are obscured, or when it is desired to float up certain tissues or parts of organs. A better picture of the cut-surface can sometimes be obtained by blotting it with absorbent paper free from lint. Organs and tissues removed from the cadaver should not be allowed to dry. Nor should they be left in water. Both conditions will quickly ruin material in so far as its after-use for microscopic study is concerned. They should be kept covered with moist cloth or paper. As the organs are removed from the body they may be quickly dipped into water and quickly rinsed, but beyond this the use of water is not advisable.

Blood and fluids within the cavities of the body should be quickly removed as soon as their character is determined. Stomach and intestinal fluids in particular should not be allowed to escape within the body-cavities. They should not be washed out, but removed by the aid of beakers and sponges. Drops of blood or other fluids upon the surface of the cadaver should be removed before they become dry. All respect should be paid to the dead body. The face and hair should be covered after they have been examined; and great care should be taken to prevent any accidental cuts on the surface; and the entire field of operation as well as the autopsy-table must be kept clean. In private practice the external genitals should be kept covered except for their examination. An abundance of large sponges and a gently-flowing stream of water under low pressure permit a clean and orderly autopsy. The use of a hose with water under high pressure is dangerous because of the accidental spattering that is sure to occur. Blood and fluids from a dead body should not be spattered about because of the great danger of spreading infection. When accidents do happen prompt cleaning up and disinfection should be carried out. Particularly in private practice is it of the greatest importance that no blood-stains be left behind.

The time required for an autopsy varies with the conditions of the individual case. A complete and well-performed autopsy under ordinary circumstances requires at least one hour, usually an hour and a half. It is true that all the organs can be removed from the body in a much shorter time, but the removal and inspection require at least the time given above, if properly done. Some cases present great difficulties and may require 4-12 hours for a satisfactory and complete examination. For a medicolegal examination 2-3 hours is usually necessary. No prosector should make more than two autopsies in one day, and, if he is making them every day, one daily is quite sufficient. The intellectual and nervous energy required for a good autopsy is so great that it is impossible for anyone to do justice to a large number made in quick succession. In many German laboratories this fact is recognized and the autopsies are assigned proportionately to members of the pathologic staff.

At the close of the autopsy the cadaver must be thoroughly cleaned and restored, as far as possible, to its natural appearance. Directions for the restoration and closure of the autopsied body will be given in a later chapter.

CHAPTER II.

THE ORDER OF THE AUTOPSY.

ORDER OF THE AUTOPSY. In so complicated a piece of work as the complete autopsy it is absolutely necessary that a definite order of procedure be followed at every autopsy, altered when necessary to suit the requirements of individual cases. In medicolegal examinations a definite autopsy order should be prescribed by law. For the average case, in fact for nearly every autopsy, I believe the following order, as given in my protocol book, to be the best one. It is based upon topographic and anatomic relationships, preservation of blood-content, ease and convenience of method, etc. As the protocol should follow this order, it is given here in full.

Autopsy-Protocol No.

1. Name: 2. Sex: 3. Age:

4. Nationality: 5. Status: 6. Occupation:

7. Day and Hour of Death: 8. Time of Autopsy:

Clinical Diagnosis:

Pathologic Diagnosis:

Prosector:

A. External Examination. General.

9. Build:	27. Muscles:
10. General Nutrition:	28. Rigor Mortis:
11. Head:	
12. Facies:	29. Panniculus:
13. Eyes:	30. Oedema:
14. Neck:	
15. Thorax:	31. Body Heat:
16. Abdomen:	32. Hypostasis:
17. Back:	
18. Anomalies:	33. Putrefaction:
19. Deformities:	34. Orifices:
20. Signs of Trauma:	Mouth:
21. Surgical Wounds:	Nose:
22. Scars:	Ears:
23. Skin:	Genital:
24. Hair:	Anus:
25. Teeth:	35. Post-Mortem
26. Mucous Membranes:	Percussion:

B. Internal Examination.
I. SPINAL CORD.

1. Dorsal Incision:	4. Inner Meninges:
2. Vertebrae:	5. Cord:
3. Dura:	6. Inner Surface of Vertebrae:

II. HEAD.

1. Scalp:
2. Periosteum:
3. Skull-Cap:

4. Dura:
5. Longitudinal Sinus:
6. Meningeal Vessels:

7. Basal Vessels:
8. Inner Meninges, Left:
9. Inner Meninges, Right:

10. Cerebrum:
11. Right Hemisphere:
12. Left Hemisphere:

13. Ventricles:
    Left Lateral:
    Right Lateral:
    Third:
    Fourth:

14. Chorioid Plexus:
15. Pineal Gland:
16. Cerebral Ganglia:
17. Peduncles:

18. Cerebellum:
19. Pons:
20. Medulla:

21. Hypophysis:
22. Basal Sinuses:
23. Basal Dura:
24. Cranial Nerves:
25. Base of Skull:

III. THORAX AND ABDOMEN. (Main Incision.)

1. Panniculus:
2. Musculature:

3. Abdominal Cavity:
4. Omentum:

5. Position of Abdominal Organs:

6. Position of Diaphragm:

7. Mammæ:
8. Costal Cartilages:
9. Sternum:

IV. THORAX.

1. Thoracic Cavity:	11. Left Lung:
2. Position of Thoracic Organs:	12. Right Lung:
3. Anterior Mediastinum:	13. Bronchi:
4. Thymus:	14. Bronchial Glands:
5. Pericardium:	15. Pulmonary Vessels:
6. Heart:	16. Great Vessels of Thorax:
7. Right Heart:	17. Thoracic Portion of Oesophagus:
8. Left Heart:	18. Thoracic Duct:
9. Cardiac Orifices and Valves:	19. Thoracic Vertebræ.
10. Coronary Vessels:	

V. MOUTH AND NECK.

1. Mouth:	9. Thyroid:
2. Tongue:	10. Parathyroids:
3. Pharynx:	11. Cervical Lymphnodes:
4. Tonsils:	12. Parotid:
5. Nose:	13. Sub-maxillary Gland:
6. Larynx:	14. Cervical Vessels and Nerves:
7. Trachea:	15. Deep Muscles of Neck:
8. Cervical Portion of Oesophagus:	

VI. ABDOMEN.

1. Peritoneum:	15. Left Adrenal:
2. Spleen:	16. Left Kidney and Ureter:
3. Large Intestine:	
4. Appendix:	17. Right Adrenal:
5. Small Intestine:	18. Right Kidney and Ureter:
6. Duodenum:	
7. Bile Passages:	19. Abdominal Aorta:
8. Stomach:	20. Iliacs:
9. Pancreas:	21. Ascending Vena Cava:
10. Liver:	22. Lymph Vessels:
11. Gall Bladder:	23. Retroperitoneal Lymphnodes:
12. Portal Vein:	24. Hemolymph Nodes:
13. Mesentery:	25. Sympathetic:
14. Mesenteric Lymphnodes:	26. Psoas Muscles:
	27. Vertebræ:

VII. MALE PELVIS.

1. Penis:	6. Prostate:
2. Scrotum:	7. Seminal Vesicles:
3. Testis:	8. Seminal Duct:
4. Epididymis:	9. Urethra:
5. Rectum:	10. Bladder:

VIII. FEMALE PELVIS.

1. Rectum:	9. Tubes:
2. Vulva:	
3. Urethra:	10. Ovaries:
4. Bladder:	
5. Vagina:	
6. Uterus:	11. Blood and Lymph Vessels of Uterus:
7. Cervix:	
8. Body:	12. Ligaments of Uterus:

IX. SPECIAL REGIONAL EXAMINATION.

1. Bones:	6. Peripheral Nerves:
2. Marrow:	
3. Joints:	7. Sympathetic:
4. Lymph Glands:	8. Organs of Special Sense: Eye:
5. Peripheral Blood Vessels:	Ear: Nose:

X. MICROSCOPIC AND BACTERIOLOGIC FINDINGS.

XI. SUMMARY OF CASE.

The organs may be inspected and opened in the body without removing them; but when weights and measures are desired they should be removed and sectioned on the table. When the spinal cord is removed posteriorly it should be done at the beginning of the autopsy, for the sake of convenience and cleanliness. If the thorax and abdomen are examined first there is a loss of solidity and resistance, making the posterior opening of the spinal canal more difficult. The head may be opened while the cadaver is face downward and the brain removed with cord attached. If the cord is examined anteriorly this should be done at the close of the autopsy after the thorax and abdomen are completely cleaned out. The head should be opened before the heart and great vessels are cut in order to avoid bleeding the sinuses and pial veins. It should be kept elevated until the heart has been examined to avoid bleeding the latter through the jugulars. The abdomen is opened before the thorax so that the position of the abdominal organs and the height of the diaphragm can be correctly noted. A complete survey of the peritoneal cavity should be made at once before the appearances are changed through the loss of blood or other fluids, or through drying or handling. The size of the liver should be estimated before the heart is cut out, inasmuch as the loss of blood through the cut inferior vena cava may reduce its size as much as one-half. The pleural cavities should be examined before its vessels are cut, as the escape of blood may alter the appearances of the pleuræ. The heart is opened before the lungs are removed, so that its blood-content may be judged. The section of the neck organs is conveniently carried out according to anatomic relationships, beginning with the tongue. In the abdomen the spleen is removed first because it is the most easily gotten out of the way. The intestines up to the duodenum may be taken next, or the adrenals and kidneys, followed then by the gastro-intestinal tract, pancreas and liver. When necessary the kidneys may be removed in connection with the pelvic organs. In the case of extensive growth of neoplasms, marked inflammatory processes, adhesions, malformations, anomalies, etc., the order must be changed to meet in the best way the demands of the situation. Such changes in the order must always be mentioned in the protocol. It is a great mistake to begin the autopsy with a local examination of a supposed fatal lesion, except in the cases of wounds, particularly in medicolegal cases, in which a most careful and minute description of the wound is necessary.

Some writers (*Letulle, Heller, et al.*) advocate the removal of neck, thoracic, abdominal and pelvic organs *en masse* and their examination outside of the body. Except in rare cases in the adult, and more frequently in the child, this method does not present any special advantages aside from the preparation of museum specimens. It may be convenient to follow it when a very short time is allowed for the autopsy, just sufficient to remove the organs so that they can be examined later. When this method is followed the order should be:

> 1. Organs should be turned over without twisting, so that their posterior aspect is uppermost. Then the examination in the following order: right and left azygos veins; thoracic duct; removal of adrenals; opening of ureters; removal of kidneys; opening of aorta, inferior vena cava, portal vein and branches, and common duct; examination of pancreas; removal of aorta as far as arch; opening of œsophagus; examination of mouth, pharynx, palate, tonsils, tongue and sublingual glands, epiglottis, larynx, trachea and large bronchi; roots of lungs, prevertebral lymphnodes, and the pneumogastric nerves.

2. Organs are then turned over again without twisting, and examined from anterior surface as follows: removal and examination of thymus and thyroid; opening of superior vena cava, termination of thoracic duct and right lymph-trunk; opening of pericardium, examination of cardiac plexus, opening of arch of aorta; section and examination of pulmonary arteries and veins and hilum of lung; examination and removal of heart and lungs; examination of diaphragm, liver, gallbladder and bile-ducts; external examination and separation of spleen, stomach, pancreas and duodenum; removal of œsophagus, stomach, pancreas and duodenum; external examination, dissection and removal of intestine to the rectum; examination of peritoneum, mesentery and omentum; separation and examination of kidneys, ureters, bladder and urethra; separation and examination of genital organs (in male, prostate, seminal vesicles, vasa deferentia and testes; in the female, oviducts, broad ligaments, ovaries, vulva, vagina and uterus).

For the ordinary clinical autopsy this method is more inconvenient and time-consuming, and offers not a single advantage over the order advocated above. I use it only in young children and in adult cases of generalized carcinomatosis, sarcomatosis, pulmonary embolism, congenital cardiac lesion, tuberculosis, aortic aneurism with tracheal or bronchial erosion and a few other rare generalized conditions. For all other cases I advise that the first mentioned order be followed, varying it as occasion demands. The autopsy should be individualized. Departures from the routine order will take place chiefly in the thoracic and abdominal cavities. It is often more convenient to remove the kidneys before taking out the intestines, to examine the liver before the spleen, or to make other similar variations in the order. The order of examination of the larger divisions of the body (head, thorax, abdomen and pelvis) should always be followed strictly; but the neck and thoracic organs, or the thoracic organs alone, may be removed *en masse* and examined outside of the body, and the same procedure may be carried out in the case of the abdominal or pelvic organs whenever advisable. Removal *en masse* with examination on the table is especially indicated in the case of the neck and thoracic organs in aortic aneurism, pulmonary embolism, congenital cardiac lesions, mediastinal neoplasms, generalized carcinoma or sarcoma of thoracic organs, etc. The same procedure is indicated in the case of the abdominal organs in generalized carcinomatosis or sarcomatosis, inflammation and tuberculosis of the abdominal organs or peritoneum, aneurism of the abdominal aorta, pseudomyxoma peritonei, etc.

In my judgment it is extremely bad practice to examine first that part of the body which the clinician believes to be chiefly affected. Still worse is it to limit the autopsy to such a regional examination. Imperfect and subjective conclusions will be avoided if the regular order is followed and each organ examined objectively. In all cases a complete autopsy should be made if permission can be obtained, and the permit for an autopsy should be regarded as one for a complete examination unless definite exceptions have been made. The examination of any organ or part should never be neglected. Many prosectors habitually omit the section of the neck-organs, intestines and genital tract when there is nothing to attract especially their attention to these parts. The examination of the spinal cord, orbits, nasal tract, ears, joints and bones may be omitted in the ordinary autopsy in the absence of especial considerations directing attention thereto; all other parts should be systematically examined. The pathologist must always maintain an unprejudiced state of mind toward the clinical diagnosis—rather a doubting mind than a disposition to accept the suggestions of the clinical opinions. The best cure for subjectivity is the complete performance of the autopsy in regular routine order, and the dictation of the protocol at the autopsy table during the operation.

CHAPTER III.
THE PROTOCOL.

THE PROTOCOL. Autopsy findings should be recorded in the form of complete, concise notes, following the order of the autopsy. Such a protocol should consist of *descriptive* statements of the pathologic changes found, as well as of all negative conditions. It must be a guarantee that all organs have been examined and that nothing has been overlooked. Herein lies the great value of the use of a protocol blank book with printed autopsy forms. When such are used and both positive and negative pathologic findings are recorded during the progress of the autopsy the chances of omission are reduced to a minimum.

The protocol must be purely objective and exact. All appearances should be so carefully described that from the protocol itself a diagnosis may be formulated. Conclusions and diagnoses have no place in the protocol until the final summing up. It is better to describe the appearance of organs than to class them as "normal" or "negative," "nothing notable," etc. The only excuse for the employment of such phrases is a lack of time for the dictation of a proper protocol, but the scientific value of the autopsy is thereby impaired. As the complete description of the normal appearances would require too much time and lessen that available for the pathologic examination, the prosector should describe briefly the chief characteristics of the normal organ, any variation in any one of these characteristics being sufficient evidence that the organ had suffered pathologic change. The description of the normal organ, however, usually offers the greatest difficulty to the beginner, and so much time may be spent upon this that the pathologic changes are slighted. However, the relatively small number of points constituting the criterion for the normal organ may be learned by experience and by the study of autopsy-protocols made by experts. The latter study is also necessary for the acquisition of the extensive protocol terminology that has been developed. A knowledge of this terminology lightens greatly the difficulties of the protocol; but its misuse leads to confusion and incorrect interpretations.

It is not a good plan to write up the protocol after the autopsy has been finished. It should be dictated during the progress of the autopsy. Only in this way can an accurate and purely objective description be obtained. The use of simple, terse English and the proper employment of autopsy terminology are also chief factors in the production of a good protocol.

The importance of following a definitely-outlined routine of procedure is very evident in the case of protocol-making. The general order of the autopsy should be followed strictly in the protocol; and all deviations from the usual method noted and described. Aside from this general order, each organ or part as it is examined should be systematically described according to the following scheme:

1. Location and relation to other parts.
2. Size and weight.
3. Shape. (Contour, lobes, edges, borders, character of surface, etc.)
4. Color.
5. Consistence.
6. Odor.
7. Cut surface.
8. Blood-content.
9. Histologic features in detail. (Capsule, surface, parenchyma, stroma, vessels, etc.)
10. General and localized pathologic conditions.

For the *hollow viscera* and *body-cavities* the following points should be systematically noted in addition:

1. Size and shape of cavity.
2. Free gas or air?
3. Fluid or solid contents? (Amount, odor, color, cloudiness, consistency, precipitation or separation on standing, presence of blood, fibrin, pus, parasites, etc.)
4. Condition of wall of cavity (serosa or mucosa).

1. **Location and Relation.** The organs and parts should be located according to the landmarks of regional anatomy. Brain-lesions may be charted upon the printed outline sheets of the different parts of the brain. Similar outline sheets may also be used for other parts of the body.

2. **Size and Weight.** The exact weights and measurements should be given in the metric terms. Organs should be weighed and measured after the removal of other tissue in which they may be imbedded (fatty capsule of kidney, etc.) or to which they are attached (diaphragm from liver, blood-vessels from heart, etc.).

The volume of the organ may be estimated by putting it into a graduated vessel containing water and noting the amount of displacement. In the absence of facilities or the time necessary to take weights and measurements an approximate estimate of size and bulk may be given by comparisons with well-known objects, such as peas, mustard-seed, pepper-corns, walnuts, apple, hen's egg, etc., but such terms are only relative and not accurate, and their use should be avoided as much as possible. That the weight and measurements of any given organ fall within normal limits cannot be taken as evidence that the organ is normal. The judgment as to the size and weight of the organ must always be controlled by a consideration of the pathologic conditions present as to the exact factor in the increase or the loss of size or weight.

3. **Shape.** The organs should be removed with the least possible disturbance of shape. If it is not possible to do this, the shape of the organ should be noted as it lies within the body. A knowledge of the normal form of the organs must serve as the basis for judgment. Comparison of pathologic alterations in form with the shape of some familiar object is permissible (horse-shoe, hour-glass, shagreen, cauliflower, mushroom, coral, polypoid, hog-backed, etc.) Borders, contours, edges, external surfaces, etc., are rounded, sharp, flatter, thinner, saccular, lobulated, smooth, wrinkled, folded, villous, polypoid, granular, nodular, fissured, etc. All possible anomalies of form exist from the very slightest deviations up to the most marked distortions.

4. **Color.** The color of an organ or part should be noted as soon as possible after its removal from the body, or, better, as soon as the cadaver is opened, since oxidation, evaporation, loss of blood, and contact with water quickly cause color-changes. Venous blood may quickly become bright red, notably in the spleen and cerebral veins and sinuses. It is not to be supposed that, even when the cadaver is opened within a very short time after death, the color is that of the living body. Certain color-changes always take place as soon as death occurs, but it is necessary to create a color-standard for the different organs as seen under the conditions of the ordinary autopsy. Injections of formalin and other undertaker's fluids destroy all color, and should not be permitted before the autopsy. Freezing likewise changes the color of many of the organs

The judgment of the color of the tissues and organs of the human body is extremely difficult because of the fact that only rarely is a pure simple color seen. Ordinarily a combination of colors is present, and the analysis of these is often not easy. If the organ is held before the eyes at a distance of about a yard an impression of a single color-unity may be obtained, but when brought nearer to the eyes the surface presents a variegated, mottled, speckled or streaked effect of many colors, sometimes running the entire range of the spectrum. The colors most frequently seen in the body are yellow, red and brown in all possible combinations and shades. Blue, gray, slate, black, green and purple are also common in combination with these three or with one another. The analysis of the color is concerned, first with the color proper of the parenchyma, secondly with the color of the blood and the blood-content, thirdly with the color of some pathologic substance contained in the tissue, as blood- or bile-pigment, carbon, melanin, etc. In describing color-combinations use the predominant color last; as, for example, a reddish-yellow-brown means that the predominant color is brown with more yellow in it than red. Innumerable combinations of these three colors exist (light brown, chocolate, yellowish-brown, brownish yellow, brownish red, etc.). The macroscopic color will not be apparent in microscopic preparations except when due to a true pigment.

The term discolored is applied to dirty, cloudy colors, particularly gray or greenish, as in gangrene. Spotted, mottled, streaked, variegated, etc., have the same application in the autopsy-protocol that they have elsewhere. The judgment of the color of an organ should be made twice: as seen through the capsule or external covering, and again on the cut surface of the organ. In the latter case the transparency, translucency or opacity of the surface should be noted with the color. Normally translucent structures become opaque as the result of inflammatory thickening, parenchymatous degenerations, leukocyte infiltrations, tubercles, post-mortem digestion, etc. An increase in translucence may be due to œdema, hydropic degeneration, amyloid, mucoid and colloid degenerations, liquefaction necrosis, anæmia, atrophy, loss of pigment, etc. (translucent, transparent, jelly-like, colloid, mucoid, lardaceous, sago, bacon, ham-fat, pearly, etc.).

5. **Consistence.** This is best estimated by placing the four fingers of the right hand beneath the edge of the organ as it lies on the board or in the body and lifting it slightly upward and inward toward the main mass of the organ. This should be done in several places, so that an idea of the general consistence of the organ is obtained. Hollow organs must be tested before and after opening, in the latter case, to get an idea of the consistence of the wall. Organs with capsules should be tested through the uncut capsule

and also on the cut surface. After the general consistence has been determined an examination of the entire organ by thumb and fingers should be made to determine localized areas of different consistence (soft: abscess, cyst, œdema, areas of degeneration, etc.; hard: amyloid, tubercles, tumors, chronic passive congestion, fibroid indurations, pneumonic areas, etc.). The size and location of such areas should be carefully noted. The presence of fluctuation, loss of elasticity, pitting on pressure, friability, hardness, etc., should be described in ordinary terms, although a comparison with familiar objects often gives a more definite impression than the simple use of adjectives describing the condition (consistence of leather, dough, mush, pea-soup, putty, wood, jelly, stone, iron, etc.). The relaxation or softness of an organ is often judged by its flattening on the board, or by its hanging down over the index-finger when this is placed beneath its middle and the organ raised, or by the jelly-like tremors of the organ when the dish containing it is agitated.

An increased friability is noted in diseased bones, muscles, pneumonic lungs, organs showing acute congestion, etc. An increase or a loss in elasticity is to be noted chiefly in the large blood-vessels, lungs, skin, etc. In describing a condition of loss of normal firmness the German School makes frequent use of the termination *malacia* (softening) in such words as *myomalacia, osteomalacia, gastromalacia, myelomalacia, encephalomalacia,* etc. When such softening is the result of postmortem autolysis or digestion, as is so often the case in the stomach (postmortem perforations), thymus, pancreas, adrenals, brain, etc., the term *postmortem softening* is more frequently used in this country. Soft tumors are described as medullary, encephaloid, etc. In all judgments as to consistence the normal differences between the organs must be considered, as well as the length of time between death and the autopsy, the cause and manner of death, undertaker's manipulations, temperature, moisture, rigor mortis, putrefaction, etc.

6. **Odor.** But little attention is paid in the average autopsy to the odors of the body, and very little has been written about their importance. This is probably due to the fact that the average individual more or less consciously or unconsciously suppresses the sense of smell. Yet a keen sense of odors and an ability to analyze them are of the very greatest importance in autopsy work. Certain infections, and other diseases as well, have peculiar and distinctive odors (small-pox, measles, colon-bacillus infections, pulmonary gangrene, diabetes, uræmia, acute yellow atrophy, leukaemia, etc.). The odor of many drugs and poisons may also be distinguished in the

tissues, gastro-intestinal tract or body-cavities (alcohol, ammonia, amyl nitrite, aromatic and ethereal oils, assafétida, carbolic acid, chloral, chloroform, creosote, ether, hydrocyanic acid, iodoform, musk, nicotine, nitrobenzol, phenacetin, phosphorus, etc.) Many foods may be recognized in the stomach by the odor (onions, garlic, cabbage, turnips, pineapple, oranges, apples, peaches, vinegar, grape-juice, caraway and anise seeds, celery, sage, cardamom, and many others). In describing odors we should compare them with natural odors or class them as sweet, sweetish, sour, bitter, pungent, sharp, heavy, yeasty, pus-like, fruity, etc.

7. **Cut Surface.** The cut surface of the organs and tissues should be examined immediately after the organ is sectioned. During the examination the organ should be moved in different planes so that the light may fall upon the surface in various angles. Color-changes, differences in reflection and refraction, minute inequalities of the surface, etc., are often brought out in this way when otherwise they might be overlooked. During the examination the surface may be gently scraped over by the blade of the large section-knife held at an angle of 45° to the surface. The character and amount of the blood and fluid exuding from the surfaces and vessels should be noted; after this has been done the cut surface may be gently washed with water and examined with regard to histologic and pathologic details. During the inspection pressure may be made upon the organs to determine still further the blood- and fluid-content. The color, moisture or dryness, consistence, reflection or "shine" (dry-shining, moist-shining, fatty shine, pearly shine, etc.), cloudiness, translucency, transparency or opacity of the cut surface must also be considered. Normal organs are never perfectly dry, although they vary greatly in the amount of moisture shown on the surface. They have, therefore, always a certain degree of reflecting power. Different parts of the cut surface of the same organ should be compared as to color, moisture and dryness. (Areas of suppuration, congestion, œdema, inflammation, recent hemorrhage, hydropic degeneration, liquefaction necrosis, etc., are more moist than normal; old thrombi, fibrinous exudates, old hemorrhages, simple, coagulation, caseous and Zenker's necrosis, dry gangrene, anæmic and hemorrhagic infarctions, amyloid, concretions of cholesterin, bile-pigment, lime-salts, urates, etc., contents of dermoid cysts and cholesteatomata, etc., are dry.) The cut surface must be described also as to its even or uneven character, finely or coarsely granular, shagreened, rough, nodular, elevated or depressed portions, fissures, folds, umbilication.

The cut surface of neoplasms is examined especially by scraping it with a dry knife held at an angle of 45°. The cells thus obtained constitute the *tissue-juice* (*"cancer- or sarcoma-milk"*). Soft medullary neoplasms yield an abundance of such cell-scrapings, hard tumors but little. The cells thus obtained may be treated according to the various methods given on Page 219, and then examined microscopically. The cut-surface of the soft parenchymatous organs (bone-marrow, spleen, thymus, lymphnodes, liver, pancreas and kidneys) also yields material for examination by this method.

8. **Blood-Content.** The blood-content of the organs should be estimated both before and after they are sectioned. This estimation should be based upon the color of the organ, condition of the blood-vessels, amount of blood exuded from the cut surface, number of bleeding-points (anæmia, hyperæmia, stasis). Capillary, arterial and venous hyperæmia should be differentiated when possible. Only rarely are evidences of arterial congestion seen in the cadaver. It is also necessary to observe the occurrence, location and extent of hypostasis and to differentiate antemortem and postmortem (lungs, brain, intestines, etc). The association with œdema and inflammation, particularly in the lungs (hypostatic pneumonia) speaks for antemortem hypostasis. A red color in parts possessing no blood-vessels (heart-valves, endocardium, intima of aorta, cartilage, etc.) indicates an imbibition of diffused hæmoglobin (hæmatin-imbibition). Changes in the color of the blood (carbon monoxide, hydrocyanic acid, and hydrogen sulphide poisoning, all poisons producing methæmoglobinæmia, icterus, leukæmia, etc.) should be described and recorded; likewise all hemorrhages, extravasations, etc.

9. **Histologic Features.** After the general points given above have been considered the histologic features of the organ should be taken up in routine. For example, in the case of the spleen, the capsule, trabeculæ, pulp, stroma, follicles and vessels should be examined; in the liver, the capsule, trabeculæ, liver-acini, blood-vessels and bile-ducts; in the kidneys, capsules, cortical surface, cortex, labyrinths and medullary rays, glomeruli, columns of Bertini, medullary pyramids, vessels, pelvis and beginning of ureter. When the organs are thus systematically examined there is but little chance that anything visible to the naked eye has been overlooked.

10. **Pathologic Lesions.** Anomalies, defects, erosions, ulcers, evidences of trauma, inflammations, abscesses, tubercles, gummata, neoplasms, parasites, and all forms of pathologic changes, local or general, must be accurately located and described. The changes

peculiar to certain diseases and infections must always be borne in mind during the examination of any organ in which such conditions are likely to be found. The relationship of lesions in different parts of the body must be recognized. Localized lesions must be described according to position, size, form, color, consistence, etc. Their nature must be recognized, their relation to other or to pre-existing conditions determined, the stage of the process estimated, and the part played in the causation of death ascertained.

In the examination of the *body-cavities* and *hollow organs,* as well as *pathologic hollow structures,* the first thing to note is the escape of gas or air under pressure. Occasionally it is best to open the organ under water to note the escape of bubbles. The odor of the gas, inflammability, etc., are to be noted. The fluid or solid contents (blood, bile, urine, féces, mucus, pus, exudates and transudates, altered secretions, food-remains, concretions, foreign bodies, parasites, etc.) are described as to their amount, color, consistence, odor. reaction, chemical nature, precipitate, presence of cellular elements, etc. The size of the cavity, monolocular or multilocular, the character of its lining (transparency, translucency, cloudiness or opacity, color, "shine," moisture, smoothness, roughness, villous or polypoid, consistence, thickening, swelling, elevations, atrophy, incrustations or deposits on the lining, etc.) are to be considered. In the case of cystic tumors (adenocystomata, dermoid cysts, cholesteatomata, etc.) especial attention should be paid to the character of the cyst-contents (mucoid, glairy, colloid, jelly-like, pea-soup-like, pultaceous, mushy, doughy, caseous, pearly, laminated, flaky, powdery, etc.).

CHAPTER IV.
THE EXTERNAL EXAMINATION.

THE BEGINNING OF THE AUTOPSY. The autopsy begins with the examination of the exterior of the body. The cadaver should be completely stripped of clothing and examined as a whole, then as to its separate parts. Time is saved and omissions prevented if a definite order is followed in the external examination, such as follows here.

1. **Identification of the Body.** In ordinary cases the name of the deceased will be given upon the autopsy-permit, and this will serve as sufficient identification. In large autopsy-services, when several cadavers may be brought in at the same time, each one should be properly tagged so that no mistake is possible. It is necessary in medicolegal cases to make a more formal identification by having the cadaver positively identified by persons having knowledge of the individual during life, or by those who first saw the body, or who took it in charge. In such cases when identification is impossible at the time of autopsy the protocol should give in full details the place, time, and conditions of discovery of the body, with an accurate description of its external characteristics, clothing, articles found on the body, surroundings, etc. Bertillon measurements and finger-markings may be taken; dental work should be carefully described; false teeth and hair, eyeglasses, etc., should be preserved, and the most careful attention should be paid to bodily anomalies or peculiarities, birth-marks, tattoo, etc. Photographs, casts, Roentgengrams, etc., may be taken. Powder-marks, blood-stains, as well as those of semen and other discharges, should be described and, if necessary, preserved. Legal names, as well as aliases, should be recorded and attested in all cases of legal significance. In fact, the only proper way to conduct any autopsy is with the assumption that the results will have legal value; and such an assumption is the best safeguard against important omissions.

2. **Sex.** This should always be mentioned in the protocol. In the case of pseudohermaphrodism the determination of the real sex may be difficult and may eventually be decided by microscopic studies. Likewise in bodies that have been burned or mutilated the question of sex becomes a matter of anatomic and histologic study.

The character of the bones, pelvis, remains of sexual organs, etc., are used as criteria to decide the question. In cases of burning, the uterus in the female and the prostate in the male may often be recognized microscopically when the head and extremities are burned off and only a charred mass of flesh and bone remains.

3. **Age.** When the true age is not known the apparent age must be estimated by considering the general appearance of the body, development, bones, epiphyses, sutures, blood-vessels, skin, hair, teeth, sexual organs, etc. Roentgengrams of the epiphyses, hands and feet may be made. The presence of an arcus senilis should be noted. Arteriosclerosis of the temporal and radial arteries may be determined by inspection and palpation. The determination of the age of the newborn will be considered in a later chapter.

4. **Nationality.** When not definitely known this may be estimated by such criteria as color of skin, finger-nails, character of hair, facies (cheek-bones, jaw, forehead, cephalic index, facial angle, eyes, etc.), hands, feet, general build, etc. For ethnologic and anthropologic data the body may be described according to the primitive type it represents (Australioid, negroid, mongoloid, xanthochroic, melanchroic, Iberian, dolichocephalic, etc., according to the different classifications).

5. **Status.** Unmarried, married, widow, widower, divorced, legal status, citizen of what country, state, county or town, etc.

6. **Occupation.** As this often throws light upon the pathologic condition present in the body, the trade or occupation should be ascertained and stated in the protocol. When no direct information is available a judgment concerning it may be made on the basis of certain conditions, occupation or industrial diseases found in the body (anthracosis, argyrosis, siderosis, silicosis, chalicosis, lead-poisoning, chronic phosphorus poisoning, nitrobenzol and other forms of poisoning, localized muscle-hypertrophy or atrophy, callus, etc.).

7, 8. **Time of Death and Time of Autopsy.** The day and hour of death and the time of autopsy should be noted. When the time of death is not known with certainty it can only approximately be estimated by the condition of the body with respect to such postmortem changes as rigor mortis, algor mortis, hypostasis, diffusion-spots, decomposition, etc. From no one of these signs of death can an absolute statement be made as to the time of death; so great a variation may occur with any one or with all of these so-called *positive signs* of death that only very relative estimates can be given.

Between the actual time of death and the appearance of positive signs of this event there exists a variable period in which death announces its appearance by *negative* signs only; the cessation of the vital functions, respiration, circulation and nervous excitability. These functions may, however, be reduced to so low a degree of strength that their existence cannot be made out by the usual methods, and a condition of *apparent death* or *"suspended animation"* may be present. Such a condition is most frequently seen in cases of cholera, hysteria, catalepsy, hypnosis, excessive fatigue, prolonged exposure to cold or to high temperatures, concussion, severe hemorrhage, action of certain poisons, electrical currents and lightning stroke, strangulation, asphyxia, suffocation, drowning, etc. The condition of apparent death may last hours or even days, but as a rule it is one of very short duration. Granting the existence of such a possibility of apparent death before absolute signs of death appear, it follows that in all autopsies made very soon after death has occurred, the prosector must bear such a possibility in mind, and satisfy himself beyond all doubt of the actual occurrence of death before beginning the autopsy.

Tests for the Determination of the Occurrence of Death. Loss of reflexes or response to stimuli are early signs. Mirror, flame or feather held before the mouth and nose, or vessel containing fluid placed on epigastrium show absence of respiration. Opening of artery, temporal or radial; if death has occurred vessel will be empty. Tests with blood-pressure apparatus are negative in dead body. Electrical tests and Roentgengrams of heart and lungs show no movement in these organs. Subcutaneous injection of ammonia; no congestion or vesicle formed in the dead body. Subcutaneous injection of fluorescin (*Icard's test*); in the living body a greenish color soon appears in skin, mucous membranes and conjunctivæ; but not in the dead body. Heat applied to the skin causes no reddening in the dead body, and, if a vesicle forms, the fluid contained in it has no albumin and the underlying skin is dry and glazed and not red. The application of caustics produces no eschar in the dead body. A steel needle inserted into the living tissues becomes quickly tarnished; in the dead body oxidation will not take place after many hours. Glazing of the eyes (if these are open) takes place very quickly after death; the eyeball collapses ordinarily, but may remain prominent in death from hanging, suffocation, apoplexy, etc. The eye loses its elasticity; the pupils can be made oval by compressing the globe (*Ripault's test*). The patch of dark discoloration on the part of the sclerotics exposed to evaporation is known as *Larcher's* *sign.* The hands held against a strong light lose the pink tinge between the fingers, and the soles and palms become yellow. A tight ligature about a finger or limb causes no reddening (*Magnus's test*). Relaxation of the sphincters occurs soon after death. It should be borne in mind in this connection that the discharge of gas and féces is not uncommon after death, that a fetus may be expelled by the increase of intra-abdominal pressure due to rigor mortis and gas-formation, that a discharge of semen or prostatic fluid almost always occurs in the adult male, that electric contractility may last several hours after death, that muscles may twitch during this period, and that atropine will dilate the pupils for some time postmortem.

9. **Build.** The body should be measured by stretching in a straight line a metal tape-measure from the vertex to the centre of the external arch of the instep, the foot being held at a right angle to the surface of the table. Giantism or dwarfism, partial or complete, asymmetrical development, etc., should be noted and the type determined (rachitic, cretinoid, congenital and acquired deformities of bones may cause dwarfism; giantism may be congenital or due to disease of the hypophysis as in acromegaly). In all cases of abnormal development of the skeleton the possibility of diseased conditions of the hypophysis, thyroid, thymus, adrenals and sexual glands must be borne in mind. In a general way the build of the body may be described as large, heavy, strong, medium, small, delicate, etc. Racial, sex and age differences should be noted. Roentgen-ray examination may here also be made use of in the determination of stages of skeletal development. Approximate estimates of the general build may be made when only part of the body is preserved. Such rules as nineteen times the length of the middle finger equals the approximate height, four times the length of the femur equals the height, the distance from the tip of the olecranon to the tip of the middle finger is five-nineteenths of the height, etc., are obviously very uncertain.

10. **General Nutrition.** The body should be weighed. Nutrition good, medium, poor, emaciated, etc. Condition of skin, muscles, panniculus, etc. Differentiate loss in fat from loss in muscle. Distinguish physiologic fat from pathologic (lipomatosis, etc.).

11. **Head.** The size and shape of the head should be noted, and any peculiarity or pathologic condition described (microcephalic, macrocephalic, dolichocephalic, brachycephalic, etc.).

12. **Facies.** Aside from individual and racial characteristics the face of the cadaver may show varying expressions (Hippocratic

facies, hepatic facies, expression of peace, pain, horror, distortion, etc.). Note all anomalies and pathologic conditions (leontiasis ossea, leonine expression of leprosy, hare-lip, etc.).

13. **Eyes.** Closed or open, shape, size, color, deep-set, changes due to death, condition and size of pupils, arcus senilis, color of conjunctivæ and sclerotics, eye-lids. The pupils are usually dilated at death, but after a short time they contract, usually unequally, and remain so for several days. Note particularly all anomalies and pathologic conditions (corneal scars, coloboma, cataract, strabismus, etc.).

14. **Neck.** Short and thick, long and narrow, thin or fat, smooth or wrinkled, scars, enlargements, marks of rope, fingers, string, evidences of strangulation, hemorrhages, abrasions, etc., other forms of trauma, cysts, enlarged glands, condition of thyroid, etc.

15. **Thorax.** Shape, length, breadth and depth, angle of Louis, epigastric angle, symmetry of sides, prominence or depressions, pigeon-breast, shoemaker's or funnel breast, rachitic rosary, character of ribs and interspaces, mammæ, degree of hairiness, eroding tumors or aneurisms, etc.

16. **Abdomen.** Depressed, scaphoid or elevated, distended, tympanitic, presence of fluctuation, symmetry, results of palpation (neoplasms), character of abdominal wall (tightly stretched or lax, wrinkled), presence of linea fusca or lineæ albicantes (pregnancy, ascites, tumor). The existence of enteroptosis or gastroptosis can often be told by inspection of the abdomen.

17. **Back.** General build and contour, bedsores, etc. Spine should be carefully examined (anterior, posterior or lateral curvatures, evidences of trauma, etc.).

18. **Anomalies.** Malformations and anomalies of any region should be thoroughly examined and carefully described. The most common ones found in adults are hare-lip, cleft palate, branchial cysts, bifid sternum, accessory ribs, malformations of fingers and toes, hypertrophy of great toe, hypospadias, cryptorchidism, pseudohermaphrodism, congenital dislocations, particularly of hip, lumbosacral meningoceles and dermoid cysts, microcephalus, club-foot and hernia, its variety, location, size and condition. Under anomalies may be considered the stigmata of degeneracy and the *homo delinquens* type. These should also be mentioned in the identification of the cadaver.

19. **Deformities.** Location, degree, character, probable cause, etc. Most commonly caused by tuberculosis, rachitis, gonorrhœa,

THE EXTERNAL EXAMINATION.

syphilis, osteitis deformans, trauma, burns, osteomalacia, tabes, muscular atrophies, gout, rheumatism, tumors, aneurism, diseases of the lung causing asymmetry of the thorax, acromegaly, etc. Most common forms are Pott's disease, spondylitis, ankylosis, spinal curvature, contractions and retractions of parts, bow-leg, knock-knee, changes in the pelvis, dwarfism, shortening of extremities, exostosis, drumstick or clubbed fingers, flat foot, loss of bones, amputations, occupation deformities, swelling of joints, tophi, Charcot's joint, hygroma, ganglion, etc.

20. **Signs of Trauma.** Location, size, character and condition of wound (bruises, bloody suffusions, hæmatoma, erosion, denudation, lacerations, punctures, crushing, blister, fractures, dislocations, bullet-wounds, marks of hanging, strangulation (abrasions in the neck caused by hanging show minute hemorrhages in and about their edges, particularly in the upper border; section of the neck shows small hemorrhages in the cervical tissues), or drowning, burns, action of corrosives (brown spots on lips), effects of electric currents, etc. In the case of powder-markings note number, direction, burning, singeing of hairs, etc. In medicolegal cases the description of traumatic lesions should be especially minute and complete. An effort should be made to distinguish postmortem from antemortem wounds. Recent wounds have clean cut walls and edges covered with blood; old wounds show reaction, vascularization, granulations, adhesion of edges of wound, or of exudate. Postmortem wounds are usually free from blood unless large veins are ruptured. Loss of the epidermis before or after death causes in the cadaver yellowish or brown, firm, leather-like spots.

21. **Surgical Wounds.** Location, size, nature of operation, state of wound, character of surgical dressings, drainage, etc., discharge from wound as blood, pus, féces, urine, etc., odor of wound, age as shown by stage of repair, evidence of infection, etc. Hypodermic marks, saline injections, blisters, venesection, cupping, exploratory punctures, recent vaccination marks, etc., should be noted.

22. **Scars.** Location, size, character, recent or old, pigmented or pale, rough or smooth, contractures, keloids, traumatic or surgical, nature of injury or surgical operation, hypodermic scars, vaccination, acne, cupping, smallpox, chickenpox, shingles, "electric belt," croton oil, burns, etc.

23. **Skin.** Color (racial differences), brown, gray or black pigmentations in Addison's disease, pellagra, syphilis, vitiligo, xanthoma, chloasma, pigmented nodes or nævi, argyria, arsenical poisoning, pernicious anæmia, xeroderma pigmentosum, chronic

jaundice, vagabond's skin, tan, following blisters, plasters, cupping, use of croton oil, Roentgen irradiation, effects of violet rays, melanotic tumors, pregnancy, etc.; bronzing in Addison's and chronic icterus; lemon yellow in chlorosis and pernicious anæmia; yellow to dark green in icterus; grayish-brown in potassium chlorate poisoning; bluish-red (cyanotic) in cardiac insufficiency; yellowish-bluish-red ("Herz-farbe") in cases of complete loss of compensation; cherry-red or rose-red in carbon-monoxide or hydrocyanic acid poisoning, rarely as the result of an erythema, although this condition usually disappears after death; dirty sallow to grayish or greenish in tumor cachexia and poisoning with H_2S; white after severe hemorrhage, cachexia of chronic Bright's disease, leucoderma, vitiligo, albinism, leprosy, etc.; red, yellow, green or brown in hemorrhages according to their age. Eruptions should be classified and described as to location, abundance, stage, etc. (macules, papules, wheals, desquamation, scales, blebs, bullæ, pustule, tubercles, ulcers, abscess, phlegmon, herpes, crusting, granuloma, etc.). With the exception of chicken-pox and small-pox the eruptions of the acute exanthemata disappear after death, as do all erythematous rashes except in rare instances. Emphysema of the skin should be differentiated from œdema. The most common lesions of the skin are acne, eczema and syphilis. Tuberculosis (lupus) is not uncommon; anthrax, favus, rhinoscleroma, actinomycosis and blastomycosis and Aleppo or Delhi boil are more rarely seen. Tinea versicolor and tricophyton (barber's itch and the various forms of ringworm) are the most common parasitic affections. In the Southern states ground-itch due to the hookworm is the most common. Leprosy should be considered in connection with individuals coming from Norway, Sweden and Finland and other leper-foci. The most common tumors of the skin are all the various forms of hæmangioma and lymphangioma (freckles, moth patches, naevi, moles, warts, birthmarks), fibroma, lipoma and squamous-celled carcinoma (horny and basal-celled types). The latter is the most common form of malignant tumor. Sarcoma of the skin is more rare; the melanotic sarcoma, arising usually in a pigmented mole, is the most common form. Next to this is the round-cell sarcoma or lymphosarcoma (mycosis fungoides, leukaemic and aleukaemic lymphocytoma, etc.). Spindle-cell sarcoma, angiosarcoma, endothelioma and other forms are less common. Sebaceous cysts (wen, atheroma, steatoma) are very common. Less frequent are molluscum contagiosum, xanthoma (endothelioma lipomatodes), myoma, myxoma, chondroma and osteoma. Adenoma sebaceum and sudoriparum are rare. Other conditions of the skin to be noted are cleanliness, elasticity, general nutrition, moisture, presence of scales, atrophy, hyperplasia (ichthyosis, horny warts, cutaneous horns, the various forms of elephantiasis), scleroderma, keloid, xeroderma pigmentosum, albinism, leucoderma, vitiligo, myxœdema, seborrhœa, alopecia, erysipelas, dermatomyositis, psoriasis, impetigo, rhinophyma, herpes, miliaria, sudamina, symmetrical gangrene, trophic changes, "goose-flesh," hemorrhages, scars, tattoo-marks, etc. The various forms of skin-diseases should be described and recorded whenever present.

The presence of petechiæ or ecchymoses in the skin (purpura) is characteristic of all the forms of essential purpura (simplex, peliosis rheumatica, hæmorrhagica, senilis, morbus maculosis Werlhofii, scurvy, Möller-Barlow disease, etc.); such skin hemorrhages occur also as the result of trauma, congenital hæmophilia, in the course of many infections (small-pox, plague, typhus, yellow fever, endocarditis, measles, scarlet fever, septicæmia, pyæmia, rheumatism, meningitis, typhoid fever), in many intoxications (snake-bite, icterus, nephritis, iodine, bromine, phosphorus, chloroform, etc.), also in severe anæmia, pernicious anæmia, leukæmia, sarcoma, carcinoma, acute yellow atrophy of the liver, hysteria, vicarious menstruation, reflex hemorrhages, stigmatization, etc. The number, size, color and location of all cutaneous hemorrhages should be recorded.

24. **Hair.** Color, abundance, distribution, character, quality, condition, length, pathologic conditions (alopecia areati, senilis, præsenilis, pityrodes, syphilitica and symptomatica, trichorrhexis nodosa, hypertrichosis, parasites, etc.). In prolonged fevers and wasting diseases the diameter of the hair is diminished. Symptomatic alopecia occurs after syphilis, typhoid fever, scarlet fever, measles, erysipelas, anæmia, Roentgen irradiation, etc. The length, color and quality of the hair as well as amount and distribution vary in different races. Hypertrichosis is often associated with degeneracy, criminal tendency, epilepsy, idiocy and certain forms of insanity. An apparent growth of hair after death may be caused by retraction of the tissues; an actual postmortem growth is not conceded by the majority of authorities in spite of the numerous tales to that effect. Loss or absence of pigment is seen in albinism, leukotrichia due to infection, Graves' disease, exposure, burns, nervous affections, fright, worry, etc. The presence on or about the body of hairs not belonging to the cadaver is a point of great importance

in medico-legal cases and one that should be thoroughly investigated as to their source. Human hair can be identified microscopically, and it is possible to recognize different specimens according to their variation in color, length, quality, etc.

The **nails** should be considered in connection with skin and hair, with reference to the following points: presence or absence, hypertrophy, atrophy, color, condition, length, development, onychia, hyperonychia, paronchyia, onychogryphosis, longitudinal and transverse ridges, fissures and cracks, opacity, brittleness, etc.

25. **Teeth.** Number, character, condition, anomalies, dental work, caries, Hutchinson's teeth, odontoma, dental osteoma, dentigerous cysts, epulis, papilloma, etc.

26. **Mucous Membranes.** Color, deposits or incrustations, eruptions, erosions, herpes, mucous patches, rhagades, ulcers, fissures, moisture, trauma, effects of corrosives, burns, pigmentation, as in Addison's disease, leukoplakia, hairy tongue, hemorrhages, tumors, etc.

27. **Muscles.** Musculature and condition of muscles (slight, athletic, well developed, poor, flabby, soft, etc.), anomalies, etc.

28. **Rigor Mortis.** Postmortem rigidity is one of the absolute signs of death. It begins usually 1-2 hours after death, the involuntary muscles and heart showing it first. Externally it shows first in the muscles of lower jaw and neck, extends downward, involving the lower extremities last and disappearing in the same order. Its appearance, however, is subject to the greatest variation, and the presence or absence of rigor mortis cannot be used as a criterion for the estimation of the length of time the body has been dead. Instantaneous rigor has been reported in suicides and in people killed in battle. Intense excitement, great muscular exertion, etc., favor its rapid appearance. It also comes on very quickly after death from rabies, tetanus, strychnine poisoning, cholera and a number of other conditions. It sometimes is delayed or absent after heat-stroke; chronic alcoholism also delays its appearance. Usually the contraction lasts 24-48 hours, but under certain conditions may persist for several days. It is prolonged in muscular individuals, after death by suffocation, rabies, strychnine-poisoning, etc. The stiffening of the muscles may be broken by application of heat or the use of force (removal of clothes from the body); when once broken it rarely returns. In a case of death from rabies seen by the writer the rigor was so strong that it required the united efforts of two men to straighten the limbs, and before the close of the autopsy the rigor had returned as strong as in the beginning. Rigidity due to undertaker's injections and freezing must not be

mistaken for rigor mortis. The possibility of rigidity due to ankylosis must also be borne in mind.

29. **Panniculus.** The subcutaneous panniculus is estimated by pinching up a fold of skin between the thumb and fingers of the right hand and the thickness determined. The amount is described as panniculus abundant, moderate, absent, etc. Estimates should be made of panniculus of upper extremities, thorax, abdomen, back and lower extremities. Pathologic conditions, such as general obesity, adiposis dolorosa, multiple lipomata, elephantiasis lipomatosa, fatty collar, etc., should be described in full.

30. **Oedema.** At the same time that the panniculus is being examined, the presence or absence of œdema (pitting on pressure) should be noted in the same regions. When present it may be described as slight, moderate, marked, extreme, localized, universal, etc. *Emphysema* of the subcutaneous tissue is shown by the presence of elastic swellings of the skin, not pitting on pressure, but giving a crepitation when palpated.

31. **Body Heat.** The absence or presence of the body heat is of great importance in giving some idea as to the relative length of time the body has been dead. The nose, ears and extremities first become cool, the liver region retaining the heat longest. The rate of cooling depends upon the external temperature and the conditions of the body. Nude bodies, cadavers exposed to water and cold, and bodies that have suffered severe hemorrhages lose their heat more rapidly. Under ordinary conditions the rectal temperature is the same as that of the surroundings in about forty hours. During the formation of the rigor there may be a slight increase in the temperature of the cadaver. An increase above the normal temperature has also been noted in the dead body immediately after death from tetanus, cholera, smallpox, peritonitis, electric currents, suffocation, gangrene, etc.

32. **Hypostasis.** After death the blood passes into the veins and very soon through gravity collects in the greatly distended veins of the lowest portions of the body, except where these are pressed upon by the weight of the body. Such a settling of the blood begins usually within 1-2 hours after death, but may take place even before death (hypostatic congestion) in cases of long-standing recumbent position, cardiac lesions with failure of compensation, wasting diseases, acute infections, death from suffocation, etc. Postmortem lividity should be described as to its extent, location and color. In anæmia the color is pale purplish red, in congestion dark purple, in cyanosis the color may be dark bluish red and the fingers, toes, ears,

etc., retain the cyanotic appearance for some hours after death; in potassium-chlorate poisoning the color is chocolate, in hydrogen-sulphide poisoning grayish green, in poisoning with hydrocyanic acid or carbon monoxide it is rose or cherry red. Fresh hypostatic patches can be made pale by pressure and when cut they will bleed freely. Hemorrhages cannot be pressed out nor will hemorrhagic areas bleed as freely as hypostatic patches. In all medicolegal cases care should be taken to differentiate bruises and ecchymoses from hypostatic patches, as in the popular mind the latter are often regarded as evidences of trauma or violence. The location of the hypostasis is of importance in showing the position of the body after death; if the anterior portion of the body is hypostatic the cadaver must have been lying upon its face for some time after death; suspension of the body for some time after death by hanging causes a hypostasis of the lower extremities. Of the internal organs the brain, lungs, stomach and coils of intestine chiefly show hypostasis. Antemortem hypostasis of the lungs is distinguished from postmortem by its deeper color, firmer consistence, more marked œdema and microscopic signs of beginning inflammation (hypostatic pneumonia). Cadaveric lividity reaches its maximum in 24-48 hours, and after this time diffusion gradually occurs. In connection with the examination of hypostatic areas the condition of the superficial vessels as to size, distention, etc., should always be noted.

33. **Putrefaction.** The first signs of putrefaction are seen in the transformation of the hypostatic areas into *diffusion spots* and *stripes* following the course of the larger veins. The color is at first a dirty red or brownish-red, but soon becomes gray or green as a result of the action of hydrogen sulphide diffusing from the intestines. Diffusion spots cannot be made pale by pressure, nor do they bleed when cut. The greenish coloration begins first over the abdomen and lower intercostal spaces, and this gradually spreads over the body, showing first in the hypostatic areas and along the veins. The abdomen then becomes distended; gas may form in the subcutaneous tissues so that the skin becomes swollen, crackles on pressure and gives off gas-bubbles when cut. The epidermis becomes loosened in spots, forming blebs containing a dirty-brown exudate, while the tissues become soft and are easily torn. The odor of putrefaction is evident. Decomposition sets in more quickly in infants, in fat and plethoric individuals, and after death from snakebite, active syphilis, plague, sepsis, heat-stroke, suffocation, acute infectious fevers, icterus, gangrene, diabetes, etc.; it is delayed by

hydrocyanic acid and other poisons. When putrefactive bacteria are present in the body, decomposition may begin immediately after death.

34. **Orifices of the Body.** The *mouth, nose, ears, anus, urethra* and *vagina* are to be examined with special regard to their condition and contents (open, closed, gaping, torn, bleeding, discharge of pus, blood, mucus, féces, stomach contents, semen, urine, foreign substances, parasites, ear-wax, etc.). In cases of suspected rape an especial examination of the orifice of the vagina or anus is indicated.

35. **Percussion and Palpation.** The external examination may be closed by the percussion of the heart, lung, spleen, liver and stomach boundaries, and by the palpation of the abdomen. The fine opportunity for control of technique, judgment as to sound, size, consistence, shape, etc., should not be lost. Rigor mortis of the abdominal muscles can be removed by kneading the muscles or by the application of hot cloths.

CHAPTER V.
THE EXAMINATION OF THE SPINAL CORD.

1. METHODS OF EXAMINATION. The spinal cord may be opened anteriorly or posteriorly. The choice of method is largely a matter of convenience or of individual skill in using certain instruments, such as the Brunetti chisels. The method of opening posteriorly is more commonly used in this country, as it requires less skill. It necessitates, however, an additional long skin incision that must be tightly stitched together to prevent leakage of blood and fluids after the restoration of the body. For this reason it is not as clean a method as the anterior opening, which requires only the one main skin-incision. In private practice the latter method is often advisable, as by it an examination of the cord can often be secured when the relatives would not consent to its removal posteriorly, on the ground of undue mutilation of the body. The anterior examination also permits a better inspection and an easier removal of the spinal ganglia and nerves.

Examination of Cord Posteriorly. For the *opening of the spinal cord posteriorly* the cartilage-knife, bone-forceps, bone-nippers and rhachiotome are necessary; in place of the latter the single saw, double chisel, Brunetti chisels or single chisel may be employed. The posterior examination of the cord should take place at the beginning of the autopsy, after the external inspection of the cadaver, before the thorax and abdomen are examined. The removal of the sternum gives a loss of resistance to the manipulations upon the back of the cadaver, and the turning-over of the body after it has been opened anteriorly is usually an unpleasant procedure because of the dripping of blood and other fluids. When it is found necessary to examine the cord posteriorly after the opening of thorax and abdomen it is better to fill these cavities with tow or excelsior, replace the sternum and sew up the anterior skin-incision before turning the body over.

The cadaver is placed face downwards, with medium-sized blocks beneath the cervical and lumbar regions, the arms being folded underneath the body. With the cartilage-knife an incision is then made through the skin and subcutaneous tissues in the median line, over the spinous processes, beginning above at the occipital prominence and ending at the lower border of the sacrum. The skin and subcutaneous tissues are then dissected back by bold slashing strokes for a distance of a hand's breadth on both sides of the spine, thus laying bare the muscles of the neck and back. The muscles may be stripped back with the skin, but the heavy flaps thus formed are very likely to fall back and cover the seat of operation. Chain retractors may be used to hold the skin flaps back, particularly in the case of a very fat individual, but usually the separate stripping of the skin and muscles is sufficient. To remove the muscles the cartilage knife is set close against the spinous processes of the uppermost vertebræ and a deep cut made on each side of the spine throughout its entire length, severing the vertebral attachments of all muscles and tendons. About four finger-breadths outside of these cuts there should now be made from above downwards on both sides another deep cut through the muscles parallel with the first two incisions. The bundles of tendons and muscles between these parallel cuts on both sides of the spine are then separated from the bones as cleanly as possible, beginning either above or at the sacral end, severing the muscle-mass at the end at which the separation begins, but leaving it attached at the other end, where it is laid over the side of the body out of the way, and replaced after the examination of the cord is completed; or the two bundles of muscle may be cut off at both ends and disposed of without further trouble. Portions of tissue clinging to the vertebræ should then be scraped or cut away with the chisel or knife.

When the vertebræ are bared the next step is the removal by saw, bone-forceps or chisel of the posterior bony wall of the spinal canal in such a manner as to expose the cord and permit of its removal without causing any damage to it, either from the instruments or from fragments of broken bone. A single-bladed saw with curved ends may be used to saw through the laminæ on both sides of the spinous processes; or even the small bone-saw (Fig. 9) may be used for this purpose. The blade of the saw should be held obliquely against the spinous processes with the sawing edge directed outward so as to cut the laminæ close to the medial borders of the ascending and descending transverse processes. The sawing is complete when the spinous processes become movable. The straight-edged chisel may be used to cut any adhesions left after sawing, and the bone-forceps may be used to cut the atlas and axis. When the laminæ have been cut through on both sides of the spinal column for its entire length, including the sacrum, the posterior ligament between the atlas and occiput is cut with the cartilage knife; and the strip of bone and ligaments loosened by sawing is torn off from above downward by grasping it in the upper cervical region with a pair of bone-nippers and jerking it off forcibly downward toward the sacrum, thus exposing the spinal canal. It may be taken off in the opposite direction by cutting the ligament between the last lumbar vertebra and the sacrum and stripping upward.

The use of the single saw is not advised, however, as it is too time-consuming. The laminæ on both sides of the spinous processes may be cut at the same time by the use of *Luer's rhachiotome* (Fig. 11). The blades are separated according to the size of the vertebral arches and are set so as to include the spinous processes and cut the outer border of the laminæ close to the transverse processes in such a manner as not to injure the cord. Since the spinal canal is broader in the cervical and lumbar regions than in the dorsal, the distance between the saw-blades must be regulated accordingly. The dorsal portion is first sawed. The sawing should be in long cuts without too great pressure, the instrument being steadied by placing the left hand on the upright bar. As soon as the spinous processes become movable on slight pressure the sawing should be stopped. Should the blades become caught in the saw-cuts great care should be taken to avoid injuring the cord while releasing them. The straight-edged chisel may be inserted into the cuts and any parts still adherent may be carefully sprung apart. This is necessary particularly in the upper cervical region. The entire posterior wall of the canal may be loosened in this way, the sacrum being also sawed, when it is desired to open this part of the canal. When all the spinous processes are movable the attachments either above or below are cut with the cartilage-knife, and the spinous processes and laminæ torn off by the bone-nippers in one piece, either toward the head or sacrum as is the more convenient.

The laminæ may be cut by a chisel instead of a saw. The straight-edged or curved single chisel, the "tomahawk" chisel, or the double-bladed chisel of *Esquirol* may be employed. The latter instrument has adjustable chisel-blades that can be set to include the spinous processes. These blades are very strong and short, and have convex cutting edges. The use of a wooden mallet (Fig. 17) is to be preferred to that of the steel hammer in driving chisels of any type. The straight, curved and tomahawk chisels are held with their cutting edges directed slightly outwards. The *Amussat rhachiotome* is a chisel-knife with a curved metallic handle, the cutting edge running along the length of the chisel. When set at an angle of 45° to the laminæ it is driven through them by means of blows from a wooden mallet delivered upon the chisel-back over the cutting edge. The *Brunetti chisels* are shown in Fig. 15. In using these to open the spinal cord posteriorly, a block should be placed beneath the abdomen so as to raise the lumbar vertebræ above the level of the dorsal. The intervertebral ligaments of the last lumbar vertebræ are then cut through with the belly of the cartilage-knife held at right angles to the spine. The laminæ and spinous process of the last lumbar vertebra are then cut out with the straight-edged chisel or bone-forceps, exposing the canal. The *right* and *left* Brunetti chisels are then alternately used, beginning usually with the "left" chisel, the blunt probe-point being introduced into the canal, while firm pressure downward is made upon the handle, while at the same time the cutting edge is driven through the outer borders of the vertebral arches by blows from a wooden mallet delivered upon the head of the handle. Great care must be taken to keep the cut at the same level throughout. It is better, however, to cut too high rather than too low. In the latter case the cord may be injured, while in the former the bone may later be easily trimmed off sufficiently without causing any damage. The arches of three to four or even more vertebræ may be cut without removing the chisel. The same thing is then done on the other side, using the "right" chisel. The loosened portion of bone and ligaments is then cut or torn off with the bone-forceps or nippers. The cut bone should not be touched with the hands because of the danger of injury and subsequent infection from the sharp spicules and splinters of bone. As the canal is opened the block under the body is pushed towards the head, the object being always to cut *down hill* and not upward. When the cervical region is reached the head of the cadaver should be firmly held by an assistant so as to give sufficient resistance to the blows of the mallet. The skilful use of the Brunetti chisels is difficult to acquire and a great deal of practice is necessary, but when once the knack is obtained the spinal canal can be opened in this way more quickly than by any other method. In private practice the noise made by the hammer upon the head of the handles of the chisels is unpleasant, and should be avoided by the use of felt or something else on the head of the chisel or mallet to deaden the sound.

Another easy and convenient way of opening the spinal canal posteriorly is the cutting of the laminæ by means of special bone-forceps designed for this purpose. The cutting-edges may engage the laminæ from without or the lower blade may be introduced into the canal as a blunt probe, while the upper blade cuts down upon it through the side of the arch. Such bone-forceps should be very strong and have long handles to give sufficient purchase, as a good deal of force is necessary to cut through the laminæ. With a good instrument the canal can be opened in this way in about 10-15 minutes. It requires much less skill than is needed for good and quick work with the Brunetti chisels, and for that reason is recommended, as is also the use of Luer's rhachiotome, for the general practitioner.

In the case of marked curvatures of the spine it may be impossible to use either rhachiotome or Brunetti chisels. The straight single chisel and small saw can be used on the concave and convex sides of the curvature respectively. In children and young adults the canal can be easily opened with the bone-forceps.

After the removal of the posterior wall of the spinal canal the peridural adipose tissue and the dural sac are exposed in the canal. The cord may now be removed with dural sac intact, and when the cord is soft this should be done, but in so doing the spinal fluid is likely to be lost; and, as it is very important to obtain a knowledge of the amount and character of this fluid, care should be taken to preserve it. With the block placed under the cervical region to keep the cervical and dorsal vertebræ higher than the lumbar the dural sac may be opened in the median line from above downward. The cervical dura is grasped with a pair of forceps and lifted so that a cut can be made in it with the small bent, probe-pointed shears. The blunt probe-point is then introduced into the subdural space and the dura cut in the median line downward toward the sacrum. With care the arachnoideal sac with its fluid may be preserved intact. What fluid there is in the subdural space will collect in the lumbar region and may be secured while the lumbar dura is cut. The fluid in the subarachnoideal space will likewise collect in the lower portion of the cord, and it is best at this stage of the operation to introduce a sterile pipette through the delicate arachnoid and draw up the fluid, preserving it for bacteriologic and microscopic examination.

The thirty pairs of spinal nerves are now cut from above downward, beginning on the right side. The cut edge of the dura or a dural fold, if the dura is left uncut, is seized with the dissecting forceps and pulled over to the left, so that as much of the nerve can be secured as possible. A long, narrow, sharp-pointed scalpel is inserted, outside of the dura, into the intervertebral foramina, as far as possible, and the nerves are cut while traction is made upon the dura to the opposite side. The same procedure is then carried out upon the left side. When all of the spinal nerves are cut, the scalpel is introduced in the spinal canal upward, as near to the foramen magnum as possible, and the cord and dura are cut transversely. The cord should be held by the dura; direct pressure with forceps or fingers upon the soft substance of the cord should never be made. If the forceps cannot be used to hold the dura with advantage, then the cord enclosed in the dural sac may be gently but firmly held in the *palm* of the left hand and lifted and drawn downward towards the sacrum with the greatest care. As the cord is removed the fibrous attachments between the dura and the longitudinal fascia of the anterior wall of the canal are cut with the small scalpel by means of oblique cuts upon the bodies of the vertebræ. Any fragments of bone impeding the removal of the cord should be trimmed off with the bone-forceps. The forcing of the cord through a tight aperture in the open canal may ruin that portion of the cord. In some cases it may be better to sever the dura and cord at the sacral end, below the cauda equina, and remove it toward the head, using the same method of holding the dura, and cutting the spinal nerves and peridural tissue. When this is done the importance of saving the spinal fluid should be borne in mind. Some prosectors prefer to sever the dura and cord above before cutting the spinal nerves, and to cut these and the epidural fascia while removing the cord. An experienced operator may save time in this way, but there is greater danger of injuring the cord. The cord may also be removed by severing the spinal nerves and vessels inside of the opened dura and lifting the cord out of the dura, but it is more likely to be damaged by this method. When the brain has been removed before the cord the dural attachments as high as the foramen magnum should be severed and the cord removed up to the point where it was severed from the brain. If it is desired to remove the cord attached to the brain, the cord is first loosened throughout its length from below up to the foramen. It is then carefully protected while the skull is opened; and after the brain-connections have been severed it is drawn up through the foramen as the brain is lifted out of the skull. After its removal from the body the cord is stretched out upon table or board and the dura opened in the median line both anteriorly and posteriorly, if the latter cut was not made before its removal from the body. If it is desired to make sections of both cord and dura for microscopic study the dura may be left uncut or attached to the cord after it has been opened in the median line. It then helps to hold the pieces of cord together after the latter has been cut. Otherwise the dura may be removed from the cord by cutting the nerve-roots and denticulate ligaments on both sides. The cord is now examined by making transverse cuts through it with a clean knife which is dipped into clean water before each cut. The cord is allowed to hang over the index-finger of the left hand while the knife is drawn across it, severing it down to the underlying pia which is left uncut to hold the pieces together. The cuts are usually begun in the cervical region and are made at the level of the spinal nerves. When the dura is left attached to the cord it may be laid back and the cord cut within it, or if it has not been opened, the cuts may be made through it and the cord at the same time, if a very sharp knife is used. Areas of softening should not be cut, but should be preserved intact for examination after fixation and hardening. If the segments of cord are left attached to the dura or pia the cord and membranes may be fixed and hardened *en masse* so as to permit future orientation.

Examination of Cord Anteriorly. After the complete examination of the neck, thoracic and abdominal organs the spinal column is divested of all remaining tissues, including the psoas muscles. A block is then placed beneath the lumbar vertebræ. With the belly of the cartilage-knife held transversely across the spinal axis the intervertebral disks on both sides of the next-to-the-last lumbar vertebra are cut down to the level of the canal. If the lumbar vertebræ are sufficiently elevated by the block placed beneath the abdomen, the cutting of the disks allows the neighboring vertebræ to spring away, so that the body of the vertebra thus separated can be cut out by the bone-forceps or chisel. The spinal canal is thereby exposed; so that the Brunetti chisels may now be used in cutting the pedicles and stripping off the vertebral bodies. As this stripping progresses upward the block is moved toward the head so that the cutting is always down hill. The chisels are driven through the pedicles of five or six vertebræ at a time; the handle is forced down until the long chisel-blade is nearly parallel with the vertebræ. At the same time the cutting-edge must be sent forward at a uniform level, just high enough to expose the canal. If the cut is too high the chisel will enter the body of the vertebra, if too low the probe-point will be pushed into the cord. When the cervical vertebræ are being cut the head of the cadaver must be steadied by an assistant. As the sections of vertebræ are loosened the intervertebral disks are cut with the cartilage-knife and the pieces of bone pulled away with the bone-nippers. When the canal is fully exposed the examination of the dura and the removal of cord and dura proceed as when the canal is opened posteriorly. The straight chisel and the bone-forceps are also used to open the spinal canal anteriorly, but the Brunetti chisels are especially recommended for this operation.

Examination of Spinal Ganglia. While these may be examined when the canal is opened posteriorly, they can be exposed with less danger of damage in the anterior examination. To expose them in the posterior examination they must either be drawn forcibly through the intervertebral foramina, or the articular processes must be cut away with the chisel.

When it is desired to remove a part of the spinal column for preservation as a specimen, the intervertebral cartilages and the cord above and below the portion to be removed are cut through with the knife, and the ribs severed with a chisel, while the adherent soft parts are cut away. The saw or chisel is then used to complete the disarticulation if necessary and the loosened portion is removed. The entire spine may be removed, if desired; and may be bisected with a band-saw. A stick of wood may be put in the place of the spine and covered with plaster-of-Paris.

After the cord and dura have been removed the inner surface of the canal should be examined. The character of the cut surface of the vertebral bodies is also noted, and the bones examined for pathologic conditions.

2. POINTS TO BE NOTED IN THE EXAMINATION OF THE SPINAL COLUMN.

1. **Dorsal Incision.** Note color of skin as it is cut, number of bleeding points, moisture, bedsores, amount and character of panniculus, color and blood-content of muscles, hemorrhages, purulent and tuberculous processes (usually infiltrations from diseased vertebræ) trichina in spinal muscles, etc.

2. **Vertebrae.** Necrosis from bedsores, surfaces smooth or rough, purulent and tuberculous processes (most common anteriorly), exostoses, curvatures, fractures, dislocations, erosions, malformations (spina bifida and supernumerary vertebræ most common), neoplasms (secondary carcinoma, primary sarcoma, myeloma and chloroma most common), actinomycosis, syphilis, rachitis, etc.

3. **Dura.** Note epidural tissue first, then dura, its thickness, color, translucency, blood-content, intradural pressure, character of inner surface (normally it is grayish-white, smooth and shining).

defects, bone-formation, organizing blood-clots, hæmatoma, gumma, neoplasm, etc. Most common pathologic conditions are chronic pachymeningitis, syphilis, tuberculosis, traumatic lesions and secondary carcinoma. Primary tumors (sarcoma) and parasites (echinococcus and cysticercus) are rare. Teratomata occur in sacral and coccygeal regions. A diffuse formation of adipose tissue is common, as is also the development of bony plates in the dura in old chronic pachymeningitis (usually syphilitic). Note character and amount of contents of subdural space (blood, pus, serous exudate, etc.).

4. **Inner Meninges.** Normally gray, transparent, delicate. Note intrameningeal pressure, contents of subarachnoid space, color, thickness and translucency of arachnoid and pia, blood-vessels, presence of blood, pus, fibrinous exudates, localized thickenings, calcification, etc. Most common pathologic conditions are acute and chronic leptomeningitis, results of trauma, hemorrhage, syphilis, tuberculosis, cerebrospinal meningitis, leprous meningitis, etc. Bony plates (osteomata) are found in the arachnoid of the majority of people over forty-five years of age. In small number and size they have no pathologic significance; they are often large and very numerous in old cases of syphilitic leptomeningitis, sometimes encasing the cord. Primary tumors (fibroma, myxoma and sarcoma) are rare. Teratoid tumors (lipoma, myolipoma, neuroma) are occasionally found in the lumbosacral region, often associated with spina bifida. Secondary carcinoma and sarcoma, and metastases of the so-called glioma of the eye are also rarely found.

5. **Cord.** Size and form. Average length about 45 cms.; weight, 30 grms.; weight of cord to that of brain, 1:48.

Anteroposterior diameter of cervical cord................0.9 cm.
Anteroposterior diameter of dorsal cord.................0.8 cm.
Anteroposterior diameter of lumbar cord.................0.9 cm.
Transverse diameter of cervical cord ....1.4 cm.
Transverse diameter of dorsal cord ....1.0 cm.
Transverse diameter of lumbar cord ....1.2 cm.

Adhesions to inner meninges, consistence (should be uniform; changes in form and consistence are often the results of postmortem changes), color (gray-white, as seen through the pia), translucency (sclerotic areas in the white matter are firmer, depressed and gray or brownish-gray in color, and more translucent when present in the gray matter), moisture, color and blood-content of cut surface, relation of white and gray matter, symmetry of parts, size of central canal, presence of cavities, areas of softening (soft, yellowish-white, loss of structure), hemorrhages, congestion, anæmia, œdema, gumma, tubercle, tumors, parasites, etc. The normal consistence of the lower portion of the cord is usually somewhat firmer than that of the upper part. The "butterfly-figure" should stand out distinctly on the freshly-cut surface; the outlines between the white and gray matters should be sharp, and the gray matter should be grayish-red in color. Normally the white matter tends to rise above the gray. Inasmuch as the cord is often injured accidentally during its removal it is important to distinguish such artefacts from pathologic softenings. This can be easily done by taking a small portion of the doubtful area and examining in the fresh state under the microscope. In true softening numbers of "fat-granule" cells and also capillary walls showing fat-degeneration are seen.

The pathologic lesions of the cord easily recognized by the naked-eye are areas of sclerosis or gray degeneration, yellow degeneration, hemorrhage, anæmia, œdema, congestion, tabes dorsalis, amyotrophic lateral sclerosis, acute poliomyelitis, syringomyelia, ascending and descending degenerations, glioma, gumma, tubercle, certain malformations, neoplasms and parasites. Other important pathologic conditions are: Malformations (myelocele, hydrorrhachis interna, diastematomyelia, etc.), atrophy, myelitis, sclerosis, effects of trauma, syphilis and intoxications, infections, tuberculosis, etc. Primary tumors are: Glioma, gliosarcoma, gliomyxoma, sarcoma (spindle-cell, myxo-, angiosarcoma, etc.), neuro-epithelioma, neuroma, diffuse gliosis, etc. All are rare with the exception of the gliomata. Metastatic carcinoma and sarcoma are relatively rare. Cysticercus and echinococcus are rare.

The thickness, color, consistence and translucence of the spinal ganglia should be noted. Atrophic nerves are smaller, more gray and more translucent.

6. **Inner Surface of Vertebrae.** The remains of the epidural tissue and the inner surface of the spinal canal should also be carefully examined, noting the consistence of the vertebræ, the character of the ligaments, fascia, periosteum, etc. The anterior wall of the canal should be smooth, the color of the vertebræ grayish-red, that of the intervertebral disks grayish-white. Caries, tuberculosis and syphilis lead to roughening of the bony wall of the canal.

CHAPTER VI.
THE EXAMINATION OF THE HEAD.
I. METHODS OF EXAMINATION.

1. **Removal of Skull-Cap.** For the section of the head the cadaver is placed upon its back with its head near the end of the table. The head may be elevated by a block placed beneath the neck, or it may be elevated and at the same time firmly held in position by the use of a special head-rest, different varieties of which are offered by instrument-makers. It is better to use the simple block of wood and to control the position of the head with the hands during the operation. The prosector takes his position behind the head of the table. The hair of the cadaver is then arranged in such a manner as to be out of the way, and protected by towels so that it will not become matted with blood and bone-dust. When the hair is short it is parted in a line extending from just behind the ears across the vertex. The shape of the head and the degree of baldness will determine the exact position of the primary incision through the scalp; sometimes it must be made farther back than the line connecting the ears in order that the incision may be concealed. In the great majority of cases it will be made as follows: The head is steadied with the operator's left hand, and turned as far to the right as possible. The point of the cartilage-knife is then inserted into the scalp, just within the hair-line, behind the left ear, and with the belly of the knife the scalp is cut through to the periosteum, in the line of the hair-part, over the vertex, and as the head is turned to the left, down to the hair-line behind the right ear, the knife, as it approaches the end of the incision being raised so as to make the point finish the cut. This scalp-incision should be made with a strong and quick drawing movement, but the knife should not be pressed so firmly against the bone as to cut through the periosteum, else hemorrhages, collections of pus, etc., may escape before they are seen.

The scalp is next loosened anteriorly by means of the hands, using the tip of the cartilage-knife occasionally to nick the fascia and thus facilitate the working forward of the anterior flap until it has been loosened as far as the supraorbital ridges anteriorly and down to the level of the beginning and ending of the incision made across the vertex. When sufficiently loosened the anterior scalp-flap is turned over the face, and stretched over the chin, where it will remain, out of the way, and with both face and hair protected. The posterior flap of the scalp is then worked back to the same level at the sides and to the lower border of the occipital protuberance posteriorly. It is then turned under between the back of the neck and the wooden block. In stripping the scalp the greatest care should be taken not to cut or tear off the periosteum. Scars, tumors, adhesions, traumatic lesions, etc., in the scalp should be carefully worked out and described as the flaps are loosened. The convex margin of the fascia of the temporal muscles is now cut with the point of the cartilage-knife and the muscles are stripped down on both sides to the level of the folded-over scalp-flaps, where they are either left hanging down out of the way or are cut off and laid aside. If they cannot be easily stripped down, they may be scraped off with the chisel. Some prosectors remove them at the same time with the scalp, but this is usually not well done. The skull now should be bare, except for the periosteum, down to the level of a line passing just above the upper margin of the orbits anteriorly, at the sides just above the aural opening, and posteriorly just below the occipital protuberance.

The periosteum is next removed over the entire cranial surface by means of the chisel, bone-scraper or dull knife. In medico-legal cases particularly it is of the greatest importance that the periosteum be removed in this way and the surface of the skull-cap carefully examined. In ordinary cases the periosteum is often left attached to the skull-cap when the external examination shows no pathologic conditions to be present.

After the examination of the periosteum and external surface of the cranium the skull-cap is removed by sawing in such a way that a space large enough for the convenient and safe removal of the brain is afforded. This may be done in several ways. A circular incision may be made through the skull around its entire circumference just above the level of the folded-over flaps of scalp. The left hand should be protected by a folded towel. The head is held firmly in the left hand and turned slightly toward the left. The saw-cut is then begun anteriorly about $\frac{1}{2}$ cm. above the supra-orbital margins, and continued around to the right, while the head is turned more and more to the left. The ear should be held down out of the way by an assistant. The saw-cut is continued then at the same level to the posterior median line just below the level of the occipital protuberance. The saw is then removed and the head turned as far as possible to the right; the saw-cut is then continued around the left side from the posterior median line until the beginning of the cut in front is reached and the circular incision is complete.

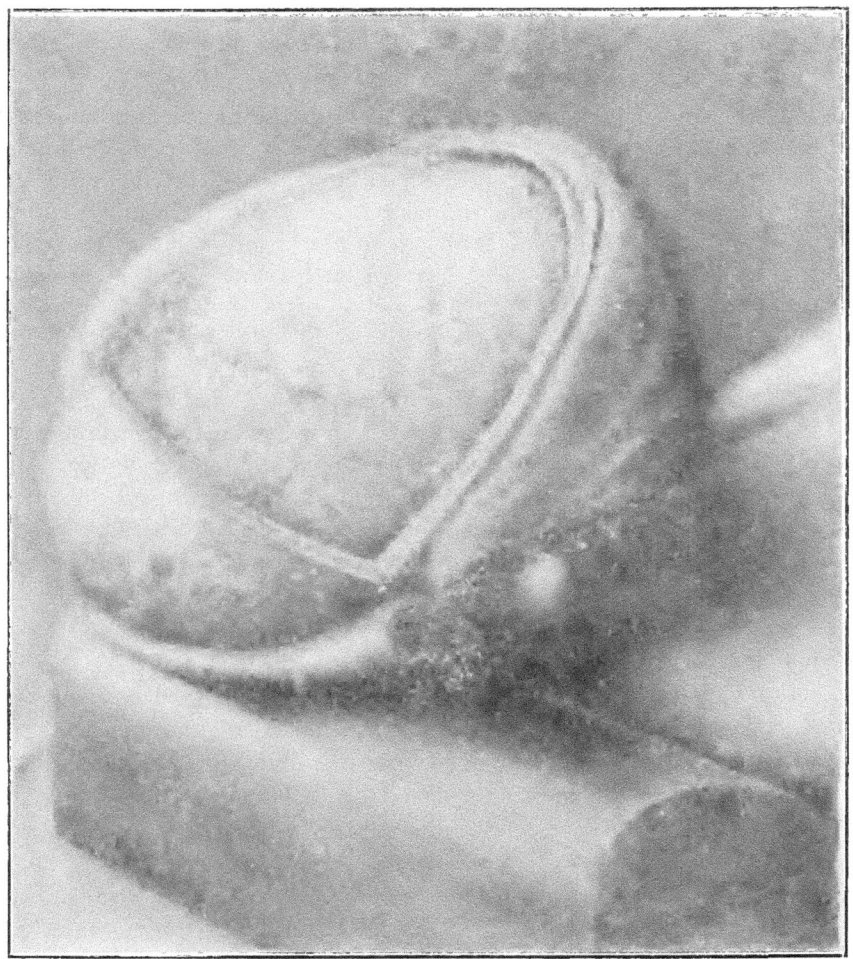

FIG. 26.—Author's method of removing skull-cap.

Another method of sawing the skull-cap is to saw in two planes, forming an angle just behind and below the ear (angular method). The anterior cut is made above the hair-line of the forehead and carried down at the sides to meet just below and behind the ear the posterior semicircular cut made at this level. A modification of this method is to make the anterior and posterior cuts join at a sharper angle in front of the ears. Both of these methods have for their object the prevention of disfigurement of the forehead. When the circular method is used a depression or ridge is often seen in the forehead, after the restoration of the body, due to the slipping of the skull-cap after it has been replaced. Such an accident may happen even when the bones are wired together, unless great care has been taken in wiring.

A more satisfactory way of opening the skull, and one that makes slipping of the skull-cap after restoration practically impossible, is the method used by the writer, and illustrated in Fig. 26. The scalp-incision and the folding back of the flaps are carried out as described above. The right half of the anterior flap of the scalp is then taken in the left hand and used to control the position of the head, the latter being turned to the left as far as possible. An oblique saw-cut is then made on the right side in a line extending from the posterior margin of the site of the posterior fontanel, over the right parietal eminence toward the right mastoid prominence. The sawing begins on the greatest convexity and is continued upward a slight distance beyond the median line, and downward far enough to cross the level of the connecting horizontal cut to be made later at a level just above the aural canal. The left half of the posterior scalp-flap is now taken into the left hand and used to steady the head while it is turned over to the right as far as possible. A similar oblique cut is then made on the left side, crossing the one made on the right, in the median line, behind the site of the posterior fontanel, and extending down across the left parietal eminence in the direction of the left mastoid prominence. While the head is still held by the left half of the posterior scalp-flap a horizontal saw-cut is begun on the left side, just above the aural canal, intersecting the oblique cut posteriorly and continued around to the front at a level just above the supraorbital ridges. When the frontal region is reached the head is steadied by holding the left half of the anterior portion of the scalp-flap. When the horizontal cut reaches the right temple the right half of the anterior flap is taken in the hand, and the head turned to the left while the cut is carried around the right temporal region to intersect the right oblique cut. When the skull-cap is removed there is formed an interlocking joint (Fig. 27) which under ordinary conditions holds the restored skull-cap firmly without wiring and without the formation of a ridge or crease on the brow, since the bone cannot slip. It is best, however, in the event of the shipment of a cadaver by rail to wire the bones to prevent any forcible dislodgement.

Whatever method is used the greatest care should be taken to saw the skull-cap without injuring the brain. The difference in thickness of different portions of the cranium must be borne in mind. Sight, sound and "the feel" are taken as guides. The outer

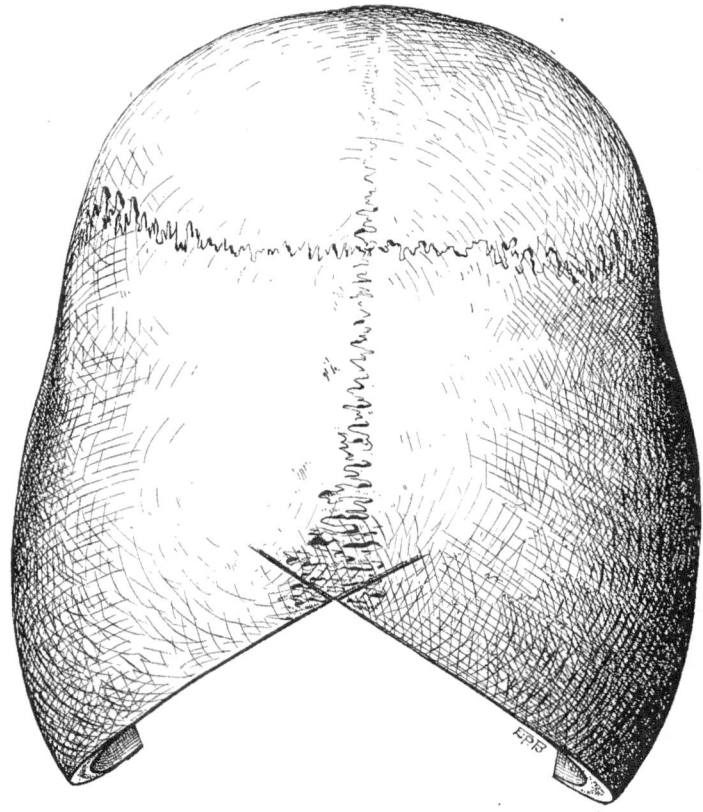

FIG. 27.—Skull-cap after removal, showing posterior interlocking joint.

and inner tables, the diploë, and the dura have an entirely different resistance and give a different sound. The saw-dust of the outer table is white, that of the diploë red, that of the inner table white. As soon as the saw strikes the dura a peculiar "rustling" or "scraping" sound is heard, and this should be taken as the warning to stop sawing. On curved surfaces it is best to begin sawing on the greatest convexity and to continue until the saw is through and then to extend the cut from this point. The sawing should be done lightly and quickly, without too strong pressure. Set the saw carefully at first, to avoid slipping. The small bone-saw is usually used for this operation; saws attached to electric or dental engines are sometimes employed. Care should be taken to bring the beginning and ending of the saw-cut into the same plane; and the oblique cuts should be symmetrical.

As soon as the sawing is completed, no matter what method is used, the T-chisel or skull-opener (Fig. 12) is used to spring off the skull-cap. The chisel-blade is inserted into the saw-cut in the right frontal region, and turned sideways with a quick, powerful movement of the right hand. Any portions of the inner table not completely sawed through (usually in the region of the petrous portion of the temporal) are thus broken, and the dura is loosened sufficiently from the inner table to allow the prosector to introduce the fingers of the right hand beneath the skull-cap in the frontal region and to hold down the dura while the fingers of the left hand inserted into the frontal saw-cut pull the skull-cap backward with a powerful tug, completely separating it from the dura, unless the dura is adherent throughout, as is the case in very young children, old people, and in certain pathologic conditions. In the latter case it may be necessary to cut the dura along the line of the horizontal saw-cut and to remove it with the skull-cap, cutting the falx as the skull-cap is lifted. In young children the dura must always be removed with the skull-cap. In the case of pathologic adhesions an attempt should be made first to separate them from the lamina vitrea by cutting them with a knife or chisel-blade inserted through the saw-cut. As the adhesions are severed the skull-cap is lifted gradually backward. Too much force should not be used in jerking off the skull-cap, else the brain may be damaged. Whenever possible the dura should be left intact, as a better judgment is thereby obtained of the intradural pressure, and there is less danger of losing the contents of the subdural space.

Some prosectors use hammer and chisel to remove the skull-cap. This is a bad method, particularly so in the case of medico-legal autopsies, as artificial fractures of the skull may thus be produced. It is safest never to use a hammer in the opening of the skull.

The skull-cap is examined as soon as taken off. If the periosteum was not previously removed it is now scraped off, and the skull-cap examined against the light. After its complete examination the operator proceeds to the removal of the brain.

2. **Removal of the Brain.** The convexity of the dura is first examined. The narrow-bladed brain-knife or long section knife (Fig. 3) is now taken in hand, and with the cutting edge directed upward the point of the blade is inserted into the anterior end of the superior longitudinal sinus and the sinus cut open as far posteriorly as the opening in the cranial vault will admit. Its walls and contents are then examined. With cutting edge outward the point of the brain-knife is then inserted through the dura just to the left of the anterior end of the falx and the dura cut around to the left at the level of the horizontal saw-cut. The knife is then inserted through the dura just to the right of the falx and the dura cut in the same way on the right side. The two halves of the dura are now loosened from the convexity of the brain by breaking the blood-vessels connecting the dura with the inner meninges. The index-finger is swept over the convexities and along the sides of the longitudinal sinus, tearing the pial veins. Pathologic adhesions should be carefully worked out. The finger is then used to raise the falx anteriorly so that the point of the brain-knife can be introduced beneath it to cut it upward and forward. The dura is then carefully examined and turned back over the brain and allowed to hang down over the occiput. The inner meninges over the exposed portion of the brain are now examined; and the brain is then removed as follows: The four fingers of the left hand are placed beneath the frontal lobes, lifting these sufficiently for the prosector to be able to cut the I, II, III, IV and VI cranial nerves, the carotids and pedicle of the hypophysis down to the tentorium cerebelli. The tentorium is then cut with the tip of the brain-knife, which is held perpendicularly, by a gentle up-and-down sawing motion, from left to right along the superior border of the petrous bones. The V, VII, VIII, IX, X, XI and XII cranial nerves are then cut as closely as possible to their exits. As they are cut the brain is lifted gradually more and more, and supported by the left hand. When all the connections have been cut except the cord and vertebral arteries these are severed by the myelotome (Fig. 4), or by the brain-knife, the point of which is put down through the foramen magnum as far as possible, and the cord and vertebral arteries severed by a transverse cut made from left to right as nearly horizontal as possible. The knife is now laid aside and the first two fingers of the right hand put beneath the two cerebellar lobes so that the medulla and portions of cervical cord fall between these fingers, which are then used to lift them upward and backward. The freed brain is now rolled over backward out of the cranial cavity upside down onto the palm

of the left hand, and is then placed upon a board, tray or dish ready for examination. If the cord has already been removed, any portion remaining is taken out with the brain. In case the cord has been freed and is to be removed with the brain it is only necessary to cut the vertebral arteries and then to lift up the brain, drawing the cord up through the foramen magnum.

3. **Section of the Brain.** (*Modified Virchow Method.*) The brain as it is taken from the cranium is placed upside down, with occipital lobes toward the prosector. The basal meninges and blood-vessels are then carefully examined. The hemispheres and convolutions are separated and the arachnoid torn by the tip of the index-finger or the handle of a scalpel; and the branches of the cerebral vessels to their deepest ramifications are thus exposed, giving a complete picture of the circle of Willis and all of its branches to the point where they enter the brain-substance. The larger vessels are opened by transverse or longitudinal cuts and their walls and contents noted. The brain is then turned over, and the meninges examined over the entire convexity. The pia and arachnoid are then removed together over the entire convex and median surfaces of the hemispheres. If the blood-vessels between the convolutions are seized with the forceps the meninges can be easily stripped off, the fingers aiding the forceps, using great care not to tear the brain substance. The meninges are removed about half-way down the outer sides of the hemispheres and are there left intact so as to hold the pieces of brain together after it has been cut, and so permit orientation. The cortical surface is then examined; if bloody, it should be washed with a weak stream of water.

The hemispheres are now separated until the corpus callosum comes into view. The left hemisphere is then held by the left hand, with the thumb on the median surface and the fingers on the outer and under sides, so that the hemisphere is turned outward and yet raised slightly at the same time, thus stretching the corpus callosum over the cavity of the left lateral ventricle. The point of the narrow brain-knife (Fig. 3) with cutting edge upward is then introduced with great care through the corpus callosum about midway between the genu and splenium and close to the gyrus cinguli (gyr. forn., Fig. 28). The corpus callosum at this point is about 2 to 3 mm. thick and it is gently nicked with the point of the knife until an opening is made into the cavity of the ventricle. The knife-point must not be allowed to slip through to damage the basal ganglia beneath. Into the small opening thus made the brain-knife, held nearly horizontal, with cutting edge upward, is introduced and the corpus callosum cut forward until the anterior horn of the ventricle is reached. The point of the knife is then passed into the horn and the knife-handle raised and turned over forward, cutting slightly outward through the frontal lobe to its apex and

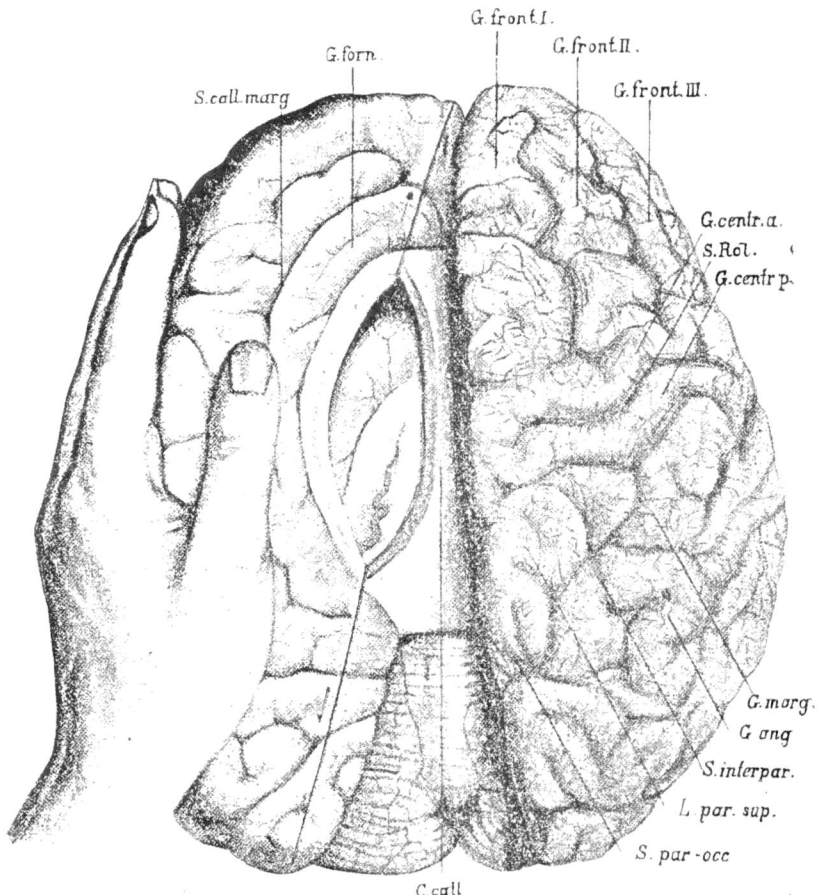

FIG. 28.—Method of examination of brain. Opening of left ventricle. Line showing direction of cuts. (After Nauwerck.)

disclosing the anterior horn. The knife is then reversed, held horizontally, with cutting edge upward, and the corpus callosum cut posteriorly from the beginning of the first cut, until the posterior horn is reached, when the point of the knife is inserted into the horn and the knife turned over toward the operator, cutting backward

72   THE EXAMINATION OF THE HEAD.

and somewhat outward through the occipital lobe to its apex and opening up the posterior horn. (See Fig. 28.) By this method the lateral ventricle is opened first at the highest point of its cavity, and the fluid contents collect in the anterior and posterior horns so that the amount and character can be easily noted.

The left hemisphere is now turned still more to the left, and

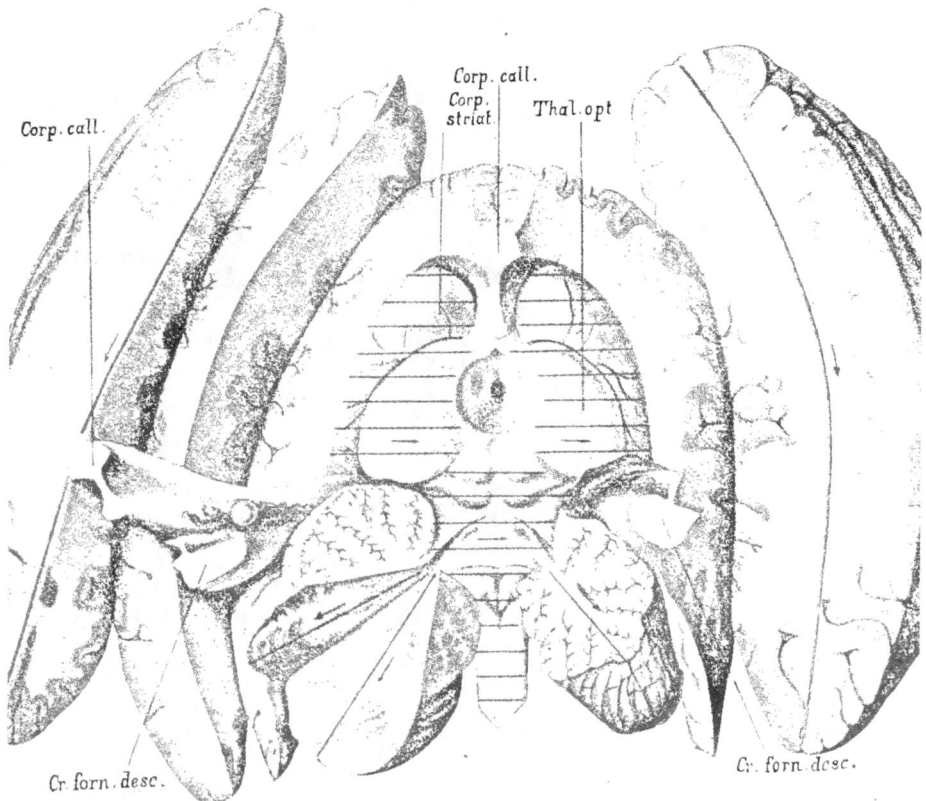

FIG. 29.—Section of brain. Ventricles opened. Lines show direction of large longitudinal incisions through brain-substance. (After Nauwerck.)

with the brain-knife a broad, smooth cut is made through it downward and outward at an angle of 45°, reaching nearly to the cortical surface, in a line connecting the cut through the frontal lobe with that through the occipital and passing along the outer borders of the corpus striatum. The left hemisphere is thus separated in the form of a prism-shaped mass having a convex under surface. (See Fig. 29.) The severed hemisphere falls back by the force of its own weight and the flat cut-surface of the cerebrum is then bisected by a cut made at right angles to it, from before backward, and extending nearly to the cortical surface. (See Fig. 29.) In the case of both of these large incisions of the hemisphere the severed parts are left connected by a small portion of cortical tissue and the pia. The knife should be perfectly dry and clean while making these cuts, and the cut surfaces should not be touched with the fingers or knife-blade, or wet with water, until they have been carefully inspected. Other straight parallel cuts may be made through the brain substance toward the cortex, the severed portions being left connected by the pia so as to permit future orientation.

The right lateral ventricle is now opened. The four fingers of the left hand are placed outside and beneath the right hemisphere with the thumb on the median surface, gently raising the hemisphere toward the left, taking care to see that the corpus callosum is not pulled over to the right of the median line. The knife is held in the right hand beneath the left one. The right ventricle is then opened in the same way as the left, beginning in the middle of the corpus callosum near to the gyrus cinguli, and opening first the anterior horn and then the posterior. The operation is somewhat more difficult on the right side than it is on the left, owing to the lack of tension in the cut corpus callosum, so that greater care must be taken to avoid injuring the floor of the ventricle. After the opening of the ventricle the right hemisphere is cut by long parallel incisions made in the same way as on the left side. (See Fig. 29.)

Some prosectors in opening the right ventricle prefer to turn the board around so that the frontal lobe points to the operator. The right hemisphere is then held in the left hand and the right ventricle opened just as if it were the left ventricle, except that the posterior horn is opened before the anterior. The method given above can be just as easily learned, and time is saved by not turning the board around twice, as is necessary in the latter case.

After the right ventricle has been opened the corpus callosum and fornix are raised by the thumb and index-finger of the left hand, putting the septum pellucidum on the stretch. The narrow brain-knife is then introduced through the interventricular foramen from the right, its blade flat, with cutting edge directed forward and upward, and the fornix and the corpus callosum are cut anteriorly, exposing the cavity of the septum pellucidum. To expose the third ventricle, the corpus callosum, septum pellucidum and fornix are then lifted up and laid back from the velum chorioides. The tela chorioidea is then, with the chorioid plexus of the third ventricle, pulled backward from over the pineal body and the corpora quadrigemina, care being taken not to tear away the pineal body. The veins entering the tela from the great ganglia are cut with the point of the knife. The right descending posterior pillar or crus of the fornix is then lifted with the thumb and index-finger of the left hand, the brain-knife on the flat side with cutting edge to the right is introduced beneath it, and the crus is cut toward the right. The corpus callosum, fornix and tela are then turned over to the left (see Fig. 29), fully exposing the pineal body and the corpora quadrigemina.

The cerebellum and medulla are now supported by the index-finger of the left hand placed beneath the latter; while the brain-knife is held nearly horizontally in the right, and a deep sagittal cut is made into the vermis exactly in the median line so as to make a small opening into the fourth ventricle. The point of the knife with cutting edge upward is then introduced into this opening and the incision through the vermis increased anteriorly and posteriorly until the two cerebellar hemispheres fall apart and the fourth ventricle is wholly opened. The point of the knife with cutting edge upward may then be introduced into the posterior opening of the aqueduct and the latter opened to the third ventricle, the pineal body being removed before the cut through the roof of the aqueduct is made. In the Virchow method the corpora quadrigemina and the vermiform portion of the cerebellum are sectioned in the median line by a cut opening up both aqueduct and the fourth ventricle. Other prosectors open the aqueduct from the third ventricle toward the fourth. The left cerebellar hemisphere is now cut through in the line of the middle branch of the arbor vitæ, exposing the dentate nucleus. Each half of the hemisphere is again bisected by a cut made at right angles to the surfaces exposed by the first cut. The right cerebellar hemisphere is then similarly sectioned.

The section of the brain now shows all of the ventricles and their relations, as well as the condition of a large part of cerebral and cerebellar brain-substance. (See Fig. 29.) All cut portions are connected with each other and it is possible to fix the entire brain as it now stands and later find no difficulty in topographic orientation. There still remains, however, the demonstration of the conditions in the basal ganglia, pons, medulla, etc. These structures are best shown by transverse cuts made across the entire brain as it lies after the opening of the ventricles. The hemispheres may be cut singly, but it is better to cut both of them at the same time, using a dry blade and drawing the knife from left to right, making identical cuts on the two sides, that the histologic features may be compared. The transverse cuts may be made in the same region as recommended in the method of Pitres (see below), or they may be made closer together. As the cuts are made the sections are separated from each other by the knife-blade and the cut surfaces examined. After the cerebrum has been cut transversely in this way the peduncles, pons, medulla and cervical cord are elevated on the index-finger of the left hand and also sectioned transversely and the cut surfaces examined. If the index-finger be placed beneath the medulla parallel with its long axis, and medulla and pons raised up the cerebellar lobes fall to the side out of the way. All transverse cuts are made from left to right and so deep that only a small portion of brain-tissue, or the basal meninges hold the parts

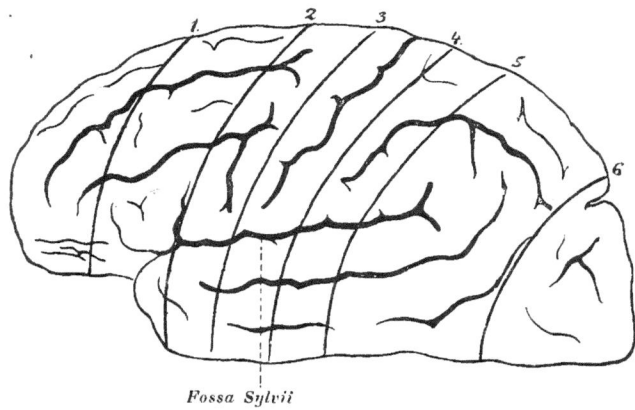

FIG. 30.—Method of Pitres. 1, *Sectio præ-frontalis;* 2, *Sectio pediculo-frontalis;* 3, *Sectio frontalis;* 4, *Sectio parietalis;* 5, *Sectio pediculo-parietalis;* 6, *Sectio occipitalis.*

together for future orientation. The brain is now completely sectioned, with all parts preserved and capable of being restored to their normal relations. The parts may be re-assembled and the entire brain put into the fixing fluid, when it is desirable to save the entire organ for microscopic study.

Other Methods of Opening Brain. For the demonstration of large localized pathologic conditions the brain may be opened by a very simple method of transverse or sagittal incisions extending entirely through the organ. The broad-bladed brain-knife should be used and the blade should be wet. The cuts should be made symmetrically on the two sides and with due reference to anatomic landmarks. They may be made either from the convexity or from the basal side.

The method of **Pitres** (see Fig. 30) is also employed for the same purpose. After the inspection of the meninges and basal vessels and opening of lateral ventricles, the brain is divided into three parts, consisting of the two hemispheres and one part made up of the cerebellum, pons and medulla. The anterior ends of the cerebral peduncles are cut transversely in front of the corpora quadrigemina, and the hemispheres are then separated by a sagittal median incision through the corpus callosum, septum pellucidum, commissure of third ventricle, substantia perforata posterior, tuber cinereum and infundibulum, the optic chiasm and neighboring optic tract having first been removed. The hemispheres are then cut as follows: The hemisphere is laid upon its median surface with the occipital lobe toward the operator. The four fingers of the left hand are then put into the central fissure and six parallel transverse cuts (see Fig. 30) are made through the hemisphere with a dry brain-knife, as follows:

1. *Sectio praefrontalis*, through the frontal lobe about 5 cm. in front of and parallel to the central fissure, exposing the cortex and medulla of the three frontal convolutions, gyrus orbitalis, and the convolutions of the median surface of the frontal lobe.

2. *Sectio pediculo-frontalis*, through the "foot" of the frontal convolutions, exposing the three frontal convolutions, anterior end of the island of Reil, gyrus orbitalis, corpus callosum, head of caudate nucleus, anterior portion of lentiform nucleus and lenticular striated portion of the internal capsule.

3. *Sectio frontalis*, through the anterior central convolution, showing the anterior central convolution, island of Reil, the temporal convolutions, corpus callosum, tail of caudate nucleus, the optic thalamus, middle portion of lentiform nucleus, the anterior portion of the lenticular part of the internal capsule, the external capsule and claustrum.

4. *Sectio parietalis*, through the posterior central convolution, showing the same, the island of Reil, temporal convolutions, corpus callosum, tail of caudate nucleus, posterior end of optic thalamus and lentiform nucleus, posterior end of the lenticular-optic part of internal capsule, the external capsule and the claustrum.

5. *Sectio pediculo-parietalis*, through the foot of the parietal convolution, 3 cm. posterior to the fissure of Rolando, showing superior and inferior parietal lobules, temporal convolutions, corpus callosum, extreme posterior portion of optic thalamus and tail of caudate nucleus.

6. *Sectio occipitalis*, about 1 cm. in front of the parieto-occipital sulcus, showing cortex and medulla of occipital lobe.

After the third cut the fingers of the left hand are taken out of the central fissure. The sections of brain as they are cut are left lying in their order with the posterior face of the cut upward. The same incisions are then made in the other hemisphere and the two series of sections compared. The cerebellum, pons and medulla are then examined as described above.

Section of Brain in Skull. When the skull-cap is removed by a circular saw-cut the brain may be cut through with the saw at the same time; or, after the skull-cap and dura have been removed, the upper portion of the hemispheres may be sliced off by a horizontal cut made at the level of the saw-cut. The portions removed are examined further by sagittal cuts. The lateral ventricles are then examined in the skull, and the remaining portion of the brain either cut transversely *in situ* or removed and sectioned outside of the cranium. This method is mentioned to be condemned.

For special neuropathologic studies a number of methods have been advised, the main purpose of which has been to preserve intact parts of the brain having

THE SECTION OF THE BRAIN.

definite anatomic relationships so that lesions may be studied by means of serial sections of the entire system involved. The methods of **Déjerine** and **Meynert** are employed for this purpose.

Method of Déjerine. After a careful examination of the cortical surface for the presence of lesions, and of the inferior surfaces of the crura for secondary degenerations, the pons is cut horizontally in a plane parallel with the inferior surface of the hemispheres and passing just above the great root of the trifacial. The brain is thus divided into two portions, one consisting of the two peduncles and superior portion of the pons, the other containing the remaining portion of the pons, the cerebellum and the medulla. The cut surfaces of the pons are examined for evidences of degeneration in the pyramidal tracts, and the hemispheres are separated after it has been determined in which one the lesion is located. If the lesion is found to be central the degenerations of importance will be found in the tracts of the internal capsule and in the region of the tegmentum. The hemispheres are then opened by horizontal incisions passing through the superior third of the optic thalamus. If the lesion is cortical the hemispheres are divided into three segments by two transverse vertical incisions, one passing just posterior to the splenium of the corpus callosum, the other just anterior to the knee. The posterior segment consists of the occipital lobe and part of the parietal; the central one contains the regions adjacent to the fissure of Rolando, the middle portion of the temporal convolutions, the basal ganglia, the cerebral peduncle and corresponding portion of the pons; the anterior segment consists of the forepart of the frontal lobe. The segments are then fixed and hardened and cut on a brain-microtome. The anterior and posterior segments are sectioned vertically transversely, the central segment is cut horizontally. By this method cortical lesions may be accurately located, and the entire course of degenerating fibres followed out.

Method of Meynert. This method aims to separate all portions of the brain possessing differences of internal structure that may be taken as indicating difference in significance, and to compare them by weight. The natural furrows or fissures are used as incision-lines, and three series of dissections are made, the first of which, here given, is the separation of the brain into three parts, the brain-mantle, brain-stem and cerebellum. The brain, with pia still intact, is placed base upward, with cerebellum toward operator. The arachnoid covering the fissure of Sylvius is cut or torn, and the island exposed. The three furrows bounding it must be plainly seen. The pia between the optic tract and uncus, as well as that in the middle portion of the transverse fissure between corpora quadrigemina and corpus callosum, is cut, and the under surface of the splenium of the corpus callosum is freed from membranous adhesions to the corpora quadrigemina and the pineal body. When the medulla with pons and cerebellum is now elevated the transverse fissure gapes open, and permits a free look into the lateral ventricles.

The brain-mantle on both sides is now separated from the brain-stem at the basal portion of its frontal end. The knife, held nearly horizontal, is introduced into the fissure between the posterior border of the orbital convolutions and the anterior border of the lamina perforata anterior; and a cut is made slightly downward, not quite parallel with the orbital surface, about 3 cm. anteriorly in the medulla of the orbital convolutions, around the under surface of the head of the corpus striatum. The temporal ends of the brain-mantle are then cut through, the knife moving externally between the temporal lobe and the island, inside between the descending horn of the lateral ventricle and the optic tract. As soon as the inner cut has been extended beyond the outer corpus geniculatum on both sides, the knife is turned downward at right angles, in a curving stroke, to cut through the junction of the occipital lobes with the stem, internally along the portion of the corpus striatum adjacent to the optic thalamus, externally between the junction of the first temporal convolution with the operculum on one side, and the posterior end of the island on the other. When this has been done on both sides the blade of the knife is turned forward in a semicircular stroke. The posterior end of the brain-stem is gradually lifted up out of the mantle by elevating the cerebellum and medulla oblongata. The upper peduncle of the arch of the brain-mantle along the upper border of the island and the outer border of the corpus striatum is severed from the stem as far as the anterior end of the upper border of the island, which bends downward into the anterior border. The peduncle of the fornix with the pedicle of the septum and the lamina of the knee of the corpus callosum are severed close above the anterior commissure, and the knife following the anterior border of the island is carried downward from the head of the corpus striatum. The remaining connections between the frontal lobes and stem are put on a moderate stretch and the incision is completed by bringing the knife back into the first cut made from the opposite direction parallel with the orbital surface over the upper surface of the stem. The three arms of the cerebellum are then severed and the brain-stem, consisting of the island of Reil, the basal ganglia, crura, pons, medulla and cerebellum, is completely freed and lifted out of the mantle.

A combination of the Meynert and Virchow methods is used by many. The lateral ventricles are opened and an incision made along the fornix into the descending horn. The stem-ganglia are then cut out and brain-mantle and stem separated. The hemispheres are then cut by frontal sections made from the anterior end as far as the central convolutions. From the central convolutions backward horizontal sections are then made; the series of sections are numbered in order and fixed and hardened for microscopic examination.

It is evident that the section of the brain can be modified to meet the individual requirements, according to the nature, location and extent of the lesion and the character of the study to be made of the latter. The brain may be fixed and hardened either before or after sectioning.

4. **Examination of Base of Cranium.** After the section of the brain the prosector returns to the head and examines the basal sinuses (see Fig. 31) by cutting them open with the point of the brain-knife or by using small shears and forceps. When cut open the walls of the sinuses should be laid back for inspection. Ordinarily the *sinus transversus, sinus petrosus superior, sinus petrosus inferior, sinus cavernosus* and the *sinus sigmoideus* are opened. The last-named is given especial attention because of the frequency of thrombosis and its involvement from carious conditions of the neighboring portions of the temporal bone. In purulent mastoid inflammation the infection often reaches the meninges by this route. The *carotids* and the *exits of the cranial nerves* (see Fig. 31) are

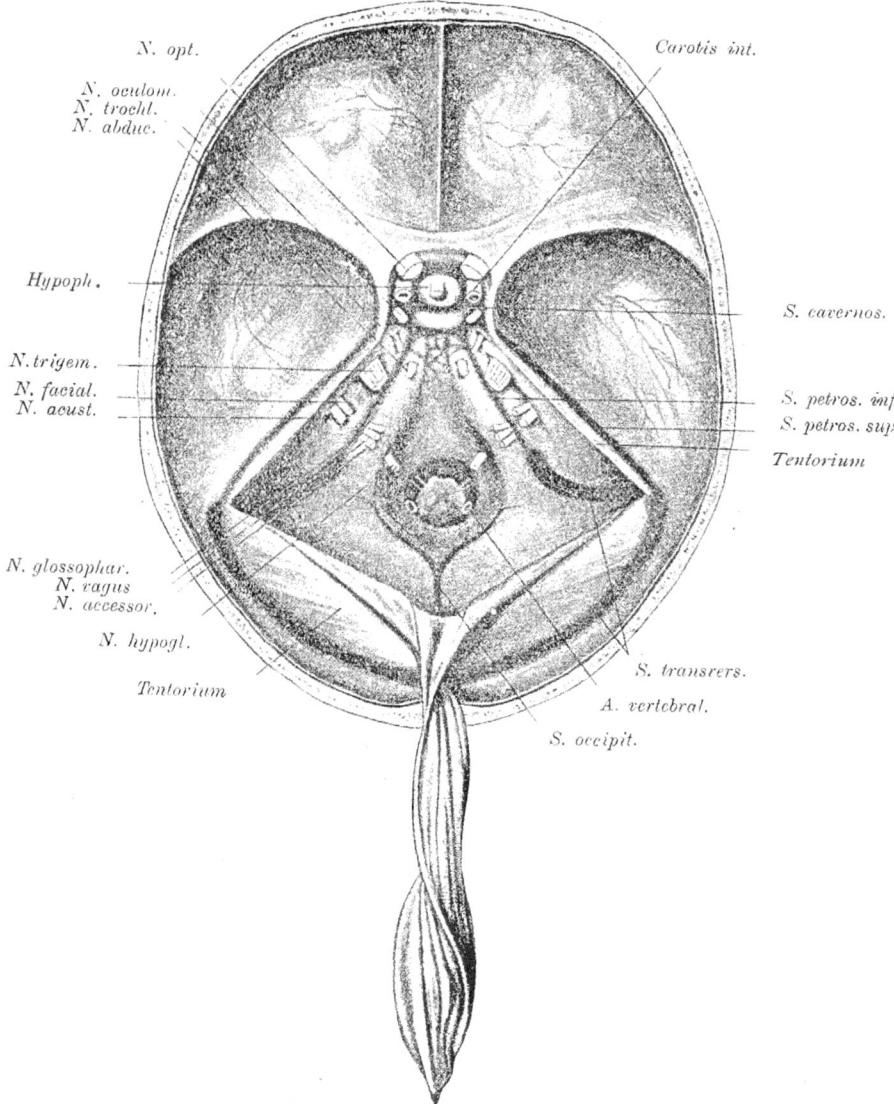

Fig. 31.—Base of cranium, after removal of brain. (After Nauwerck.)

then examined. The *hypophysis* (see Fig. 31) is then removed by making semicircular cuts through the overlying dura mater around the gland and then lifting it out of the sella. This is best accomplished by means of the small scalpel and forceps. It is sometimes necessary to chisel away the overhanging bony parts in order to remove the hypophysis without damaging it. When removed it

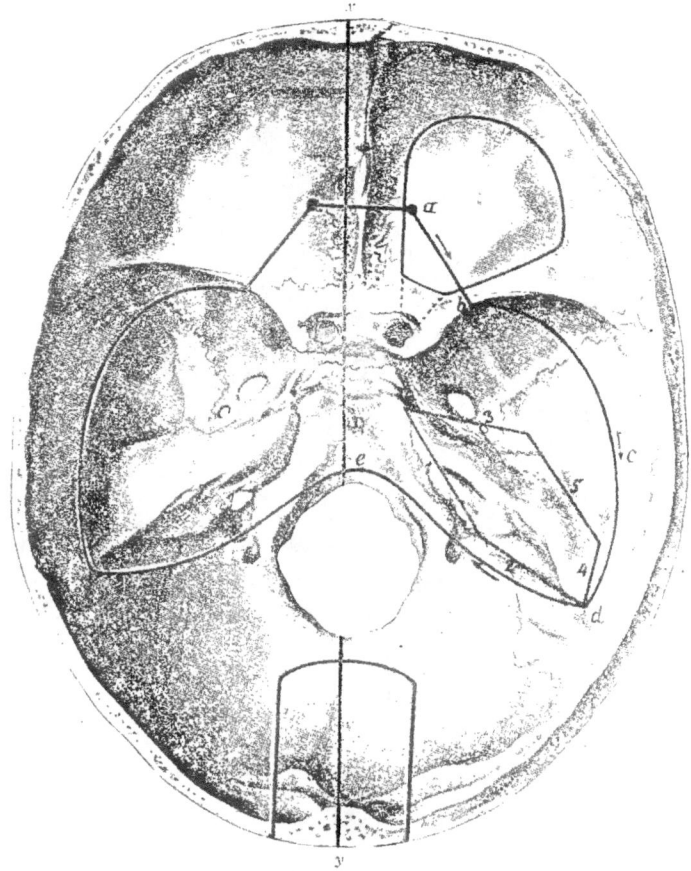

Fig. 32.—Incisions for examination of orbit, ear and nose. x y marks line of incision for exposing nasal tract according to method of Harke.

may be sectioned by a sagittal cut made either to the left or right of the pedicle.

The basal dura is next removed by means of forceps and knife, chisel or dura-forceps. The bones are then carefully examined for fractures, caries, etc. Particularly in cases of middle-ear disease, meningitis, etc., should the dura be removed from the temporal bone and the latter carefully examined.

5. **Examination of the Orbit.** When the eye-ball cannot be enucleated anteriorly the orbit may be opened by removing its roof with small bone-chisel and hammer according to the lines of incision given in Fig. 32. The dura is, of course, first removed. The bony plate covering the orbit is thin and easily splintered, so that the chisel should be very carefully used. The pieces of bone should be removed with the forceps. The optic foramen and the superior orbital fissure may be opened at the same time. After the removal of the roof of the orbit the orbital fat and muscles are dissected away until the optic nerve and eye-ball are exposed. The sclera is then seized with the forceps and the eye-ball pulled back and cut quickly around its equator with sharp shears or scalpel. The head should be held so that the eye looks downward, so that when cut the vitreous humor falls out, leaving the retina well spread out over the posterior half of the bulb. If the retina is

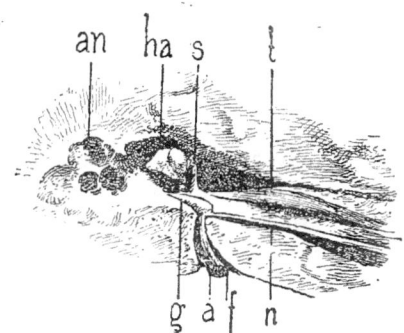

FIG. 33.—Tympanic cavity after removal of tegmen. an, mastoid antrum; ha, hammer-anvil articulation; s, tendon of musc. tens. tymp.; t, musc. tens. tymp.; g, genu of facial nerve; a, auditory nerve; f, facial nerve; n, nerv. petros. superfic. major. (After Politzer.)

thrown into folds it may be straightened by blowing into it or filling it with water. After the retina has been examined it may be washed off from the chorioid, leaving it attached around the papilla. The pigment-layer remains attached to the chorioid, and when the latter is examined for the presence of tubercles it should be removed. When removed for microscopic studies the eye should be placed at once in a suitable fixing fluid.

6. **Examination of the Ear.** The dura is removed from over the temporal bone and the *tegmen tympani* cut off with chisel and hammer as indicated in Fig. 32, *1, 2, 3, 4, 5*, thus exposing the tympanic cavity as shown in Fig. 33. When the tegmen tympani is very hard and compact the hammer and chisel are used to remove

that portion of the tegmen lying laterally to the eminence formed by the upper semicircular canals. As the ear-ossicles lie immediately beneath the roof of the tympanic cavity care should be taken not to injure them with the chisel, and this can be best accomplished by beginning to chisel so far posteriorly that the tegmen of the mastoid antrum is first cut away, and from this opening the cut is extended carefully until the tegmen tympani is removed. When the tegmen of the tympanic cavity is very thin and porcelain-like, as is often the case, it may be most quickly and expediently removed by means of the pointed bone-forceps. A complete view of the tympanic cavity is obtained by removing the coverings of the mastoid antrum posteriorly and the bony canal anteriorly after first drawing out the musc. tensor tymp. from the canal. The mastoid process may be opened with the saw or with chisel and hammer. The labyrinth may be exposed by cutting anteriorly with the chisel held horizontally in such a way as to spring off the upper half of the bony labyrinth, exposing the vestibule and cochlea. The superior and posterior semicircular canals come off, and from their open spaces the membranous semicircular canals can be lifted out with the forceps and then examined in water.

The external auditory canal may be opened and the outer surface of the ear-drum examined by carrying the anterior flap of the scalp downward and forward until the entrance into the bony canal is reached. The external ear is then cut off close to the bone, using slight pressure so as to avoid tearing out the lining of the canal or injuring the tympanum. The anterior bony wall of the canal, and a part of the lower, are then carefully chiseled away until the membrane is exposed. Any bony projections on the thicker upper or lower wall of the canal may be trimmed off to give an unobstructed view. When pathologic changes are present upon any part of the wall of the canal the latter should be opened from the other side so as to expose the condition fully.

For the *removal of the auditory apparatus and its examination outside of the body* a number of methods are advised. The temporal bone may be resected by extending the scalp-incision halfway down the neck along the anterior edge of the trapezius. The anterior flap with the external ear is carried forward as far as the middle of the zygoma and below to the angle of the lower jaw. The posterior flap is carried backward to the middle of the occipital bone. All soft parts are cut as closely to the bone as possible. A saw-cut is now made across the posterior cranial fossa, beginning just behind the mastoid process and extending to the median line of the clivus half-way between the anterior border of the foramen magnum and the sella turcica. The sinus sigmoideus is thus included in the part to be removed. A second saw-cut is then made across the middle cranial fossa, in a line nearly parallel with the transverse diameter of the skull, cutting the middle of the zygomatic arch, the anterior portion of the squama, the great wing of the sphenoid and the pterygoid process, to the tuberculum sellæ. The median ends of the two saw-cuts are then united by a chisel-cut in the median line of the sella and clivus. All bony connections remaining are then cut with the chisel. The soft parts are then cut, beginning with those attached to the mastoid process; the loosened bone is then raised and pulled anteriorly so that the posterior capsule of the maxillary joint can be cut and the jaw-bone disarticulated. All remaining soft parts of neck and nasopharynx are now cut and the temporal bone with the complete ear-apparatus and neighboring portion of nasopharynx is removed. When both temporal bones are removed the saw-cuts should not be carried to the median line, but should stop at the borders of clivus and sella, and then united on each side by sagittal chisel-cuts made along these borders, leaving the clivus and sella as a firm connecting bridge between anterior and posterior portions of the skull. The resected bone may now be examined by means of a saw-cut made perpendicularly through the apex of the eminence of the superior semicircular canals and parallel with the crista of the petrous bone. The tegmen should be removed before the saw-cut is made and the covering of the tympanic cavity and the outer wall of the external auditory canal also removed. The tendon of the tensor tympani is cut and the anvil-stapes articulation severed so that the saw-blade passes between the drum, hammer and anvil on one side and the head of the stapes on the other without damaging or displacing the ossicles. This can be accomplished by pushing outward the drum with hammer and anvil so that the saw-blade can pass between the anvil and the head of the stapes. The bone should be held in a vise and a fret-saw used. On one side of the cut will be seen the drum, hammer, anvil and anterior portion of the mastoid cells; on the other the stapes, wall of the labyrinth and posterior half of the mastoid cells. The Eustachian tube may be easily worked out from the tympanic cavity or from the pharyngeal opening.

A sagittal section of the middle ear may be made, giving pictures as shown in Figs. 34, 35. The temporal bone is resected as above, the tegmen tympani removed and the bony covering of the Eustachian tube removed with hammer and chisel until the tube is exposed from its pharyngeal opening to the isthmus. The temporal bone is then divided into an outer and an inner half by cutting the roof of the tube with fine straight scissors from the pharyngeal mouth to the bony portion and then cutting the membranous floor of the canal likewise. The bony canal, the floor of the tympanic cavity

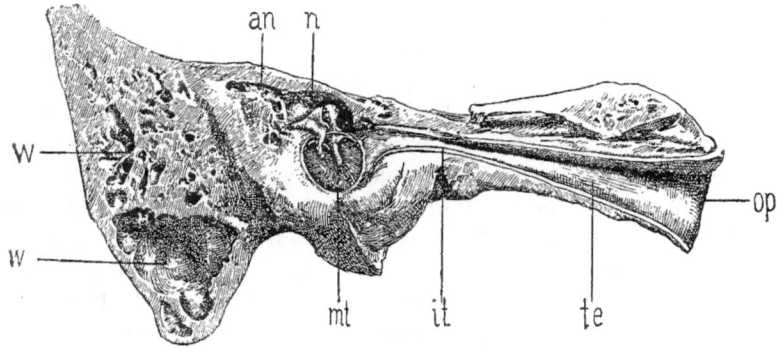

Fig. 34.—Sagittal section through left middle ear, outer half. an, mastoid antrum; n, niche of the hammer-anvil body; op, mouth of Eustachian tube; te, Eustachian tube; it, isthmus of tube; mt, tympanum; ww, mastoid cells. (After Politzer.)

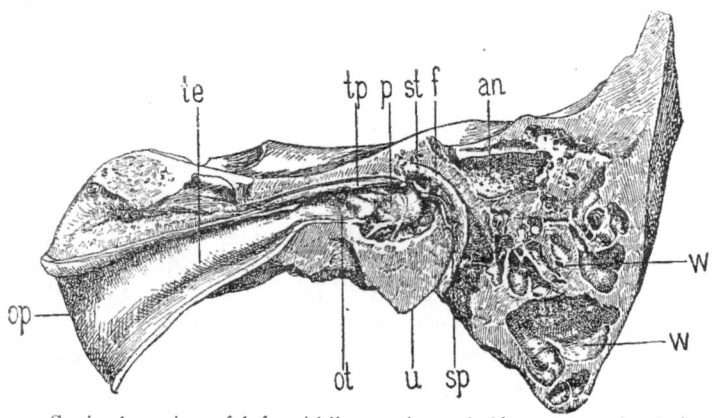

Fig. 35.—Sagittal section of left middle ear, inner half. op, mouth of Eustachian tube; te, Eustachian tube; tp, musc. tensor tymp.; p, promontory; st, stapes; sp, musc. staped; f, facial nerve; an, mastoid antrum; ww, mastoid cells; ot, ost. tymp. tubæ; u, lower wall of tympanic cavity. (After Politzer.)

and the mastoid process are then cut sagittally with a fine fret-saw, passing between the lower annular segment of the sulcus tympani and the inner wall of the tympanic cavity. By altering the direction of the saw-cut the Eustachian tube may be removed in connection with either outer or inner portion of the temporal bone.

Other methods of examining the ear are shown in Fig. 32. The tympanic cavity and labyrinth may be removed intact by cutting with a chisel having a cutting edge 3 cm. broad, in the lines *1, 2, 3, 4, 5*, as shown in Fig. 32. The cut *1* is made with the chisel held nearly horizontal and parallel with the base of the skull. Cuts *2, 3, 4* and *5* are made vertically. Great care must be taken not to splinter the bone. A small chisel can be used to connect the ends of the cuts. Soft parts are cut away with the chisel. An elevator is then introduced into cuts *1* and *2* and the part lifted out by cutting the remaining soft parts and the articulation of the lower jaw. The portion removed contains the inner section of the external auditory canal, tympanic cavity, ear-drum, a portion of the mastoid cells, the entire labyrinth, auditory and facial nerves.

Politzer's method of removing the auditory apparatus in connection with the nasopharynx and the Eustachian tubes is also shown in Fig. 32 by the lines *a, b, c, d, e*. Two drill-holes are made in the floor of the anterior fossa at *a*, 1 cm. to the right and to the left of the crista galli, extending vertically through the nasal cavity to the under surface of the hard palate. A fine key-hole saw is then introduced through the right drill-hole, and the base of the skull is then sawed in the lines *ab, bc, cd* and *de* as indicated in Fig. 32. Symmetrical cuts are then made on the left side following the same lines and the two drill-holes connected by a transverse saw-cut. Any remaining bony connections are then cut with a wide chisel. In order to cut the bony bridges in the region of the nasopharynx it may be necessary anteriorly to use the Hey-saw through the mouth-cavity as well as from the cranial side. To facilitate the removal of the loosened portion two parallel saw-cuts are made in the occipital bone 3 cm. to the left and right of the median line, extending nearly to the posterior edge of the foramen magnum and connected below by a slightly rounded cut as shown in Fig. 32. A long-armed chisel can now be used conveniently through the opening thus made, for horizontal manipulations upon the base of the skull, while the loosened portion of the base is lifted with the bone forceps or nippers set in the posterior saw-cut *e* and the *sella turcica*. As the bone is raised the posterior and lateral pharyngeal walls are cut with the cartilage-knife, the posterior wall of the capsule of the maxillary articulation on both sides severed, the jaw disarticulated, and all muscular and membranous connections cut, until the preparation is completely freed. The auditory apparatus and the Eustachian tubes can now be examined by any one of the methods given above.

7. **Examination of Nose and Neighboring Cavities.** Of all the methods advised for the examination of the nasal cavities the method of *Harke* (Fig. 32) is the easiest and gives the best views of the nasal tract. After the brain has been removed the scalp incision is carried downward to the middle of the neck on both sides, following the anterior edge of the trapezius, as for the removal of the temporal bone. The anterior flap is then carried forward as far as the bridge of the nose and the edges of the orbits, and the flap pulled down over the face. The posterior flap is carried back as far as the upper cervical vertebræ, removing the muscles with the scalp.

The head of the cadaver is now raised and firmly held by an assistant or clamped in a head-holder; and with the large meat-saw the occipital bone is sawed through in the median line, cutting first the squama and then the clivus. The saw is then set anteriorly into the frontal bone, to the left or right of the septum, in order not to injure the septum narium. (Fig. 32.) The sawing then proceeds through the sella turcica, body of the sphenoid, ethmoid and frontal bones until the base of the skull is divided into halves. The cartilage-knife is then introduced through the foramen magnum and the basal ligaments cut. The right and left sides of the skull posteriorly are then taken in the two hands and with a quick, powerful tug forced outward until the nasal bones, hard palate and alveolar processes break apart. The two halves of the base of the skull then open like a book, turning on an axis, running through the inferior maxillary articulation and the occipito-atloid ligaments. If there is too great resistance in the region of the foramen magnum, the anterior and posterior arches of the atlas may be cut with a chisel.. The sphenoidal sinus, septum narium, frontal sinus and the nasal cavity on one side of the septum with the nasopharynx are thus exposed, and their walls and contents may now be examined. Material for bacteriologic examination should be secured before further cutting is done. The septum may then be removed with forceps and scissors, the nasal cavity on the other side examined, the nasopharynx inspected, and the antrums opened with small bone-forceps. After the examination is complete the halves of the base are brought together and fastened with copper wire anteriorly and posteriorly, taking care that the anterior wire will not be visible through the skin of the forehead.

8. **Examination of Face.** When the anterior flap of the scalp is carried down to the edge of the orbits and half-way across the lower jaw as advised above for the removal of.the temporal bone, the *parotid* region may be examined. The *upper* and *lower maxillary bones* are best examined after the removal of the neck-organs. A transverse incision is made in the skin of the neck low enough to be concealed by the clothing, and connecting with the longitudinal scalp-incisions. The facial flap is then dissected upward with great care as far as the infraorbital edges, exposing the maxillary bones, from which the soft parts must be so carefully removed that restoration of the face can be made. For the examination of the anterior nasal-cavities the upper lip must be separated from the bones.

II. POINTS TO BE NOTED IN SECTION OF HEAD.

1. **Scalp.** Note wounds, hemorrhages, inflammations, scars, parasites, neoplasms, number and location of bleeding-points on section, color of different portions, adhesions to periosteum or cranial bones, etc. Most common pathologic conditions are wounds, hemorrhages, wens, lipoma, squamous-celled carcinoma, syphilis, tuberculosis, favus, pediculi, trichophytia, angioma and round- and spindle-celled sarcomata. The temporal muscles should be examined for hemorrhages, œdema, purulent inflammations and trichinæ. The postmortem hypostasis of the back of the head should not be regarded as pathologic.

2. **Periosteum.** Subperiosteal hemorrhages, purulent infiltrations, adhesions, indurations, chronic inflammation with new-formation of bone, and neoplasms are the most common pathologic conditions.

3. **Skull-Cap.** The measurements (circumference, 49-65 cms.; long. diam., 18 cms.; trans. diam., 13-15 cms.), form, asymmetry, character of surface (normally smooth and moist), color of cranial bones, character of sutures and fontanels (easily traced?), supernumerary sutures and bones, consistence (softened in craniotabes, purulent inflammations, syphilis, neoplasm), new-formations of bone, perforations (syphilis, neoplasms, Pacchionian granulations, purulent inflammation), elevations, depressions, fractures, areas of erosion or absorption, thickenings of external surface (crater-like due to organized cephalhæmatoma, chronic periostitis, neoplasm or gumma), radiating scars or indurations (syphilis), red, soft, spongy thickenings (rachitis). The temporal and frontal regions are most frequently the seat of syphilitic (corona veneris) and rachitic changes (frontal and temporal bosses, square forehead, etc.) Note ease or difficulty in sawing, relation of external table, diploë and inner table, measure thickest and thinnest portions, character and amount of diploë, weight of skull-cap (heavy in sclerosis, light in atrophy), dural adhesions, examine by transmitted light (color, blood-content, presence of pus in diploë may be shown by greenish or yellow color), smooth or rough inner table, erosions (rough, more or less reddened), grooves of meningeal vessels, Pacchionian erosions, hyperostosis, exostosis, osteoma, osteophytes (not uncommon in pregnant women, also in hydrocephalus, acromegaly), atrophy (old age, craniotabes, hydrocephalus), sclerosis (syphilis). In marked cachexias (cancer of stomach) the inner table often shows a high degree of erosion and atrophy.

4. **Dura.** Collections of pus may be found between skull-cap and dura in purulent inflammations of scalp or diploë. Rupture of middle meningeal artery or its branches, with or without fracture of the skull, gives rise to hemorrhagic extravasations in same location. Old hemorrhages may be partly organized. In young infants the dura is adherent to the skull-cap and cannot be separated. In youth and adult life it is adherent only along the longitudinal sinus and about the blood-vessels; in old age it becomes more adherent. Extent, location and strength of adhesions should be noted. The normal dura should be grayish-red, smooth, symmetrically stretched, so that a small fold only can be taken up by the fingers in the frontal region, and just translucent enough to show the outlines of the convolutions and the pial vessels. An increased tension is caused by exudates, tumor, abscess, hydrocephalus, hemorrhage, congestion, œdema, etc. Diminished tension occurs in atrophy of the brain, especially marked in the frontal region, where the dura may be wrinkled and loose. Perforations of the dura by Pacchionian bodies are very common along the longitudinal sinus in late life, and should not be regarded as pathologic. Small osteomata are not uncommon in the same place and in the falx; they may be very numerous in acromegaly, late syphilis and cachectic conditions. Changes in the color of the surface of the dura may be due to hemorrhage, purulent or syphilitic inflammation, old thickenings, etc. Thickenings are more easily seen from the inside surface of the dura; they appear as hard, tendon-like, opaque areas. The normal inner surface is smooth, grayish and moist-shining. In pachymeningitis it may be dry, dull, roughened, and covered with blood, pus or fibrin. The most frequent pathologic condition on the inside of the dura is the organizing or encapsulated hemorrhage (pachymeningitis hæmorrhagica chronica, hæmatoma duræ), so common in chronic alcoholics. Miliary tubercles of the dura are common in meningeal tuberculosis. A gummatous pachymeningitis is not infrequent in late syphilis. Pachymeningitis fibrosa is also common in old syphilitics. Actinomycosis occurs in connection with actinomycotic encephalitis. The primary tumors of the dura are fibroma, osteoma, fibro-endothelial tumors (psammoma) and angiosarcoma, etc. Secondary carcinoma or sarcoma is rare.

5. **Longitudinal Sinus.** Character of walls and contents. Thrombosis, with purulent or gangrenous inflammation, is the most important condition. Note mouths of superior cerebral veins.

6. **Meningeal Vessels.** Note grooves, rupture, thrombosis, hemorrhage, infection, amount of blood, symmetry of distribution,

etc. Traumatic rupture of middle meningeal is the most important condition.

7. **Basal Vessels.** Anomalies in size and distribution, thickness and character of vessel-walls (sclerosis, atheroma, aneurism, calcification). Thrombosis, embolism, aneurism, sclerosis, atheroma, calcification, obliterative endarteritis due to syphilis, are the most common conditions. The changes in the middle cerebral arteries are of especial importance in cases of apoplexy, softening, etc.

8. **Inner Meninges.** The arachnoid, subarachnoid space and pia are usually considered together. The arachnoid bridges over the sulci, the pia dipping down following the brain substance. The contents of the subarachnoideal space are best seen, therefore, between the convolutions. The inner meninges are gray, delicate and transparent; the pial veins show plainly, the arteries are empty and lie deeper, while the more superficial veins are uniformly filled with blood. Sclerotic arteries run more superficially and are more prominent. The removal of the skull-cap often gives rise to the presence of air-bubbles in the pial vessels, and this should not be mistaken for any pathologic condition. Hypostasis likewise should not be regarded as a pathologic condition. Normally the membranes are moist; in increased intracranial pressure (tumors, hydrocephalus, hemorrhages) they are dry and dull. Inflammation is shown by a loss of transparency of the membrane and by the presence of exudate in the subarachnoideal space. Old thickenings are white and opaque. The amount of fluid in the subarachnoideal space may be so great as to cause the arachnoid to bulge out over the sulci. Note character of exudate (purulent, fibrinous, serous or hemorrhagic). In purulent meningitis greenish-yellow or yellowish-white collections of thin pus are found in the meshes of the arachnoid; in fibrinous inflammation the exudate is grayish or milky white. The normal fluid (cerebrospinal) of the subarachnoideal space is clear and small in amount. It is increased in œdema and congestion, as well as in serous inflammations. In inflammatory conditions the membranes are dull and cloudy and the fluid more or less turbid. Pathologic adhesions may exist between dura and inner meninges, and between the latter and the brain-substance. In the latter case the meninges do not strip easily, but pull off portions of the cortex. Over tumors, gummata, areas of softening, the meninges may be so adherent that they cannot be separated from each other. In old syphilitics, alcoholics, cachexias of old

age, etc., the pia may be thickened, white and opaque (leptomeningitis chronica fibrosa). Aneurisms of the pia vessels are of great importance in cases of meningeal hemorrhage. They may be very small (size of pea) and often are found only after very careful search. Atheroma, infective emboli, etc., are also causes of meningeal hemorrhage. Meningeal tubercles are very common and often hard to recognize. They are usually best seen over the basal meninges. Often they can be demonstrated by stripping off the meninges and floating the membrane in mercuric chloride or formalin fixing-fluids. After a few minutes' fixation the tubercles appear as minute grayish or opaque points, the membrane often appearing as if sprinkled with fine sand or powder. The Pacchionian bodies of the arachnoid must not be mistaken for tubercles. They are grayish in color, and most abundant along the longitudinal sinus. The meninges over the two hemispheres should be compared as to transparency, thickness, blood-content, amount of fluid in arachnoideal space, etc.

The most important pathologic conditions of the inner meninges are anæmia, hyperæmia, stasis (asphyxia), œdema, hemorrhages (stasis, anthrax, aneurism, atheroma, infective emboli), serous, purulent and fibrinous inflammation (pyogenic cocci, bacillus pneumoniæ, pneumococcus, bac. coli, diplococcus intracellularis), chronic leptomeningitis (syphilis, alcoholism, toxæmia, etc.), tuberculosis, syphilis (gummatous meningitis), blastomycosis, actinomycosis and neoplasms. The last named are not common. Cholesteatoma, hæmangioma, lymphangioma, endothelioma, fibroma, osteoma and lipoma represent the benign tumors found here. Primary sarcoma is the most common tumor, usually angiosarcoma, perithelioma, cylindroma, round-cell-, spindle-cell- or myxosarcoma. Secondary sarcoma and carcinoma occur. Animal parasites are cysticercus and echinococcus.

8. **Cerebrum.** Weight of brain as a whole 1,200-1,400 grms. (15-50th year). Cerebrum averages 1,039 grms. in the female, 1,155 grms. in the male. A weight of 1,100 grms. may be taken as the minimum normal, and 1,700 grms. as the maximum for the brain as a whole. The relation of the brain-weight to that of the body is 2-100. In old age there is a loss of weight. Sagittal diameter 15-17 cm., transverse 14, vertical 12.5 cm.

Examine the convexity, comparing hemispheres, noting convolutions and sulci (size, number, symmetry, etc.) Atrophy of the gyri is shown by increased width of sulci and the narrower, sharper gyral apex. With increased intracerebral pressure the gyri are flattened and broader, and the sulci smaller. Note color and consistence of cortex, adhesions with pia, areas of fluctuation, induration, depressions, yellow softening, recent and old hemorrhages, effects of trauma, tumors, tubercles, gummata, etc. Examine median surfaces, note arching of corpus callosum. On section of the brain note *color* (pale in anæmia, red in capillary hyperæmia; hemorrhages, areas of softening, tumors, tubercles, gummata, sclerotic areas, abscesses, etc., all show color variation from the normal gray or white); *consistence* (soft in degeneration and abscess, hard in sclerosis), *moisture* (normally is moist-shining; moisture increased in œdema, inflammation, abscesses, soft tumors, recent degenerations; dry in old caseous tubercles and gummata, and in anæmia), *blood-content* (number of bleeding-points, distinguish from punctate hemorrhages), *character of cut surface* (normally smooth, sclerotic areas, abscesses and areas of softening are uneven and depressed, hard tumors and sclerotic blood-vessels are elevated above the surface). The absolute and relative size of cortex and medulla, and the distinctness of the boundary between them, should be noted.

Hemorrhages may occur in any part of the brain, and may be large or small. Rupture into a ventricle is always fatal. The large hemorrhages are due to rupture of a diseased artery; small punctate hemorrhages throughout cortex are usually embolic (fatty embolism). Old hemorrhages are brownish in color (pigment). Areas of softening are usually the result of embolism, thrombosis or sclerosis. They are usually yellow, yellowish-white or brownish-yellow or red.

9. **Ventricles.** Contain about a teaspoonful of clear fluid. This may become purulent, cloudy, hemorrhagic, fibrinous. Note size of ventricles and horns. (Fluid increased and ventricles dilated in hydrocephalus.) Character of ependyma (normally gray-red, delicate; may be pale or red, indurated, thickened, roughened (chronic ependymitis), hemorrhagic, etc. Compare floors of lateral ventricles as to symmetry (corpus striatum large in hemorrhages), color, etc. Adhesions are found most frequently in posterior horns. A fine granulation of the ependyma is caused by miliary tubercles. Large solitary tubercles may be found in the ventricles. Do not mistake postmortem softening of ependyma for pathologic changes. In the third ventricle note the presence of any abnormal contents, character of wall, symmetry of corpora quadrigemina, etc. Look for same changes in fourth ventricle as in lateral. Lining is gray-white and delicate; floor should be gray-white, firm, and show anatomic structures. Gray sclerotic areas are often present in

floor. Solitary tubercles, tumors (glioma, neuroepithelioma, gliosarcoma, sarcoma), dermoids and cysticercus-cysts may be found here. Examine aqueduct of Sylvius for abnormal contents.

10. **Chorioid Plexus.** The tela chorioidea is normally delicate and translucent. Note color (red, pale, cloudy), swelling, purulent infiltration, condition of blood-vessels, tubercles, etc. Psammoma, sarcoma, papillary epithelioma, carcinoma, fibroma, angioma, cholesteatoma, cysticercus and echinococcus may be found in the tela and plexus. Cysts due to œdema are very common, also aneurismal dilatations of the vessels. In cases of hydrocephalus the veins of Galen should be examined for thrombi or compression from without. In acute hydrocephalus the plexus is deep red; hyperæmic, its vessels distended with blood.

11. **Pineal Gland.** The most common pathologic findings are: psammoma, adenoma, teratoma, sarcoma, formation of cysts (hydrops cysticus glandulæ pinealis), hypertrophy, abscess (purulent meningitis), metastatic tumors. In all cases of giantism especial attention should be paid to the pineal gland as well as to the hypophysis.

12. **Cerebral Ganglia.** Color, consistence, moisture, blood-content, hemorrhage, degeneration, sclerosis.

13. **Peduncles.** As above.

14. **Cerebellum.** Cerebellar cortex is 2 mm. thick, grayish-red in color. Note irregularities in thickness, color, consistence, blood-content, moisture. Compare hemispheres. White substance should be shining and moist. Abscesses, tubercles (solitary or conglomerate), gummata and neoplasms are the most common pathologic conditions.

15. **Pons.** Consistence firm normally. Note blood-content, relation of white and gray stripes, hemorrhage, degenerations, cysts, neoplasms, etc.

16. **Medulla.** Color grayish-white, consistence firm. Note blood-content, hemorrhages, degenerations and cysts (syringomyelia).

17. **Hypophysis.** Cysts are common, also calcareous concretions. Adenomatous hyperplasia is the most common tumor (acromegaly, obesity). Carcinoma, sarcoma, lipoma and teratoma are rare. Gumma and tubercle occasionally occur; even when the gland is wholly destroyed, acromegaly does not result. Epithelial tumors of the infundibulum may occur in association with hypoplasia of

the genitals. In diseases of the thyroid the condition of the hypophysis should be especially considered.

18. **Basal Sinuses.** Note contents (marantic and infective thrombi), especially in middle-ear disease and meningitis. Distinguish postmortem clots from thrombi, the former being dark-red, soft and moist, and are not adherent to the walls. The walls of the sinus should be gray, delicate, and shining.

19. **Basal Dura.** Note same conditions as in dura covering convexity.

20. **Cranial Nerves.** Examine and trace to exits. Note atrophy, degenerations, compression, indurations, thickenings, neoplasms (neuroma), etc.

21. **Base of Skull.** After the removal of the basal dura the bones of the base should be smooth and gray-yellowish-red in color. Look for fractures, caries, roughened areas, exostoses, collections of pus, hemorrhage, neoplasms, etc.

The most important pathologic conditions of the brain are congenital defects or malformations (hydrocephalus, microcephalus, etc.), anæmia, hyperæmia, œdema, hemorrhage (traumatic, spontaneous, capillary, apoplexy), embolism, thrombosis, arteriosclerosis, aneurism, anæmic infarction, encephalomalacia (white, yellow and red softening), pigmented scars, atrophy, secondary degeneration, encephalitis, (non-purulent, purulent, hemorrhagic, syphilitic, metastatic, chronic), sclerosis (diffuse, disseminated, focal, hypertrophic), tuberculosis, syphilis, actinomycosis, blastomycosis, rabies, primary neoplasms (glioma, neuroglioma ganglionare, angiosarcoma, spindle-cell sarcoma, polymorphous-cell sarcoma, perithelioma, endothelioma, angioma, myxoma, fibroma, osteoma, teratoma, lipoma), primary epithelial tumors of ventricles, pineal gland and hypophysis (adenoma, cholesteatoma, papillary epithelioma, carcinoma), metastatic tumors (all forms of carcinoma and sarcoma, malignant chorioepithelioma), cysts, parasites (cysticercus, echinococcus) and traumatic lesions (commotio cerebri, contusio cerebri, hemorrhage, red softening, puncture and shot-wounds, infected wounds, traumatic abscess). Especial examination of the brain should be made in all cases of acromegaly, epilepsy, cretinism, congenital idiocy, degeneracy, criminal tendency, insanity, chorea, caisson disease, locomotor ataxia, paralysis agitans, syringomyelia, spastic paralysis, infantile paralysis, hereditary ataxia, rabies, all forms of paralysis, motor or sensory disturbances and neuritis.

3. POINTS TO BE NOTED IN EXAMINATION OF EYE.

The fat-tissue in the orbits should be yellowish-white; from it the red muscles and the white nerves should be easily distinguishable. On section of the eye-ball the vitreous normally is clear and the retina uniformly grayish-black and smooth. The most common and important conditions to be looked for are phlegmonous inflammations, purulent panophthalmitis, orbital hemorrhage, thrombosis of ophthalmic vein and sinus cavernosus leading to pachy- and leptomeningitis, neoplasms of orbit, wall of orbit, eye-ball or lachrymal gland (melanosarcoma, glioma, gliosarcoma, neuroepithelioma, various forms of sarcoma, angioma, lipoma, adenoma, carcinoma), affections of individual muscles (myositis, atrophy), atrophy of optic nerve, choked disk, retinitis, choroiditis, iritis, glaucoma, etc.

4. POINTS TO BE NOTED IN EXAMINATION OF EAR.

Note condition of scalp (hyperæmia, œdema, hemorrhage) about ear, condition of external canal (dry, moist, character of contents), condition of periosteum, particularly over the mastoid process (normally grayish-red), condition of bone after removal of periosteum (normally smooth). Inflammatory œdema, purulent infiltrations in the soft parts, collections of pus beneath the periosteum, roughness of bone beneath elevated periosteum, presence of pus or blood in external auditory canal, perforations of drum, etc., should be noted. Normally the drum should be grayish-white and shining. Note contents of middle ear, Eustachian tube, condition of ossicles, mastoid cells and bone. Lining of middle ear should be grayish-red and smooth; the cut edges of bone should be uniformly grayish-red. When infiltrated with pus they are brown or greenish. The mucous membrane is deep-red or greenish in purulent inflammation; yellow, creamy pus, often of very offensive odor, may be found in middle ear, Eustachian tube or external canal. Note character of perforations; old ones have smooth and thickened edges. The most important pathologic conditions are: otitis media purulenta, inflammation of mastoid cells, caries of mastoid process, sinus-thrombosis (leading to meningitis or pyæmia), otitis media tuberculosa, granulomatous polypi, cholesteatoma, sclerosis, congenital anomalies, foreign bodies, parasites, neoplasms (chiefly of external ear).

5. POINTS TO BE NOTED IN EXAMINATION OF NOSE.

The normal mucosa of the nasal tract is light grayish-red. Note character of contents of the cavities (mucus, blood, pus, dry clots or scabs), congestion, hemorrhage, erosions, ulcerations, diphtheritic membrane, diffuse or localized thickenings of the mucosa (polypi), adenoids, exostoses, caries, foreign bodies, parasites (maggots) and neoplasms (sarcoma, fibroma, carcinoma). The most important conditions are acute and chronic catarrhal inflammations, ozæna, croupous or diphtheritic inflammations, syphilis, atrophy or hyperplasia of the mucosa, polypi, and more rarely tuberculosis. Syphilis causes inflammations and gummatous infiltrations of the mucosa, gummatous periostitis, foul-smelling necrosis of the bony portions (ozæna syphilitica). Dense hard fibromata developing from base of skull may fill up the nasopharynx or erode the cranial base and press upon the brain. Softer sarcomatous growths may arise from the hypophysis, or from the lymphoid tissue of the mucosa. Squamous-celled carcinoma is not infrequently primary in the antrum and thence invades the nose. Primary malignant tumors of nasal tract not common. Leprosy, glanders, blastomycosis, and rhinoscleroma are more rarely seen.

CHAPTER VII.
MAIN INCISION: THORAX AND ABDOMEN.
I. METHOD OF OPENING TRUNK.

1. **The Main Incision.** After the examination of the cranium has been completed, the skull-cap is replaced and the anterior flap of the scalp drawn up over it, to hold it in place until the close of the autopsy. The head is then wrapped in a towel to protect the face and hair.

The prosector then stands at the right side of the cadaver (if left-handed, on the left side), the body being brought as near as possible to the edge of the table. The cartilage-knife is then held in the palm of the right hand and with it an incision is made through the skin in the median line of the body, extending from just below the thyroid cartilage to the base of the penis in the male, and to the anterior commissure in the female, passing to the left of the umbilicus. If pathologic conditions (hernia, surgical wound, tumor, etc.) are present in the median line the main-incision should deviate to right or left as expedient. The incision in the suprasternal notch is made with the point of the knife, the thumb and fingers of the left hand being used to put the skin of the neck on a stretch. Over the sternum the knife is held horizontally and the tissues cut to the bone. As soon as the epigastrium is reached less force is used, and the cut should not be deeper than through the skin and subcutaneous tissue over the abdominal portion of the incision. At the end of the incision the knife is raised vertically and the cut finished with the point of the knife. The incision is then carefully deepened in the epigastrium, just below the ensiform, until a small opening is made through the peritoneum into the abdominal cavity. To determine the presence of gas within the peritoneal cavity the peritoneum should first be nicked with the point of the knife to make a very small opening through which the escape of any free gas within the cavity can be easily noted. When bacteriologic examinations of the peritoneal fluid are to be made, the incision should be extended down to the peritoneum, which should then be seared, and the fluid secured by means of a sterile pipette forced through the seared portion. If it is more expedient to secure the

THE MAIN INCISION. 97

fluid through an incision, the opening should be made with a sterilized knife and the fingers should not be put into the cavity, but are used to lift up the abdominal wall at the sides of the incision.

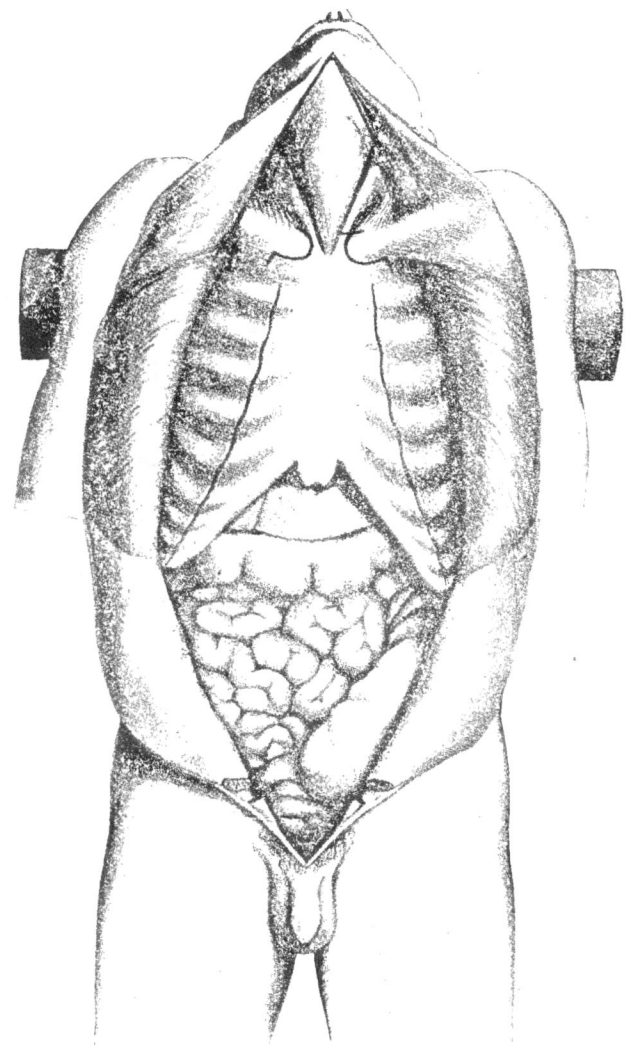

FIG. 36.—The main incision completed. Lines show incisions through costal cartilages, and for disarticulation of sterno-clavicular joints. (After Nauwerck.) The incision in the neck is begun higher than is usual in this country.

In cutting through the peritoneum great care should be taken not to injure the stomach or intestines, which, often greatly distended, are pressed tightly against the peritoneum. If the opening is made just below the ensiform the knife, should it slip through unexpectedly, usually strikes the liver without causing any damage.

The abdominal incision is now extended downward to the pubis. The first and second fingers of the left hand are introduced into the peritoneal cavity and used as directors to lift up the abdominal wall and to keep the intestines from the knife, the latter cutting between them in the line of the first incision through the skin and subcutaneous fascia. When the main incision is complete the knife is introduced into the abdominal cavity with cutting edge directed outward and the abdominal muscles are divided on either side just above the pubis by cuts extending outward to the skin. (See Fig. 36.) Care should be taken not to cut the latter. These transverse cuts made from the peritoneal surface permit the opening of the peritoneal cavity to the necessary extent, so that transverse incisions through the skin are not necessary.

> The main incision is carried to the left of the umbilicus and then back to the median line, in order not to injure the umbilical vessels, the ligamentum teres of the liver, or a concealed hernia or persistent omphalomesenteric duct. In the case of the newborn the incision to the left of the umbilicus is extended to the pubis in an oblique line diverging from the median line. After the examination of the umbilical vessels through the main incision a second diverging cut is made from just above the umbilicus, passing to its right, across the umbilical vessels and hepatic ligament down to the pubis, forming a triangular flap including the umbilicus, urachus and umbilical arteries.

The abdominal flaps are now held back and a thorough inspection of the cavity made, noting particularly the position of the abdominal organs, contents of cavity, condition of peritoneum and appendix, occurrence of perforations, etc. The position of the diaphragm is then determined on both sides, by passing the right hand up under the ribs to the highest part of the dome of the diaphragm and then pressing outward against the chest-wall so that the height can be estimated by rib or interspace.

The skin and muscles are now stripped from the thoracic wall on both sides of the median incision, beginning first on the right. (See Fig. 36.) The right flap of the abdominal wall is taken in the left hand just above the umbilicus and turned over the right lower border of the ribs, and pulled forcibly upward and outward to the right, putting the peritoneum, the ligamentum teres of the liver and abdominal muscles upon a stretch over the edge of the ribs. These are then cut by the cartilage-knife in an incision extending from the median line along the edge of the ribs deep down into the flank.

OPENING OF THORAX.

The loosened flap of skin and muscle is then pulled over to the right with the left hand, while the right hand holds the cartilage-knife, with its cutting edge turned obliquely to the surface of the ribs, and makes long, sweeping cuts from above downward, severing the thoracic muscles and fascia as closely as possible to the costal cartilages and ribs. The skin and muscles are thus stripped off from below upward until the right side is laid bare as far back as the anterior axillary line and to the middle of the clavicle above. (See Fig. 36.)

In stripping the muscles from the ribs it is necessary only to do it sufficiently to show the costal cartilages and their articulations with the ribs. Too clean dissecting is not necessary. On the other hand, careless slashing cuts should be avoided, as they might cut through into the pleural cavity.

The right mammary gland is next examined. The index-finger of the left hand is put upon the nipple, the skin-flap turned over, and an incision made from the inner surface, extending through the gland to the nipple. Parallel incisions may then be made. The axillary glands may be examined by carrying the skin and muscle flap farther down into the axilla. The thoracic wall is then laid bare on the left side, in exactly the same way as on the right, except that the right hand works underneath the left, as the latter pulls the flap over to the left. When the left side is stripped, the left mamma is examined in the same way as the right.

The thorax is now opened, beginning with the right second costal cartilage. This is cut with the belly of the cartilage-knife about $\frac{1}{2}$-1 cm. from the costal articulation so as to leave as much of the cartilage attached to the sternum as possible. (See Fig. 36.) The cut is made with a rocking motion so that the knife-blade will strike upon the next lower cartilage instead of going through into the thoracic cavity. The cartilages and intercostal muscles are cut in this manner in succession down to the tenth, the cut flaring outward below with the outward curve of the costal articulations. The cartilages forming the lower edge of the ribs are left uncut at this time. When the first opening into the pleural cavity is made attention should always be paid to the possible escape of gas or air (pneumothorax). When pneumothorax is suspected the opening may be made through a little pocket of water formed by holding up the skin-flap and filling the hollow with water. A similar incision is then made through the cartilages on the left side from the second to the tenth. The lower right edge of the ribs is now lifted with the right hand, and the cartilage-knife, held on the flat, with cutting edge toward the abdomen, is put through the opening of the incision through the cartilage and through the diaphragm, and the last cartilages cut by a stroke made outward and slightly upward to avoid injuring the abdominal organs. The last cartilages on the left side are then cut by putting the blade of the cartilage-knife, held on the flat with cutting edge outward, through the diaphragm from the abdominal side, into the incision through the cartilages, and cutting through the lower edge of the ribs in the same manner as on the right.

The lower part of the sternum and cartilages is then lifted in the left hand and the diaphragm trimmed off closely beneath it. Still lifting the sternum the tissues of the anterior mediastinum are cut close to its under surface, care being taken not to cut the pericardial sac. The sternum is thus freed up to the cartilage of the first ribs and the sternoclavicular attachments. With the sternum lifted as high as it is possible to do so without breaking it the cartilages of the first ribs are now cut with the blade of the cartilage-knife turned outward to avoid cutting the large vessels and flooding the part with blood from the distended veins. This is possible since the cartilages of the first ribs extend farther outward than those of the second ribs. (See Fig. 36.)

After the first costal cartilages have been cut on both sides, the sternum is lifted nearly perpendicularly and twisted slightly toward the right so that the capsule of the left sternoclavicular articulation can be put upon a stretch. The latter is then opened from below until the joint is exposed. With the sternum still pulled firmly upward and toward the right the left sternoclavicular articulation is completely severed, the left sternocleidomastoid and other muscles and fascia attached to the sternum are cut from left to right; and the sternum, twisted over to the right, is disarticulated in the same manner from the right clavicle, and the right sternocleidomastoid cut. The freed sternum is now examined. It may be cut through in the median line with the saw, or cuts made into it with knife or chisel.

Ossification of the cartilages of the ribs is very common in late middle life and old age, more rarely in younger persons. The first cartilages, particularly the left one, and the lower ones usually show it in the most marked degree. It may be impossible to cut them with a knife, and the hand-saw must be used. Ankylosis of the sternoclavicular articulation is also not rare, and it is sometimes necessary to saw through the clavicles. The sternoclavicular articulation and the cartilage of first rib may also be opened from above downward with a long, narrow-bladed scalpel, the incision following the articular surfaces.

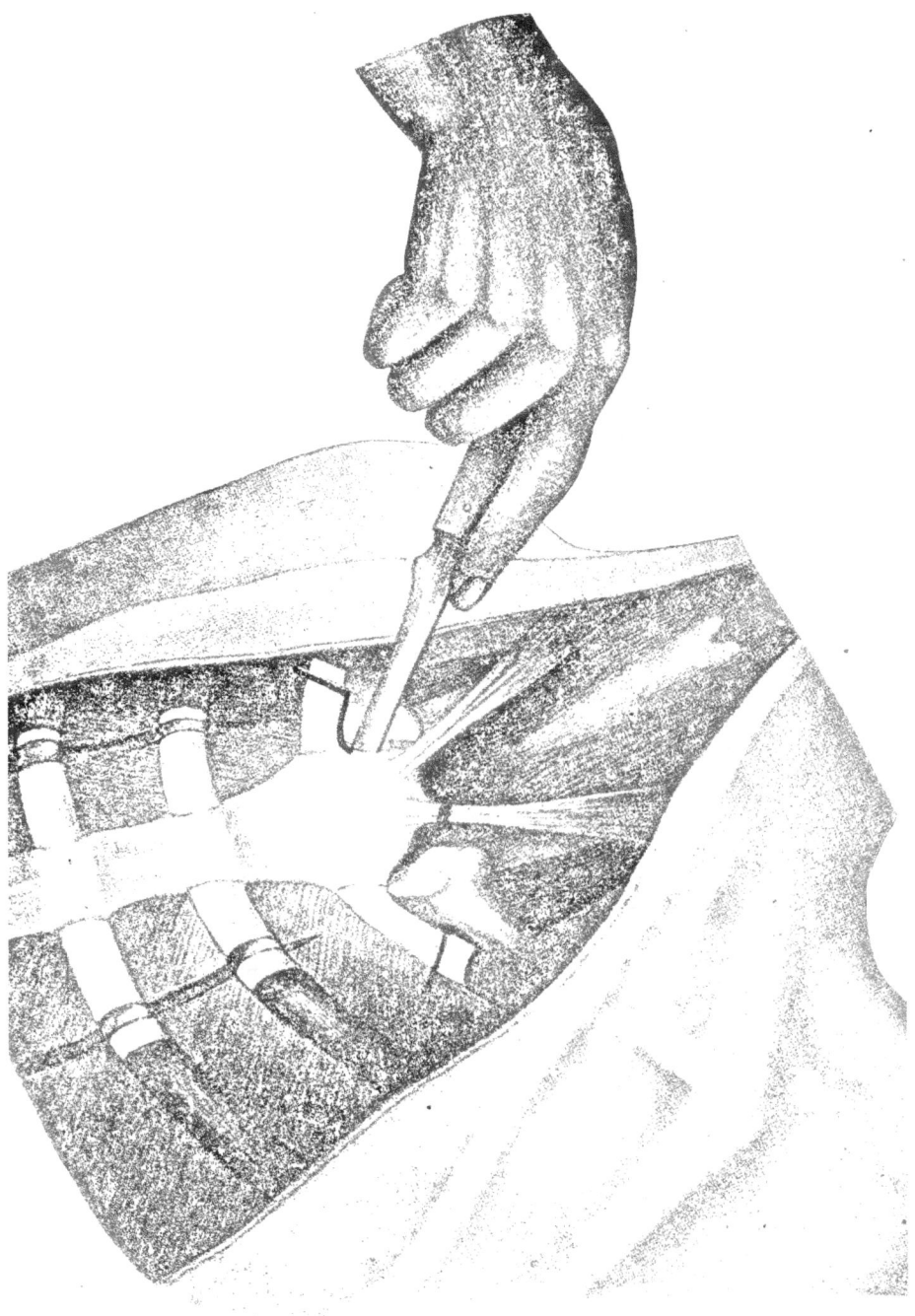

Fig. 37.—Method of disarticulating sternoclavicular articulation and cutting cartilage of first rib from above. (After Nauwerck.)

Many prosectors prefer this method. (See Fig. 37.) The location of the joint and the direction of the incision may be ascertained by moving the arm and shoulder of the cadaver. The sternocleidomastoids may be cut when the skin-flaps are stripped off. In case bacteriologic examination is to be made of the contents of the pleural cavity the incisions into the cavity should be made with a sterilized knife, or the material for culture may be obtained by means of a pipette introduced through a seared interspace.

2. POINTS TO BE NOTED IN THE MAIN INCISION.

1. **Panniculus.** Note thickness at different points in the incision, color (straw-color, rosy or almost white in early life, orange or reddish-yellow in atrophy or old age, brown in severe anæmias), moisture (œdema, serous or purulent inflammation, transfusion; the latter should not be mistaken for pathologic œdema), dryness in atrophy, long-continued fevers, cachexias, etc., number of bleeding points (passive congestion, hypostasis), hemorrhages (recent, old, pigmented).

2. **Musculature.** The muscles of the neck, thorax and abdomen are examined with reference to the following points: size (atrophy, hypertrophy), color (normally bright brownish-red, may be paler than normal, deep brown, yellow or grayish), consistence (pale muscle usually tears easily, brownish muscle usually tears less easily), moisture (moist in œdema, inflammation, and as a result of transfusion; dry in anæmias, severe diarrhœas, long-continued fevers), translucency (increased in Zenker's necrosis, fatty infiltration, fatty degeneration, atrophy, anæmia; diminished in cloudy swelling and simple necrosis), blood-content (anæmia, hyperæmia), hemorrhages (trauma, surgical, hypodermic injections, toxic, infective, hæmatoma of abdominal rectus in typhoid fever), inflammation (acute, chronic, focal, diffuse, primary, secondary, abscess, fibroid, etc.), bony formations (myositis ossificans), parasites (trichina the most common, especially frequent in muscles of neck and in the intercostals and diaphragm, small whitish, oval bodies looking and feeling like grains of sand; echinococcus and cysticercus are more rare), neoplasms (not common, the spindle-cell fibrosarcoma or "recurrent fibroid" of abdominal wall the most frequent form). Zenker's necrosis (hyaline, waxy or "fish-flesh" degeneration) is of frequent occurrence in the abdominal muscles in typhoid and other severe fevers and intoxications. Anomalies of sternal and pectoral muscles are not rare.

3. **Abdominal Cavity.** Watch carefully for the escape of gas when the first cut through the peritoneum is made. A lighted match may be held over the opening, or the skin incision may be

filled with water and the peritoneum opened through the water, noting the escape of bubbles. The odor (sour, sweetish, yeasty, fécal, putrid, etc.) should be noted. Abnormal contents of the peritoneal cavity are to be measured and described as to color (amber, greenish-yellow, color of bile, red, bloody, brown, gray, creamy, milky, opalescent, etc.), consistence (thin, clear, watery, serous, pea-soup-like, gruel-like, creamy, jelly-like, colloid, semi-solid, etc.), odor (fécal or foul, due usually to the presence of the colon bacillus; acid or yeasty in perforation of stomach; fruity in diabetes, acute hemorrhagic pancreatitis; odor of ether, chloroform, alcohol, etc.), contents (blood, bile, féces, stomach-contents [distinguish perforations due to postmortem digestion], fibrin, fat, chyle, pus, foreign-bodies, mucin or pseudomucin, parasites) and reaction (acid, alkaline). Non-inflammatory ascites occurs in portal stasis, hepatic cirrhosis, thrombosis or compression of portal or splenic veins, chronic passive congestion, chronic valvular lesions with incompensation, nephritis, severe anæmia, obstruction or rupture of thoracic duct, etc. The fluid of transudates is usually clear, odorless, alkaline, low specific gravity (below 1.016), small albumin- and fibrin-content, few flocculi, and relatively small number of white cells. Inflammatory exudates are turbid, often foul-smelling, usually acid, specific gravity over 1.016, high albumin-, fibrin- and urea-content, numerous thick flocculi and numerous cells. In early peritoneal tuberculosis the fluid may be clear and resemble that of a transudate. Milky and opalescent fluids are found in diabetes, lipæmia, new-growths of the peritoneum, obstruction or rupture of thoracic duct or receptaculum. Hemorrhagic exudates may be traumatic (rupture of spleen, liver, intestines, extrauterine pregnancy, etc.), inflammatory (severe acute peritonitis), or due to new-growths or tuberculosis of the peritoneum, extreme portal stasis, perforation of gastric or typhoid ulcers, severe intoxications, chronic icterus, etc. Red effusions may be due to diffused hæmoglobin. In such cases there is no settling of the color, and coagulation may not occur. When red cells are present settling takes place on standing. Rupture of gall-bladder or bile-ducts may lead to presence of free bile in the peritoneal cavity. Postmortem diffusion of bile through the gall-bladder wall should not be mistaken for a pathologic condition. In normal conditions there is just enough fluid in the peritoneal fluid to make the surfaces moist, and about a teaspoonful in all may be collected from the flanks and pelvis. The amount may be greatly increased just before death in all cases of slowly progressive cardiac weakness.

Note character of peritoneum (normally moist-shining, grayish, translucent, cloudy, dry, lustreless, thickened, hyaline ("iced" or "Zuckerguss") in chronic inflammation.

4. **Omentum.** Note position of lower border, amount of fat, condition of blood-vessels, dry or moist-shining surface, adhesions (to appendix, cæcum, oviducts), indurations, contractions (edges rolled up), character of lymphnodes, cysts, tubercles, secondary tumors, snared-off tumors from ovary or uterus (parasitic cysts, fibroids), encysted foreign bodies, etc.), exudates on surface, fat-necrosis, accessory spleens, encysted parasites, hernia, etc. Most common pathologic conditions are inflammation (secondary to appendicitis, salpingitis, etc.), metastic carcinoma and tuberculosis.

5. **Position of Abdominal Organs.** Note situs viscerum inversus, gastro-enteroptosis, displacements due to spinal curvatures and deformities, and hernia, anomalies or malformations, locate organs by usual landmarks (edge of ribs, ensiform, umbilicus, etc.), position of lower and left borders of liver, gall-bladder, spleen, pylorus and fundus of stomach, appendix, colon, etc. Malposition of transverse colon especially common. Note volvulus, ileus, invaginations, etc. Examine stomach and intestines carefully for perforations. Differentiate postmortem perforations and those due to pathologic conditions. (Edges of postmortem perforations soft, slimy, without evidences of disease.) The appendix should also be carefully examined at this time. Note also peritoneal surface (color, thickness, translucency, tubercles, adhesions), color and blood-content of all abdominal organs before acted upon by exposure to air. In the female examine pelvic organs. Do not mistake postmortem perforations of stomach or intestine, postmortem imbibition and diffusion of bile in region of gall-bladder, postmortem contraction of intestines, dilatations of lymphatics with lymph or chyle, agonal transudates, accessory spleens, etc., for pathologic conditions.

6. **Position of Diaphragm.** Normally fourth rib or interspace on right, fifth rib on left, higher in the young, lower in old age. Raised in conditions of increased abdominal pressure (pregnancy, ascites, enlargement of liver or spleen, subdiaphragmatic abscess, dilatation of stomach, urinary or gall-bladder, tumors of any abdominal or pelvic organ, especially ovarian cysts, etc.), low in increase of intrathoracic pressure (pleuritic effusions, pneumothorax, pericardial effusion, hypertrophy of heart, tumors, aneurism, etc.).

7. **Mammae.** Condition varies according to age, pregnancy, lactation, etc. In resting glands the structure is lobulated, connective-tissue white with yellow fat between; in the white connective-tissue are small grayish-red nodules of gland-tissue ("breast-grains"). During lactation the fat disappears entirely or to a large extent, the entire organ consisting of a more homogeneous grayish-white glandular tissue, distinctly granular on section, and resembling the section of a salivary gland. Note size of ducts, presence of secretion (colostrum or milk) on pressure, congestion, œdema, abscess, fistula, caseous tubercles or gummata, cysts (milk, "soap," "butter," senile, new growths), neoplasms, atrophy, hypoplasia, hypertrophy, accessory nipples, parasites (echinococcus). The most common tumors are adenofibromata and carcinomata. Tuberculosis is not rare. In the male breast hypertrophy has been noted in association with malignant chorioepithelioma of the testis; and in the female with pseudopregnancy and tumors of the genital tract. Adenofibroma, gumma and tuberculosis are the most common conditions of the mammæ in males.

8. **Costal Cartilages.** Note color (ochronosis), degree of ossification, anomalies, separations, fractures, caries, tuberculosis, alteration in shape (pigeon-breast, emphysema, Pott's Disease, erosions of tumors or aneurisms, rickets, etc.). The costochondral edges are thickened as a result of rachitis (rachitic rosary). In old age the costal cartilages may undergo the so-called "asbestos-like" degeneration, becoming yellowish- or grayish-brown, streaked with shining whitish granules, with calcification or ossification and new-formation of blood-vessels. Degeneration cysts (senile) are not infrequent, and the cartilages sometimes appear as if soaked with oil, soft and translucent. Fibroid or calcified areas may be present. Spaces and clefts within the cartilage may be filled with new-formed bone-marrow.

9. **Sternum.** Note shape (pigeon-breast, "shoemaker's," rounded, scaphoid, bifid, anomalies of ensiform, etc.), fractures (in marked osteoporosis the bones may break during removal), erosions (aneurisms, tumors), tuberculous and syphilitic caries, gummata, perforations, etc. Under surface of sternum should be smooth, shining, translucent and grayish. In chloroma the under surface may present a uniform greenish layer ½-1 cm. thick. Bone-marrow of sternum is normally red and lymphoid in character; may be green in chloroma, pyoid in leukæmia, hyperplastic in severe anæmias. Sclerosis and osteoporosis of sternal bones are not rare. In the former condition the marrow may be entirely absent; in the latter hyperplastic.

CHAPTER VIII.
THE EXAMINATION OF THE THORAX.
I. METHODS OF EXAMINATION.

1. **Thoracic Cavity.** As soon as the sternum is removed the anterior mediastinum and the **pleural cavities** are examined, noting first the **position** and **relation** of the **thoracic organs**, quantity and character of mediastinal fat, the contents of the pleural cavities, pleuritic adhesions, etc. Pleuritic exudates should be removed before they have become mixed with blood from the cut vessels or heart; and the pleural surfaces should be examined before their appearance has been changed by exposure to the air or to fluids. Pleuritic adhesions should be broken or cut, beginning with the left side and then on the right, and the entire surface of both lungs wholly freed.

2. **Thymus.** The thymus is then examined by means of transverse cuts; or, when large, is dissected from below upward, turned up onto the neck, and removed later in connection with the neck organs. When no traces of thymic tissue are visible to the naked eye the thymic fat should always be cut transversely and examined for the presence of small lymphoid nodules. In the case of hypertrophic thymus the question of pressure upon the trachea becomes of very great importance, and, to settle this, the trachea should be opened above the sternum before the thymus is removed; or the thymus may be taken out in connection with the trachea and both sectioned horizontally at the same time. In cases of sudden death, in which the thymus may be an etiologic factor, it is safest to examine the trachea from above the sternum before the thorax is opened, or to fix the whole body (infant's or child's) in formalin and then to remove thymus with trachea, and examine by means of transverse sections.

> The heart is examined before the lungs chiefly for two reasons: Its blood-content can be more accurately determined, and the blood caught in the pericardial sac, so that when the pulmonary vessels are cut in the removal of the lungs there is no gush of blood into the pleural cavity.

3. **Pericardial Sac.** This is next examined with respect to the degree of intrapericardial tension. Its anterior wall is then picked up at about its middle by the thumb and index finger of left hand,

and the point of the long section-knife, with cutting edge outward, is pushed through the pericardium and a small slit made into the sac. The escape of gas or air should be noted at this time. A sterile pipette may now be introduced and the fluid contents of the sac secured for bacteriologic examination; or before the pericardial sac is opened the pericardium may be seared with a hot iron and a sterile pipette pushed through it into the cavity. The longitudinal incision through the pericardium is now extended upward to its attachment to the great vessels, and through the opening thus made the character and amount of the pericardial fluid are determined. The incision is then extended to the left at its lower end by cutting the sac-wall toward the apex of the heart. Through the three-cornered incision thus made the heart is lifted out of the sac and the surfaces of the parietal and visceral layers of the pericardium examined. Localized adhesions of the pericardium may be cut or torn, extensive or complete adhesions may be separated when this is possible; if this cannot be done, the pericardial layers are cut with the heart wall.

4. **Section of the Heart.** The heart may be examined either in the body or outside. The choice of several methods may be taken, and the one most convenient and easy of performance is advised, rather than a method based upon such considerations as the direction of the blood-current in the normal body. The chief essential is to expose completely the interior of the heart with the least possible disturbance of anatomic relationships, and to accomplish this in the simplest and easiest way. Such a method must leave the heart in such shape that it can be reconstructed for histologic study or utilized as a museum specimen. This can be accomplished by a modified *Rokitansky* method, as follows:

The heart is first carefully inspected as it lies in the pericardial sac. The apex is then lifted in the left hand and the posterior wall inspected. The heart is then drawn up over the right edge of the ribs, so that the left border of the heart presents uppermost as the line of greatest convexity. The point of the narrow brain-knife (amputation-knife), with cutting edge upward, is then inserted through the wall of the left ventricle at the apex, just to the left of the septum, and the knife pushed into the cavity until the point can be forced through the ventricular wall just below (ventricular side) the left auriculoventricular ring, and the ventricle-wall is then cut upward (as the heart is held) to the apex, in the line of greatest convexity, exposing the cavity of the left ventricle. The knife is laid aside and the ventricle is explored with the fingers of the right hand and the size of the mitral opening estimated. Before the fingers are introduced through the valvular openings the flaps should be carefully examined to see that no vegetations, thrombi, etc., are in danger of being loosened by them. With the opening of the heart-chambers the blood, if fluid, may pour out into the pericardial sac and flood the pleural cavity if not prevented by sponging or by removing it by means of a beaker. The knife is then introduced on the flat through the mitral opening into the left auricle in a line continuing the first incision with the junction of the left pulmonary veins. (See Fig. 38.) The

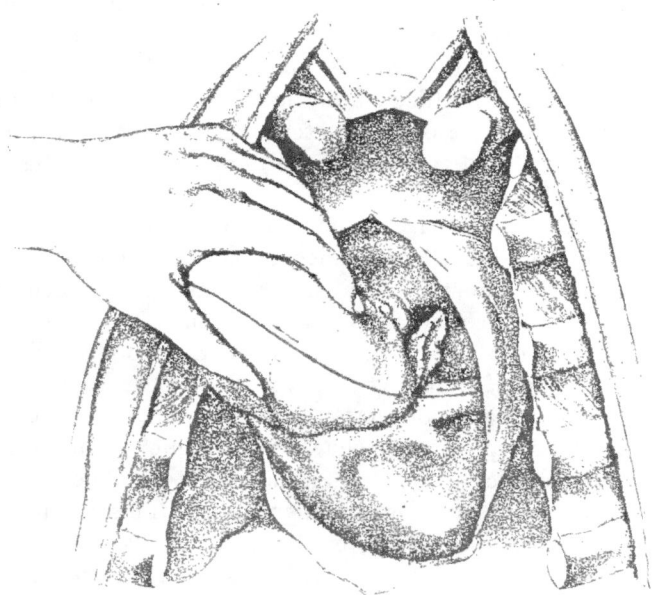

Fig. 38—Section of left ventricle and auricle, when heart is examined in the body. (After Nauwerck.)

knife is then turned with cutting-edge upward, the point thrust through the upper left pulmonary vein or between the left pulmonary veins, and the auricular wall is cut upward (downward anatomically) to meet the first incision below the mitral ring. The incision should pass between the mitral segments. The left auricle, mitral ring and flaps and the greater portion of the left ventricle are thus exposed and should be inspected.

The heart is then taken in the left hand and held by the anterior flap of the left ventricle, with the fingers inside the ventricle and the thumb on the outer surface of the anterior wall of the left ventricle, and lifted up vertically out of the pericardium. The brain-knife held perpendicularly, with cutting-edge to the right, is pushed through the right ventricular wall just to the right of the septum, carried across the cavity of the ventricle, to engage again in the ventricular wall in the line of greatest convexity, just below (anatomically) the right auriculoventricular ring, and the wall is then cut upward to the apex. The right ventricular cavity is thus opened, the fingers are introduced to explore the tricuspid ring, and the cavity and contents are inspected. The knife, held flat, is then carefully introduced through the tricuspid opening into the right auricle, the cutting edge outward, and its point thrust through the wall of the auricle midway between the superior and inferior venæ cavæ, and the auricular wall and tricuspid ring are cut upward toward the apex to meet the first incision into the right ventricle. If sufficient care is taken the incision will fall between the anterior and posterior cusps. Right auricle, tricuspid flaps and ring, and the right ventricle are thus exposed for inspection.

The heart is then drawn downward and allowed to lie flat in the pericardial sac, and the pulmonary artery is then explored with the fingers of the right hand. While the anterior wall of the right ventricle is held by the thumb and index-finger of the left hand the knife is then introduced, on the flat, along the right side of the septum, into the pulmonary artery; the edge is turned upward and the point pushed through the wall of the artery, about 3 cm. beyond the ring, and a cut made toward the apex through the anterior wall of the artery, pulmonary ring and anterior wall of right ventricle, just to the right of the septum. The pulmonary artery, ring, pulmonary flaps, and right side of auricular and ventricular septum are now inspected. In cutting the pulmonary ring care should be taken to make the incision between the two anterior cusps.

With the heart still lying flat in the pericardial sac, the aortic opening is explored by the index-finger of the right hand and the size of the ring estimated. The knife is then introduced on the flat, into the left ventricle, along the left side of the septum, through the aortic opening and as far as possible into the aorta. It is then turned, with the cutting edge upward, and the point pushed through the anterior wall of the aorta. The heart is then drawn downward and slightly raised by the left hand, holding it at the apex by the two flaps of the right ventricle. The knife is then drawn from above downward toward the apex, cutting in succession the anterior wall of the aorta, across the pulmonary artery, through the aortic ring, and the anterior wall of the left ventricle, just to the left side of the septum. By dissecting away the pulmonary artery from the aorta the incision through the former may be avoided. (See Fig. 41.) When desired this cut may be brought down through the septum instead, but if the bundle of His is to be studied in serial sections the cutting of the septum should be avoided. The enterotome or long straight shears may be used for all the incisions except the first ones made into the ventricles. For these the knife is necessary. The incision through the aortic ring usually cuts the anterior segment, but by making the cut more to the right the incision will pass between the anterior and the right posterior flaps.

Before the valvular orifices are cut it is often expedient to test the adequacy of the valves by means of water or air. The hydrostatic test is employed to the best advantage in the case of the pulmonary and aortic valves, either by pouring water into the vessels, or by immersing the heart in water and then lifting it up quickly. In the case of the auriculoventricular valves the air-test is carried out by inserting the nozzle of a bellows through an opening made in the ventricular wall and noting the effect of blowing and suction. Graduated cones or balls may be used for more accurate measurement of the orifices, or they may be measured after they have been cut.

If sufficient care is exercised in cutting the valvular rings the incision can be carried between the flaps without injury to the latter. This is often desirable in cases of valvular lesion, endocarditis, etc. In such cases the valvular rings may be left uncut, the line of incision being broken by the auriculoventricular ring, when the mitral and tricuspid valves are concerned. The pulmonary and aortic rings may also be left uncut; the incisions are stopped at the rings, and then begun again in the vessel-walls beyond the valves.

When bacteriologic examinations of the heart-contents are to be made the wall of the auricles or right ventricles can be seared with a cautery and a pipette introduced through the seared area; or the heart can be opened with a sterile knife, care being taken not to introduce the fingers into the opening or to permit the entrance of water.

Excellent preparations for the museum or for demonstration purposes can be made by distending the heart with alcohol or formalin. Blood and blood-clots should first be washed out. When fixed the heart may be sectioned in various planes, leaving the segments attached by the epicardium posteriorly, or openings may be cut in the walls. A very good picture of hypertrophy and dilatation is obtained by making a transverse cut through the ventricles midway between apex and base. Alterations in the form and position of the ventricular septum are best seen by this method.

After the opening of the heart and the inspection of the orifices, valves and auricular and ventricular septa, the coronary vessels should be examined by transverse cuts, or opened by fine probe-pointed scissors, beginning at their origin in the aorta. The auricular septum should be carefully examined for possible defects. While this is being done the wall should not be put on the stretch, but should be lax. The auricular appendages should be cut open from the auricles and examined for thrombi, which are of not infrequent occurrence in them. The mouths of the coronary veins and the veins of Thebesius should be examined also. The cardiac muscle is examined by parallel, vertical or horizontal incisions. The papillary muscles should be cut longitudinally from apex to base. The cardiac plexus and the ganglion of Wrisberg should be examined before the heart is removed.

When the heart is in a state of rigor mortis the contraction should be made to pass away by kneading or by the application of heat, before the organ is opened, or before any measurements are taken. After the heart has been opened it may be removed for weighing.

The heart may be removed first and then opened outside of the body. The organ is grasped in the left hand and lifted vertically and upward toward the head as far as possible, putting all of the attachments on the stretch. The vessels are then cut from below upward, first the inferior vena cava, then the pulmonary veins, the superior vena cava, pulmonary artery and lastly the aorta. (See Fig. 39.) The vessels should be cut as closely as possible to their exits through the pericardium, and care must be taken to get out the auricles entire.

After removal from the body the heart is placed upon the board with its anterior surface up, and the apex toward the operator. It may then be opened by the same method given above, by inserting the point of the brain-knife into the left ventricle just to the left of the septum, and cutting first the wall of the left ventricle along its left border as far as the mitral ring, exploring the mitral orifice, and then cutting it and the auricular wall into the upper left pulmonary vein with the long shears. The right ventricle, right auricle, pulmonary artery and finally the aorta are opened in succession, using the enterotome for all cuts except the first opening

112 THE EXAMINATION OF THE THORAX.

of the ventricle. The first incisions into the ventricles can be made very conveniently by holding the heart vertically with apex up, and the ventricle to be opened toward the prosector. The brain-knife is held vertically and its point inserted into the ventricle, just to the right or left of the septum, according to the ventricle to be

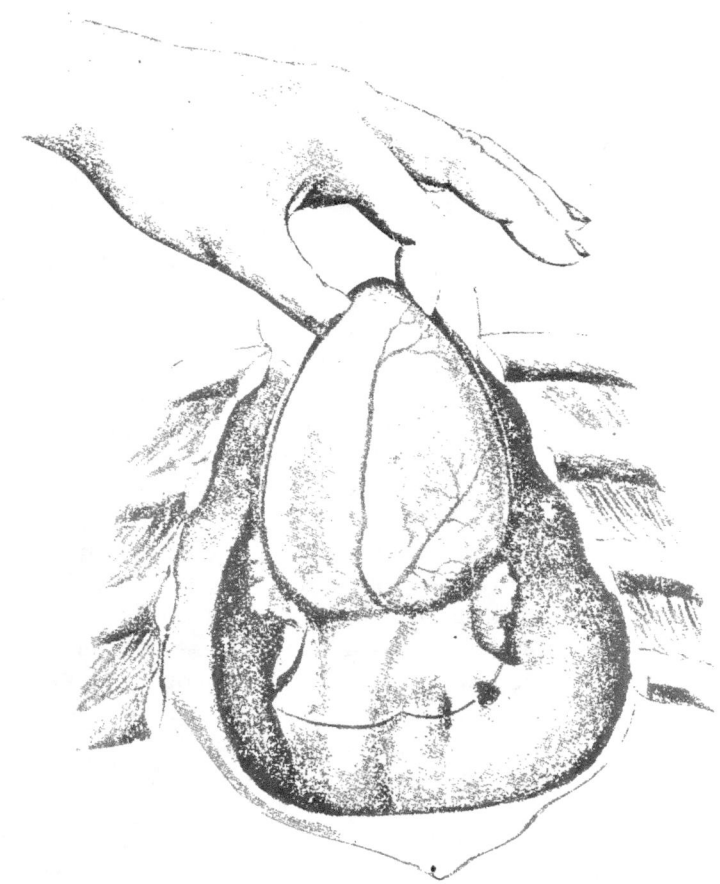

FIG. 39—Removal of Heart. Dark line shows incision through vessels. (After Nauwerck.)

opened, then carried across the cavity and pushed through the ventricular wall below the auriculoventricular ring, and the wall is then cut toward the apex. The remaining incisions are most easily made with the enterotome when the heart is held flat on the board with its anterior surface up. When the heart is opened outside of the body the Virchow method of opening in the direction of the blood-stream may also be used. (See below.)

Under certain conditions other methods must be employed for the examination of the heart. In cases of suspected aneurism, pulmonary embolism, patent ductus arteriosus, etc., the thoracic organs should be removed *en masse* and dissected on the table. They may be removed in connection with the neck-organs or alone. In the latter case the trachea is cut transversely above the sternum, the fingers of the left hand introduced into the trachea, and, while traction downward is being made with force, the œsophagus and cervical vessels are cut transversely, the trachea and vessels stripped down to the level of the clavicle, and the subclavian vessels cut on both sides. The thoracic organs are then stripped from the vertebræ down to the diaphragm and cut off just above the latter.

The pulmonary artery may be examined *in situ* before the heart is opened by thrusting a sharp-pointed scalpel through the wall of the artery just beyond the valves and cutting upward to the branches going to the right and left lungs. This incision may be extended downward through the pulmonary valve and the anterior wall of the right ventricle, and the right side of the heart first exposed.

Virchow Method. The heart is rotated toward the left side of the cadaver so as to bring the venæ cavæ into view, and is held by the index-finger and thumb of left hand. An incision is then made in the wall of the right auricle, beginning midway between the two cavæ and extending downward as far as the right auriculoventricular ring, in the direction of the right ventricular ridge. The tricuspid is examined from above. The tricuspid ring may be left uncut and an incision made in the ventricle-wall, beginning just below the valve and extending downward along the right ventricular ridge to the septum, or the incision may be carried down in the same line passing through the tricuspid ring. The long narrow-bladed knife or the enterotome is introduced into the right ventricle and an incision made from the middle of the first incision, just above the insertion of the anterior papillary muscle, through the pulmonary orifice into the pulmonary artery, passing between the two anterior leaflets of the pulmonary valve. The heart is now drawn up on the right edge of the ribs so that the left ventricular border presents uppermost. The left auricle is then opened by an incision beginning in, or just below, the lowermost pulmonary vein and extended in the direction of the left ventricular ridge as far as the auriculoventricular ring. Beginning just below the ring an incision is made through the entire length of the left ventricular ridge as far as the apex and to the septum, which lies usually beyond the apex. A second incision is then made in the left ventricle from the apex, extending through the anterior ventricular wall close to the septum, parallel to the descending branch of the anterior coronary artery and about 1 cm. from it, and passing through the aortic opening between the anterior and the right posterior cusps. This is the more easily accomplished if the pulmonary artery has been dissected away from the aorta, so that the incision can be carried well over to the right. (See Fig. 41.) As the chambers of the heart are opened the contents should be inspected, clots removed, and the valvular orifices examined from the upper side. The coronary arteries are then opened with the fine probe-pointed scissors. When the heart has been removed from the body it may be opened on the board by following the method as given above. The heart is held very conveniently for the Virchow incisions by putting the four fingers of the left hand beneath it and the thumb on the anterior surface; complete pronation puts the heart in the position for opening the right side; complete supination gives the position for opening the left side.

Nauwerck Method. By this method the left auricle, left ventricle, right auricle and right ventricle are opened in succession. The heart is seized in the

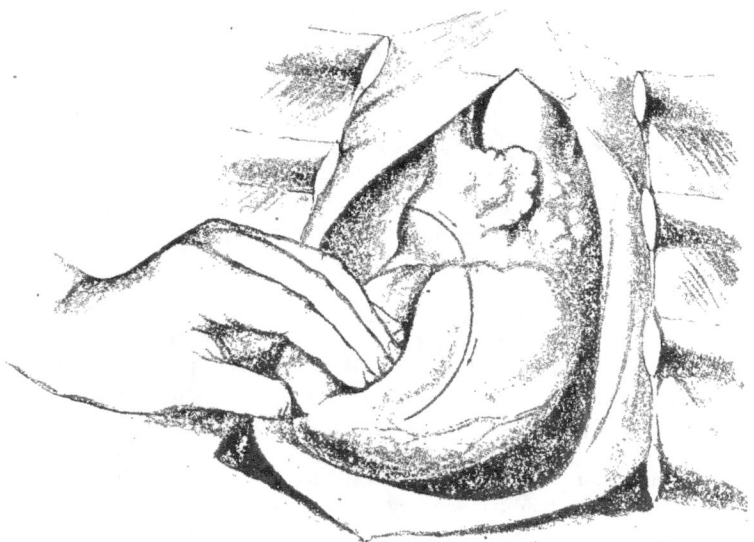

FIG. 40—Section of right auricle and ventricle, according to Nauwerck.

left hand, and without rotation is drawn upon the right edge of the ribs. Beginning in the upper left pulmonary vein or between the veins an incision is made through the wall of the auricle to the sulcus circularis, avoiding any injury to the coronary vessels. Beginning below the mitral ring an incision is carried along the left ventricular ridge to the apex. The left auricle and ventricle are then cleared of blood and the mitral opening examined. The heart is then put back into its natural position; the left thumb is placed in the apex of the left ventricle and the four fingers passed over the right border of the heart to its posterior surface, rotating the heart to the left until the right auricle is brought uppermost. (See Fig. 40.) Then an incision is made through the wall of the right auricle, beginning midway between the superior and inferior venæ cavæ and extending to the tricuspid ring, then begun again 1 cm. below, is carried along the right border of the heart, or slightly anterior to it, as far as the septum. (See Fig. 40.) The contents of right auricle and ventricle and the tricuspid valves are now inspected. The heart is then removed from the body by lifting it up vertically as far as possible and cutting the vessels from below upward as close as possible to their exits through the pericardial sac. The hydrostatic test is then applied to the aortic and pulmonary valves by pouring water into these vessels, or by immersing the heart in water and then lifting it out. The heart is then laid flat on the board with apex toward the operator. The enterotome is introduced into the right ventricle and through the pulmonary

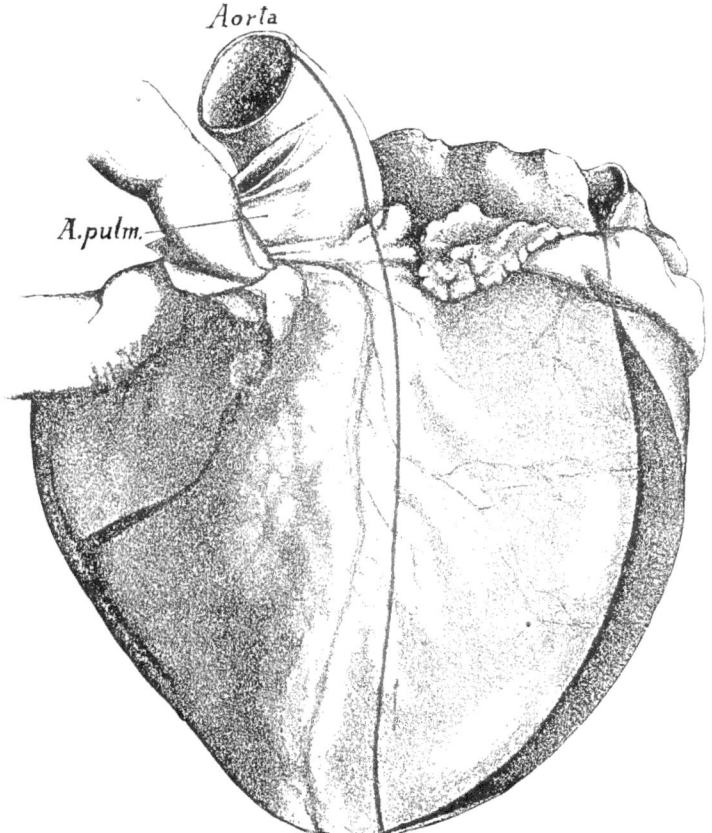

FIG. 41—Incision for opening of aortic ring; same for all methods described in text. (After Nauwerck.)

orifice and an incision made through the anterior wall of the right ventricle, beginning just above the anterior papillary muscle at about the middle height of the ventricle, and cutting through the pulmonary conus and pulmonary valve well to the left, close to the septum, following the narrow ridge of fat at the base of the artery so as to pass between the left anterior and posterior segments. The heart is then rotated on its vertical axis so that the right auricle is turned toward the prosector, and the tricuspid ring is opened with the intestinal shears. The auricular appendage is then cut open from the auricular incision. The heart is then held in its former position and an incision is made in the anterior wall of the left ventricle just to the left of the septum, from the apex through the aortic ring and the left wall of the aorta, while the pulmonary artery is pulled to the right. (See Fig. 41.) Care must be taken not to damage the right border of the base of the mitral; the cut should pass half way between the pulmonary orifice and the left auricular appendage, cutting the left aortic flap. If it is desired to save the cusps the pulmonary artery may be dissected from the aorta and the incision carried between the right posterior and the anterior valve-flaps. The heart is again rotated toward the right and the mitral ring is cut with the enterotome, which is introduced from the left auricle into the left ventricle. The left auricular appendage is then cut open. The heart-wall is then examined by means of parallel vertical or horizontal incisions. The papillary muscles are cut longitudinally from apex to base. The coronary vessels and their branches are then examined, partly from the aorta and partly from the incisions through the muscle.

Prausnitz Method. The heart is removed and held in the palm of the left hand and two vertical incisions are made on either side of the septum, parallel with it, and extending from base to apex. Two other incisions are then made from base to apex on the outer borders of the ventricles, connecting at the apex with the first incisions. The ventricles are opened by the triangular flaps of the anterior wall thus formed, these flaps being attached at the base of the heart. The contents of the cavities are examined and removed; the valvular orifices and flaps are examined, and the pulmonary and aortic rings are cut through with the shears by extending the two incisions made on each side of the septum, taking care to pass between the cusps.

The heart can also be opened with the long shears alone. The openings of the two cavæ in the right auricle are connected by an incision. The auricular appendage is opened by a second cut. The shears are then put through the tricuspid ring, and this with the right ventricle is cut, the incision following the right ventricular border. The pulmonary orifice is then opened by a cut made along the right side of the septum. The left heart is opened through the pulmonary veins, cutting first the auricle-wall, then the mitral ring and ventricular wall to the apex. An incision is then made along the left side of the septum, through the aortic orifice into the aorta.

5. **Section of the Lungs.** The general inspection of the pleural cavities and pleural surfaces is made as soon as the thoracic cavity is opened, as indicated above. If a pneumothorax is present the pleural cavity on the affected side is filled with water, the neck organs are exposed and a tube inserted into the trachea. When air is forced through this bubbles will escape from the perforation and the opening can be easily located. When extensive or complete pleural adhesions are present, so that they cannot be separated, it becomes necessary to remove the costal pleura in connection with the visceral layer. This is accomplished by loosening the costal pleura and subpleural fascia at the cut edge of the ribs

SECTION OF THE LUNGS.

with the blade of the knife, until the fingers and, finally the hand, can be worked in between the costal pleura and the chest-wall, gradually separating the two until the entire lung is freed with both layers of pleura adherent. Firm adhesions at the apex may have to be cut with the knife. Similar adhesions with the pericardium or diaphragm may make it necessary to cut out the adherent portion with scissors or knife and remove it in connection with the lung. When the pleural adhesions are very firm upon the right side the prosector may find it most convenient to stand at the left side of the cadaver and from this position separate the right costal pleura from the chest wall. An assistant may be of great service in pulling the thoracic wall outward. The edge of the ribs or cartilages may be covered with a towel or the skin may be drawn over it to protect the hands. In extreme cases it may be necessary to saw the ribs and remove them in connection with the lungs. Sometimes the adhesions may be separated more easily if the neck-organs are first removed down to the clavicle, and then, in connection with the lungs, are removed *en masse*, by means of powerful tugs, from above downward. The apical and posterior adhesions may be torn fairly easily in this way when ordinary manipulations in the thoracic cavity have no effect upon them.

When the pleural surfaces are free the **left lung** is lifted out of the cavity onto the right edge of the chest-wall, pulling it forcibly over to the right so that its posterior surface becomes uppermost. In this position the lung may be sectioned by one or more main incisions made with the long section-knife, cutting the organ from apex to base, down upon the ribs in the direction of the main bronchi and vessels. After the examination of the cut surfaces the organ may be returned to the cavity. It is better, however, to remove the lung, and section it outside the body. This is done by cutting the mediastinal pleura, pulmonary vessels and main bronchus with the cartilage-knife, while the lung is held upon the right edge of the thoracic opening, holding the knife so that its blade strikes the edge of the costal cartilages.

The lung, when free, is placed upon the board with its hilus downward and base toward the prosector. (See Fig. 42.) It is then held in the left hand, as shown in the illustration, the thumb holding the lower lobe, the index-finger between the lobes with its tip upon the main bronchus, the other fingers holding the upper lobe. With the long section-knife held slightly obliquely toward the anterior edge the main-incision is now made in one sweeping cut from apex to base, along the line of greatest convexity, down upon the main-bronchus and its chief branches and the large vessels. Care should be taken not to cut off the bronchi of the two lobes from the main bronchus. Incisions parallel to the main one may be made, if desired. Usually it suffices to go carefully over the remaining part of the lung, feeling it carefully for airless solid areas; if such are present they may be sectioned separately. The

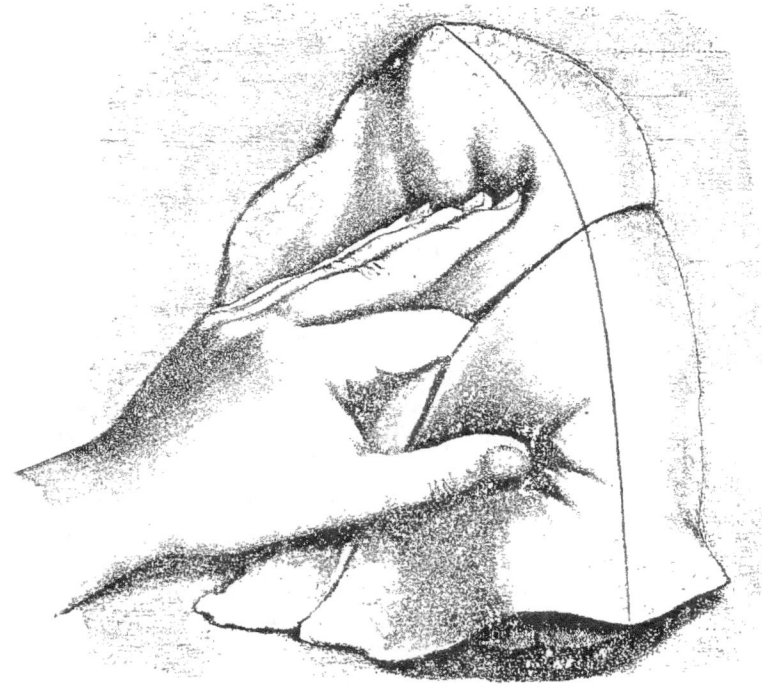

FIG. 42—Section of left lung. (After Nauwerck.)

bronchi are then opened from the cut surface by means of the probe-pointed scissors, cutting as near to the pleura as possible. The sound or director may be used with advantage in opening up cavities from the bronchi. The position of the lung should be so changed that the bronchi always extend away from the prosector in a straight line. The portion of the lung containing the uncut bronchus should be left hanging over the left hand to put it on the stretch, thereby facilitating greatly the opening of the bronchus. The **pulmonary vessels** are opened with fine probe-pointed scissors from the cut surface. The bronchial lymphglands are then sectioned with the knife.

SECTION OF THE LUNGS. 119

The **right lung** is then lifted up out of the thorax onto the right side of the thoracic opening, and is either sectioned in this position, or the mediastinal pleura, pulmonary vessels and bronchus are cut from below upward with the knife, its edge being directed against the ribs. When freed the lung is placed on the board, root downward and apex toward the prosector. (See Fig. 43.) The index-finger is put between the upper and lower lobes, the thumb holds

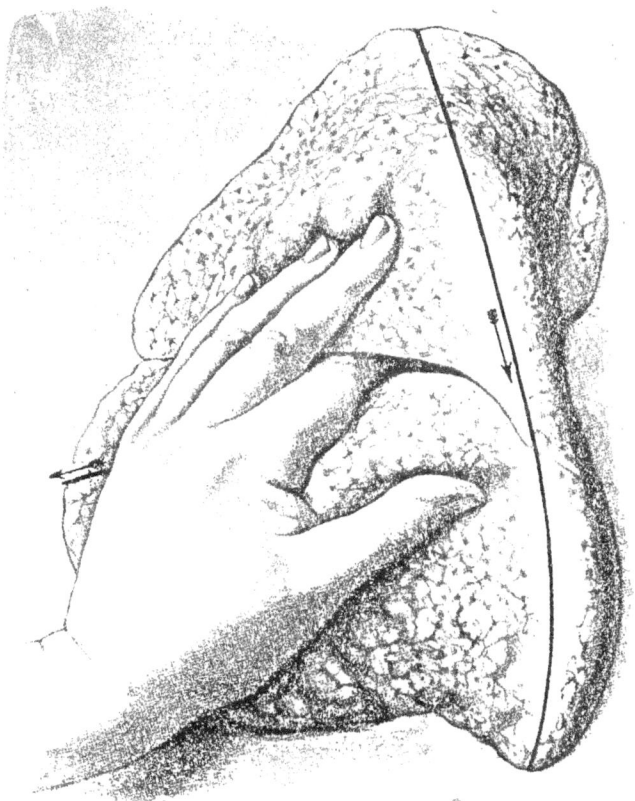

FIG. 43—Section of right lung. (After Nauwerck.)

the upper lobe, the other fingers are spread out over the surface of the lower lobe. The main-incision is then made in a sweeping cut, from base to apex, along the line of greatest convexity, the knife-blade being held slightly obliquely toward the anterior border (see Fig. 43), cutting down upon the main bronchus and its first division. Other parallel cuts may be made. The middle lobe is then sectioned by a sagittal incision on its anterior surface, directed toward its anterior border. The **bronchi, pulmonary vessels** and **bronchial lymphnodes** are then opened as in the case of the left lung.

Bacteriologic examinations may be made from smears or cultures made from the cut surfaces; or, to avoid contamination, the surface may be seared with a hot iron and the material obtained by means of a sterile pipette pushed through the seared surface into the lung-tissue.

The lungs may also be removed by drawing them downward and outward, away from the root, while the bronchi and pulmonary vessels are cut, the knife being directed against the vertebræ, care being taken to avoid cutting the aorta and œsophagus. The lungs are then lifted up toward the middle line, while the mediastinal pleuræ are cut. The section of the lungs may be carried out, if so desired, from the root, the main bronchus and then all of the branches as far as the pleuræ being opened up by means of the probe-pointed scissors. Other incisions may be made if desired.

As mentioned above, it is sometimes more convenient to remove the thoracic organs *en masse*, either alone, or in association with the neck organs. When this is done the dissection follows the method of Letulle (see above), or the organs may be separated and sectioned according to the methods just given.

The section of the heart usually precedes that of the lungs, in order that the blood-content of the former may be more correctly estimated. Under certain conditions it may be more convenient or expedient to section the lungs first, beginning with the left one.

When the neck-organs are not removed the section of the thorax closes with the examination of the **aorta, oesophagus, thoracic duct** and **thoracic vertebrae**. The blood-vessels and œsophagus are opened with the curved scissors, from above downward, the contents noted, and the walls examined. The thoracic duct is best dissected out from the right side, by cutting along the right side of the aorta and turning the latter over to the left. The duct is more easily recognized at its lower end. It may be inflated with the blow-pipe, or opened with a probe and fine probe-pointed scissors. Sometimes the duct can be most easily found by removing the left lung and then turning the right lung over into the left pleural cavity. The posterior mediastinal tissues are put on a stretch, so that the duct can be recognized through the pleura. For the examination of the left subclavian vein the left clavicle should be removed.

II. POINTS TO BE NOTED IN THE EXAMINATION OF THE THORAX.

1. **Thoracic Cavity.** Presence of gas or air (pneumothorax, infections with colon bacillus, gas-forming bacillus, proteus, etc.), relative degree of pressure, odor, etc. Measure contents of each pleural sac; note character of fluid (clear, turbid, bloody, chyliform, chylous, purulent, fibrino-purulent). Normally the pleuræ are moist-shining, smooth, grayish, transparent; only a few drops of fluid found in the cavities. In cases of slowly progressive cardiac insufficiency large amounts of clear fluid may collect in the cavities just before death. Non-inflammatory collections of fluid also occur in general œdema. In these conditions the pleuræ are not cloudy or dull, while in the case of inflammation the pleural surfaces are dry, cloudy, dull-shining, injected, rough or covered with fibrinous or purulent exudate. Examine pleural surfaces particularly for evidences of inflammation, recent and old tuberculosis, primary and secondary neoplasms (carcinoma).

2. **Position of Thoracic Organs.** Locate anterior borders of lungs, apex and borders of heart. The normal lung collapses after the removal of the sternum. How much of the pericardial sac is left uncovered by the lungs?

3. **Anterior Mediastinum.** Note character of connective-tissue, amount and color of fat-tissue, number and size of lymph-nodes, occurrence of œdema or emphysema. An artificial œdema may be caused by the injection of large quantities of salt solution in the pectoral region just before death. An artificial emphysema may be produced by the removal of the sternum. The condition of the large veins in the upper portion of the mediastinum should be noted before the heart is removed. Are they lax, moderately full, or distended? Secondary tumors, hemorrhages, abscesses, œdema and emphysema are the most common pathologic conditions.

4. **Thymus.** The writer believes that the weights usually given for the thymus in the newborn are too high, and that 7-10 grms. represents the usual normal weight. A gland weighing 20 grms. or more must be regarded as enlarged. The organ reaches its fullest development at the end of the second year. Atrophy begins then, developing slowly up to the age of puberty, after that more rapidly. In adults the thymus normally consists of a mass of adipose tissue containing lymphoid nodules, in some of which corpuscles of Hassall persist to old age. Postmortem softening

should not be mistaken for abscesses. The most important pathologic change is hypertrophy. Pressure of the enlarged gland upon the trachea, nerves or great vessels may cause thymic stridor, asthma, or thymic death ("lymphatic constitution"). Enlargement of the thymus may occur in "status lymphaticus," exophthalmic goitre, cretinism, myxœdema, Addison's disease, acromegaly, myasthenia gravis, epilepsy, scorbutus, rachitis, tonsillar hyperplasia, adenoids, congenital syphilis, Hodgkin's disease, leukæmia, anencephaly, anæmia, acute infections, or it may exist as an independent affection. Oedema, congestion, inflammation, tuberculosis, neoplasms, etc., may also cause an enlargement. Absence of the thymus has been observed. Primary and secondary forms of atrophy in association with marasmus occur in children. Note relation of size of thymus to condition of child; atrophy of the organ is usually coincident with marasmus. Inflammation, tuberculosis, cysts, primary and secondary neoplasms, gummata, etc., are not common.

5. **Pericardium.** Note tension of sac, fluctuation, adhesions, thickness, character of inner surface, contents (amount, color, odor, presence of fibrin, blood or pus, gas). Normally there are about 5-10 c. c. of clear yellow fluid in the sac. Both peri- and epicardium normally are moist-shining, smooth, grayish and transparent. Large amounts of clear watery fluid may collect in the pericardial sac in slow death in cases of chronic valvular lesions, chronic nephritis, bronchitis and emphysema, but the surface of the peri- and epicardium remains smooth and shining. In inflammatory increase of the pericardial fluid the serous surfaces are dull, cloudy or dry, and may be covered with a layer of fibrin, the fluid is more or less cloudy and contains flakes or strings of fibrin, or may be purulent. The fibrinous exudate may be very extensive and from the movement of the heart be drawn out into bands, threads or villus-like prominences (cor hirsutum or villosum). Pericarditis is common in acute rheumatism, septicæmia, pyæmia, puerperal fever, osteomyelitis, pneumonia, and as a terminal infection in cardiac and renal disease. Tuberculosis is one of the most common causes of purulent, fibrinous and hemorrhagic pericarditis, particularly of the cor villosum. Examine surfaces for tubercles. The presence of blood in the pericardial exudate points usually to tuberculosis or malignant neoplasm, but in small amount may be found in various infections and intoxications. The age of the pericarditis may be judged by the amount of organization of the exudate,

adhesions, thickenings, etc. "Milk spots," "soldier's spots," "tendinous patches" or "friction scleroses" represent hyaline thickenings of the pericardium due to old pericarditis. Total synechia or atresia of the cavity may occur. As the result of calcification of an old pericarditic exudate the heart may be surrounded by a calcareous sheath ("stony heart," "petrified heart"). Hæmopericardium results from the rupture of the heart, aorta, pulmonary artery or coronary vessel. Petechiæ of the peri- and epicardium are found in pyæmia, septicæmia, hæmophilia, scurvy, severe anæmia, leukæmia, chronic nephritis, and death from suffocation and various intoxications. Pneumopericardium may be due to perforating wounds, or to perforations from lungs, stomach or œsophagus, or to infections with gas-forming bacilli. Malformations are rare (diverticula, ectopia). Tuberculosis is usually secondary. Gummata are rare. Actinomycosis is usually secondary to actinomycosis of the neck or lungs. Primary neoplasms are rare. Secondary carcinoma and sarcoma (especially lymphosarcoma) are more frequent. Cysticercus, trichina and echinococcus are rare.

6. **Heart.** Note more carefully its position, whether displaced to right or left, location of apex, borders, etc. Relative size compared to cadaver's right fist, which is usually a little smaller than the heart. Weight and measurements:—(The heart should be weighed after it has been opened, and its cavities freed from blood and clots.)

Average weight in adult male, about 300-350 grm.
Average weight in adult female, about 250 grm.
Normal limits, 200-350 grm.
Weight of heart to body-weight in adult male, 1:169; in the female, 1:162.

Circumference at base of ventricles 25.8 cm., length of ventricles 8-9 cm., breadth 8.5-10-5 cm., thickness 3-3.6 cm.; minimal measurements are for the female. Auricles are 5-6 cm. in length. Compare ventricles as to size.

Note form (long, cylindrical, pyramidal, broad, short, round, etc.) In hypertrophy of the left ventricle the heart is longer and more cylindrical; in hypertrophy of the right it is broader and more rounded. Normally the apex is formed by the left ventricle, the sulcus longitudinalis running to the apex and nearly dividing the heart into halves. In hypertrophy of the right ventricle the apex is formed by this ventricle, the sulcus longitudinalis passing to the left of the apex; in hypertrophy of the left ventricle the longitudinal sulcus runs to the right of the apex. What part of the heart lies anteriorly? (Normally a large part of the right ventricle.)

The consistence of the organ, particularly that of the ventricles, should be noted (firm, flabby, soft, etc.). Condition of the heart-chambers (empty, contracted, dilated, full). Rigor mortis should be removed by kneading or by the application of heat. The amount of subepicardial fat, its color, translucency, occurrence of serous atrophy, œdema, subepicardial hemorrhage, etc., are to be noted. In marasmus a serous or mucoid degeneration of the subepicardial fat is not uncommon. The subepicardial fat increases with age, and is normally most abundant along the grooves and blood-vessels, particularly the auriculoventricular grooves and on the right ventricle. Normally the color of the heart-muscle of the ventricles should be seen through the epicardium. The fat is increased in obesity, chronic alcoholism, chronic anæmia, tuberculosis, etc. When the fat-infiltration is so marked that the muscle cannot be seen the condition is known as adipositas or obesitas cordis, or in extreme cases as *lipoma cordis capsulare*.

7. **Right Heart.** Note amount of blood contained in right chambers (over-distended in death from asphyxiation, pneumonia, etc.), also its consistence (thick, thin, watery), color (light, dark, red, yellowish, chocolate, purplish), blood-clots (size, color, cruor, lardaceous clots, chicken-fat clots, pus-like clots, consistence, moisture), presence of free fat, gas or air, diffusion of hæmoglobin, presence of bile-pigment in blood. Note also amount and character of blood in venæ cavæ. The size of auricular and ventricular cavities should be estimated, noting condition of trabeculæ and papillary muscles (atrophic, flattened, hypertrophic, fatty, fibroid, calcification). The musculature of the ventricular walls is examined as to its thickness (normally the right ventricle wall is 4-5 mm. thick). Postmortem contraction should not be mistaken for hypertrophy. The color of the heart-muscle normally is pinkish in infants, flesh-red in adults, and brownish-red in old age and in atrophy following compensatory hypertrophy (brown atrophy). Under normal conditions the muscle is translucent. In cloudy swelling the heart-muscle appears cloudy and opaque as if cooked. Fatty degeneration appears as yellowish, opaque patches or streaks ("tiger-heart"), particularly in the papillary muscles and trabeculæ. In severe intoxications the process may be diffuse, and the entire musculature appear cream-colored or yellowish and opaque. The consistence may be firm, flabby, soft, putty-like; localized areas may be caseous. Infarcted areas are soft when fresh (myomalacia

cordis). The consistence is increased in atrophy, fibroid heart, chronic interstitial myocarditis, syphilis, etc. Cloudy swelling and fatty degeneration make the heart muscle softer and more friable. In postmortem decomposition the heart as a whole becomes soft. Normally the endocardium should be gray, delicate, thin and transparent. The chordæ tendinæ are long, narrow and delicate. Note thickenings of endocardium and chordæ tendinæ, presence of thrombi (dry, brick-red, yellowish or gray, firmer than clots and adherent to the endocardium, often show simple softening, which should not be mistaken for pus; may be parietal, polypoid, valvular or free). The endocardium may be stained diffusely yellow (bile) or brown (methæmoglobin). Creamy or yellowish opacities of the intima are due to fatty degeneration.

8. **Left Heart.** Note same things in left side of heart as on right. In cardiac paralysis left ventricle is filled with blood if rigor mortis has not set in. Left ventricle wall is 10-15 mm. thick normally; may become 30 mm. thick in hypertrophy. Papillary muscles and trabeculæ may be markedly hypertrophic, but in the greatly dilated heart (aortic insufficiency) may be much flattened. The septum of the ventricles may share in the hypertrophy of either ventricle and when hypertrophic bulges into the cavity of the unaffected side. Examine wall of left ventricle, particularly near the apex, for infarcts, fibroid patches, aneurismal dilatation, rupture, fatty degeneration, thrombi, etc. Look particularly for pathologic conditions involving the atrioventricular bundle.

9. **Orifices and Valves.** Orifices should measure as follows:— Tricuspid (12-12.7 cm.), mitral (10.4-10.9 cm.), pulmonary (8.9-9.2 cm.), aorta (7.7-8 cm.). Rough measurements may be taken with the fingers, tricuspid admitting three, mitral two, pulmonary one and a half, aorta thumb. The orifices may be measured by graduated cones, or in the ordinary way after the heart is sectioned. Normally the edges of the valve-flaps should be delicate, smooth and thin. Examine for vegetations, thrombi, induration, thickening, contractions, ulcerations, tears, perforations, defects, calcification, atheroma, valvular aneurism, etc. Note thickening, contraction, adhesion, shortening, etc., of the chordæ tendinæ. When the tendons are long, narrow and thread-like, and without adhesions, the probabilities are that a lesion of the mitral orifice was not present.

10. **Coronary Vessels.** Walls should be uniformly delicate and thin, and the intima should be delicate, gray and transparent. Note contents of arteries and veins. Examine arteries especially

for thrombi, emboli, arteriosclerosis, atheroma, calcification, obliteration of lumen, thickening of wall, loss of elasticity, opacity of intima and increased tortuosity of course.

The most important pathologic conditions of the heart are:— endocarditis (ulcerosa, maligna, verrucosa, simplex, chronica fibrosa, sclerosing), valvular insufficiency and stenosis, hypertrophy, dilatation, atrophy, fatty infiltration, fatty degeneration, cloudy swelling, anæmic infarction, calcification, acute and chronic myocarditis, abscess, fibroid heart, cardiac aneurism, rupture, thrombosis, embolism, malformations (septum defects, patent ductus arteriosus, stenosis or atresia of orifices), tuberculosis (not rare, in association with tuberculous pericarditis, or general miliary tuberculosis), syphilis (gumma not common, localized or diffuse interstitial myocarditis the most common manifestation), actinomycosis, cysticercus, echinococcus, trichina and neoplasms (primary rare, in part congenital, fibroma, lipoma, angioma, myxoma, rhabdomyoma; secondary sarcoma less rare than secondary carcinoma, most common forms are melanotic sarcoma and lymphosarcoma).

11. **Left Lung.** Weighs 350-500 grm. *Size* (voluminous, collapsed, compare lobes); *form* (edges rounded, sharp, nodular, saccular or cystic, contractions, depressions, emphysematous enlargements); *pleura* (examine again more closely. Circumscribed dull-shining or cloudy areas point to some pathologic condition of the lung beneath. Look for evidences of healed tuberculosis, particularly in the pleura of the apices. Secondary carcinoma of the pleura is very common. Primary tumors are rare; endothelioma and sarcoma are the most common forms. Small circumscribed areas of pigmentation usually represent old tubercles); *color* (depends upon degree of anthracosis, blood-content and condition of pleura, areas showing especial color should be examined closely; most common colors are pinkish-gray normally, grayish, slaty, black, red, brown, dark-red to black); *size of air-cells* (normally can be seen with naked eye, best seen at apex and borders, about size of pin-points, when larger than the head of a pin they are emphysematous); *lobules* can also be seen with naked eye, usually polygonal in shape, 2-3 mm. in diameter; *consistence* (estimate by going over entire lung, pressing the lung-substance between thumb and fingers; air-containing lung is soft, elastic and crepitates; airless areas are hard, firm and do not crepitate).

On the cut surface the following points should be noted: *Blood-content* (anæmia, hyperæmia, hypostatic congestion), *color of cut-surface, air-content, exudate* (serous, purulent), *consistence* (hard, soft, elastic, caseous, brittle, crumbling), *character of surface* (smooth, granular, nodular, cavities). Cavities should be described according to their position, size, shape, contents and character of their walls.

12. **Right Lung.** Weight 420-620 grms. Note size, form, color, surface, size of air-cells, lobules, consistence, blood-content, air-content, exudate, consistence and character of cut-surface, as in case of left lung.

Evidences of healed tuberculosis are found in practically all adult lungs in the form of localized thickenings or puckering of the pleura, especially at the apices, hyaline or anthracotic nodules, encapsulated, caseous or calcified tubercles. Old scars and indurations are firm, hard and usually black in color. Caseous areas are smooth, dry, white or grayish, and opaque. Very young tubercles are elevated, grayish and translucent. Atelectatic areas are depressed and bluish-red in color. Areas of hepatization are red or gray, elevated, granular, crumbling, moist in early stage, dry in caseous hepatization. In bronchopneumonia the areas of hepatization are usually sharply circumscribed. Metastatic abscesses lie usually beneath the pleura, are usually multiple and distributed over both lungs. Bronchopneumonic areas are usually found in the dependent portions, particularly in right lung. An abundance of foamy, watery fluid on the cut-surface indicates œdema; when very bloody there is usually a marked stasis or beginning hepatization present. In atelectasis and fibrinous hepatization the exudate from the surface is not foamy. Emphysematous areas are white or grayish-white and are most frequently found along the borders. Large air-spaces are often found along the interlobular septa (interstitial emphysema), particularly in children following trauma, croup, whooping-cough, etc. In chronic passive congestion the lung is firmer than normal, deep-red or brownish in color. Hemorrhagic infarcts lie usually beneath the pleura, are wedge-shaped, with base toward pleura, firm, smooth on section, or granular, and when fresh are nearly black; older ones are lighter and brownish. Cavities in the lung occur in tuberculosis, embolic and primary abscesses, actinomycosis, gangrene, bronchiectasis, primary and secondary tumors, etc. Gangrenous areas have diffuse borders, are gray or greenish in color, with central softened areas, with ragged borders and stinking smell. In bronchiectatic cavities the smooth mucosa of the bronchus passes directly into the wall of the cavity. Primary carcinomata of the lungs appear as cavities having a white medullary wall, or as medullary strands running along the bronchi. Tuberculous cavities have caseous walls, are more or less encapsulated, and usually show younger tubercles in the neighborhood of the wall. Antemortem hypostasis is usually darker and firmer than postmortem, and is usually associated with inflammation (hypostatic pneumonia).

The most important pathologic conditions of the lungs are:— Anomalies (anomalous lobes common, infradiaphragmatic accessory lungs, agenesia, congenital bronchiectasis), atelectasis (fœtal, compression, obstruction, paralytic, etc.), emphysema (acute, chronic, vicarious, senile, atrophic, hypertrophic, interstitial, gangrenous), hyperæmia, stasis, brown induration, hypostasis, œdema (universal, stasis, hypostatic, atelectatic, acute, chronic, terminal), hemorrhage, hemorrhagic infarction, thrombosis, embolism, fatty embolism, pneumonia (croupous, atypical, bronchopneumonia, acute and chronic interstitial), abscess, gangrene, tuberculosis (acute miliary, caseous pneumonia, peribronchial, tuberculous bronchopneumonia, indurative, fibroid, phthisis pulmonum), syphilis (gumma, white pneumonia), actinomycosis, neoplasms (primary adenoma, lipoma, papilloma, chondroma, osteoma, sarcoma, carcinoma and teratoma are rare; metastatic sarcoma and carcinoma are common; malignant chorioepithelioma is not infrequent), parasites (echinococcus, cysticercus, hook-worm embryos, pentastomum and distomum pulmonale).

13. **Bronchi.** Note size, contents, thickness of wall, color and thickness of mucosa. Normally the bronchi are empty, and the mucosa grayish-red. In pulmonary œdema they contain clear, foamy fluid; in bronchitis they may contain a mucous, mucopurulent, purulent, fibrinous, hemorrhagic or putrid exudate. In acute bronchitis the mucosa is red; in chronic bronchitis the mucosa may be red or brownish, and thickened or folded. Material from the stomach may enter the bronchi postmortem and cause a postmortem digestion of the mucosa or wall.

The most important pathologic conditions of the bronchi are:— Inflammation (acute and chronic catarrhal bronchitis, fibrinous, putrid, atrophic, obliterans), bronchial asthma, tuberculosis, syphilis, stenosis, bronchiectasis, perforation (aneurisms, abscess, carcinoma, tubercles, etc.), bronchial calculi, foreign bodies, neoplasms (adenoma, papilloma, carcinoma, chondroma, osteoma), parasites (cysticercus, echinococcus, hook-worm embryos, distomum pulmonale, pentastomum).

14. **Bronchial Glands.** Note size, pigmentation (gray, dark-gray, black), consistence, character of cut-surface, caseation, fibroid induration, calcification, œdema, congestion, abscess, neoplasm. Tuberculosis and secondary neoplasms are the most common conditions. Lymphosarcoma is the most frequent primary tumor.

15. **Pulmonary Vessels.** Character of walls and contents. Normally the intima is smooth, grayish-white and translucent. Fatty degeneration of the intima is not rare (acute infections and intoxications); atheroma and aneurismal dilatation are infrequent. Occasionally parietal thrombi and thickening of the wall due to organization of a thrombus are seen. The pulmonary arteries are normally empty or contain soft cruor or agonal white clots. These are not adherent to the wall, do not fill the lumen and are soft and moist. Emboli fill the lumen as if forced into it (at the branchings of the artery they form "rider's" emboli); they are more dry and brick-red, brownish or grayish in color. Occasionally they may be unrolled into long fibrinous strands. Older emboli may show more or less organization and adherence to the vessel-wall. In air-embolism the pulmonary arteries contain a mixture of blood and air looking like a stiff-beaten white of egg of red color. Large emboli of liver-tissue or liver-cells may be found in the pulmonary arteries after traumatic rupture of the liver. Fat-emboli of the smaller arteries can be recognized by the naked-eye. Thrombosis of both pulmonary arteries and veins is very common in chronic valvular lesions, pneumonia, terminal infections, burns of the skin, poisoning with hemolytic agents, etc.

16. **Great Vessels of Thorax.** Note size of lumen, condition of walls, particularly of intima, and the contents. Circumference of thoracic aorta 4.5-6.0 cm., thickness of wall 1.5-2 mm. Test elasticity of wall by stretching; note if it retracts and becomes shorter than the œsophagus, which was cut at the same level. Note consistence of wall (stiff and hard in sclerosis and calcification). Normally the intima of the aorta is smooth, grayish-white and semitranslucent; the wall is elastic. Fatty degeneration, sclerosis, atheroma and aneurismal dilatations are the most common pathologic findings. Fatty degeneration shows itself in yellowish spots or streaks, more opaque and slightly elevated. Sclerotic areas are hard, white and tendon-like. Atheromatous "plaques" and "ulcers" are white or yellowish, elevated, rough, scaly, with loss of substance, often more or less calcified. Thrombi are frequently formed upon such atheromatous patches. Hemorrhage into the intima may occur (aneurysma dissecans). Radiating or linear sclerotic

folds and depressions in the intima, with or without dilatation of the lumen, usually result from syphilis (mesaortitis). A dirty brownish discoloration of the intima is due to an imbibition of diffuse hæmoglobin, usually postmortem. In chronic icterus the intima may be bile-stained. Thrombosis of the aorta is not common. Congenital or acquired stenosis at the isthmus is rare. Tuberculosis of the aorta-wall is also very rare.

17. **Thoracic Portion of Oesophagus.** Note size (stenosis, dilatation, diverticulum), contents (food, stomach-contents, blood, pus, foreign-body), thickness of wall, color of mucosa (normally grayish-white), neoplasms (carcinoma), perforations, erosions (aneurism, abscess, neoplasm), inflammation. Anomalies, tuberculosis, syphilis, actinomycosis and neoplasms (with the exception of carcinoma) are rare. The most common location of carcinoma is toward the cardia. Thrush is the most common parasite. Varices of the œsophageal veins are common, and from these fatal hemorrhages may occur. In the thoracic portion they are usually the result of collateral distention to offset a portal stasis (hepatic cirrhosis, Banti's disease, thrombosis of splenic or portal veins). The passage of stomach-contents through the cardia into the œsophagus may cause a postmortem softening or perforation of the œsophageal wall.

18. **Thoracic Duct.** Note size, contents and character of wall. Tuberculosis, malignant neoplasms, obstruction, rupture and purulent inflammations are the most important pathologic conditions. In miliary tuberculosis the thoracic duct may be the primary focus or the avenue by which the bacilli enter the blood. The duct also plays an important part in the dissemination of malignant tumors and infections from the abdominal cavity and pelvis. Chylothorax and chylopericardium are usually caused by the blocking of the thoracic duct by malignant neoplasms (lymphosarcoma, carcinoma), or by rupture of the duct.

19. **Thoracic Vertebrae.** Note surfaces of vertebræ (normally smooth), curvatures, softening, erosions, exostoses, neoplasms, fractures, dislocations. Tuberculosis, curvatures and malignant tumors (secondary carcinoma, primary sarcoma, myeloma, chloroma) are the most common conditions. Aneurismal erosions are not rare.

CHAPTER IX.
EXAMINATION OF THE MOUTH AND NECK.
I. METHODS OF EXAMINATION.

1. **Removal of the Neck-Organs.** The block is left beneath the neck, and the chin pulled upward by an assistant, so as to put the skin of the neck on a tight stretch. If the main-incision cannot be extended to the symphysis of the chin, the cartilage- or long section-knife is run up beneath the skin in the median line to the point of the chin, and, with the blade held nearly flat, the skin is loosened from the tissues of the neck, first on the left side, then on the right, as far back as the mastoid processes and the spinal column and to the ends of the clavicles. Great care should be taken not to cut through the skin. The long section-knife, with blade flat, is then pushed through the floor of the mouth, to the left of the median line, taking care not to damage the tongue, and with the blade of the knife closely hugging the inner border of the lower jaw, the floor of the mouth is cut through as far as the angle of the jaw. The knife is then turned with its cutting edge toward the right and a similar cut made through the floor of the mouth as far as the right angle of the jaw. The knife must be held at right angles to the floor of the mouth to avoid cutting the tongue. When the mouth is open the course of the knife can be seen, but usually the mouth is tightly closed in rigor mortis. When cutting the floor of the mouth it is better to make short sawing movements with the knife than to attempt to cut it with one sweeping cut. Instead of cutting from the median line the knife may be inserted at the right or left angle of the jaw and the cut extended upward to the chin and thence toward the other angle. (See Fig. 42.)

As soon as the floor of the mouth is opened and the tongue loosened from the lower jaw the left hand is introduced beneath the skin, through the incision, into the mouth, and the tongue seized by thumb and middle finger, and drawn forcibly downward, while the other fingers are used to lift up the skin from the knife. The long section-knife, with cutting edge turned toward the left, is then introduced in the median line, along the left hand, until its point reaches the hard palate, taking care to work the point back slowly until it reaches the border between soft and hard palate. This must be done by feeling rather than by sight. The block under the neck is then pushed up under the head and the chin thrown forward so that the point of the knife is directed at right angles against the cervical vertebræ. The soft palate is then cut

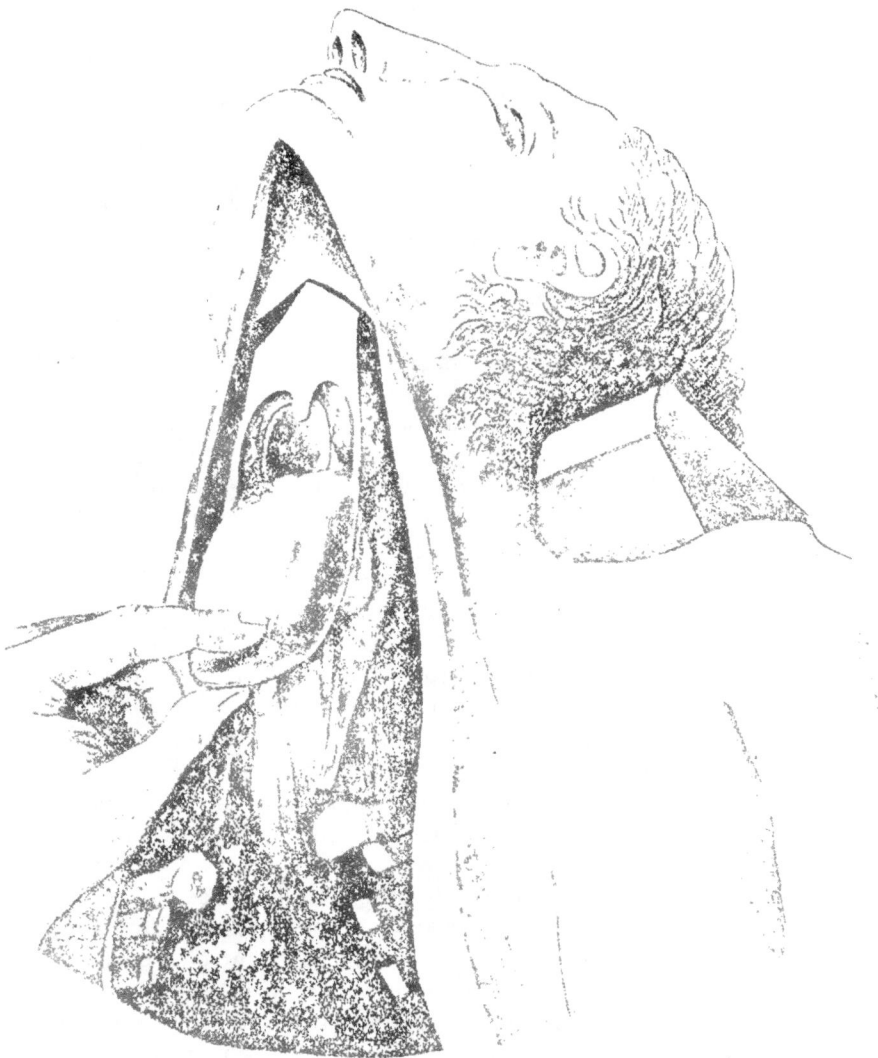

FIG. 44 — Removal of neck-organs, when skin-incision is carried to the chin. The same cuts through the soft palate are made, when the knife is pushed up beneath the loosened skin of the neck. (After Nauwerck.)

to the left, while the tongue is pulled firmly downward and toward the right, putting the uvular arch on a stretch so that the knife passes around the left tonsil. The knife is then turned and the same cut made on the right, severing the right faucial pillar and tonsil, while the tongue is pulled downward and to the left. The point of the knife is then pushed back to the pharyngeal wall and the latter is cut from right to left by a strong, firm stroke directed at right angles to the surface of the upper cervical vertebræ. The cut through the pharyngeal mucosa should be at the level of the boundary between the laryngeal and nasal portions, at about the height of the axis. While this cut is being made firm traction should be kept up on the tongue, pulling it downward, and alternately to the left and right. The loose retropharyngeal and retro-œsophageal fascia tears easily and the mouth organs can now be pulled so far downward that first transverse and then oblique cuts through this fascia can now be made upon the vertebræ, severing the vagi, carotids and jugulars, and working from above downward, until the mouth and neck organs can be lifted up through the skin-incision and the entire mass of the neck-organs separated from the spinal column as far as the clavicles. Pulling the mass toward the right, the left subclavian vessels and fascia are severed by a cut directed downward and outward beneath the clavicle. Traction is then made toward the left and the right subclavians cut beneath the clavicle. If the thoracic organs have been removed the œsophagus and aorta may now be stripped down to the diaphragm and there cut off, or the neck-organs may be cut off at the level of the bifurcation of the bronchi.

The organs, having been removed, are placed on the board, œsophagus upward, and the tip of tongue toward the prosector. The **tongue** is then cut in the median line and the cut surfaces examined. Transverse cuts may be made when indicated. The **uvula** is then lifted up and examined; and the **tonsils** and **palate** next examined, the former by means of longitudinal incisions. The intestinal shears are now introduced through the fauces into the œsophagus and the left pillar cut between the uvula and the tonsil. The posterior wall of the **pharynx** and that of the **oesophagus** for its entire length is then cut in the median line, and these structures examined. After the examination of the larynx from above, the long blade of the intestinal shears is introduced into the **larynx** and **trachea,** and these are cut in the posterior median line into the right bronchus. The œsophagus is pulled to the left (prosector's right) out of the way. The left bronchus is opened by a special incision to avoid cutting aorta and œsophagus. The larynx is now lifted up and held in both hands with the thumbs on the horns of the thyroid cartilage, and the fingers outside, and the larynx opened by forcibly bending back or breaking the cartilage, so that the entire interior of the larynx can be examined without touching the mucosa.

The neck-organs are now turned over, with the aorta toward the prosector and the tongue pointing away. The right and left lobes of the **thyroid** are opened by oblique cuts running from above downward and inward, and the isthmus is cut sagittally. The **parathyroids** must be dissected out behind and below the thyroid, along the course of the terminal branches of the inferior thyroid artery. The **parotid, submaxillary** and **sublingual glands** and the **cervical lymphnodes** are opened by longitudinal cuts. The **aorta, carotids, jugulars** and their branches are opened with the curved or probe-pointed scissors. The **vagus, superior** and **inferior laryngeal nerves** and the **cervical sympathetic ganglia** are to be examined when the case requires it. The examination of the neck-organs then closes with the inspection of the **muscles** of the neck and the **cervical vertebrae**.

If permission cannot be obtained for the complete removal of the mouth-organs, the neck-organs may be removed by cutting them transversely against the vertebræ between the hyoid bone and thyroid cartilage and then stripping them from the vertebræ and removing them as in the method given above. The skin-incision in such cases need not be carried higher than the collar-line, the skin of the neck being loosened by a subcutaneous dissection.

When permission is withheld for the removal of the neck-organs they may be examined *in situ*, by freeing the skin of the neck by a subcutaneous dissection, cutting the lobes and isthmus of the thyroid in place and then opening the trachea and larynx by an anterior median incision. The salivary glands, parathyroids, cervical lymphnodes, vessels and nerves can all be examined by this method without removing the organs as a whole.

In cases of aortic aneurism, corrosive poisoning, carcinoma of œsophagus, trachea or bronchi, it is best to remove the neck-organs in connection with the thoracic, removing first the neck-organs down to the clavicles and then stripping all down to the diaphragm, where they may be cut off and examined outside of the body. In cases of poisoning it is often necessary to remove the œsophagus in connection with the stomach. The mass of neck- and thoracic organs are removed as far as the diaphragm and then allowed to lie over the edge of the thorax or are turned down over the abdomen so that the œsophagus is upward and the tongue toward the prosector. The œsophagus and aorta are then separated from the other organs and left in the thorax to be examined later in connection with the abdominal organs.

If the thoracic duct was not examined when the thoracic organs were, it may be examined after the section of the neck-organs is finished, but it is more easily found after the method given above by turning the right lung over into the left side of the thorax and then looking for it in the neighborhood of the diaphragm, on the right side behind the aorta and between it and the azygos vein. It runs upward toward the left to the body of the last cervical vertebra, then over the left subclavian artery downward to the left innominate vein.

II. POINTS TO BE NOTED IN EXAMINATION OF THE MOUTH- AND NECK-ORGANS.

1. **Mouth.** Contents (blood, mucus, stomach-contents, foreign-bodies, etc.), color of mucosa (normally grayish-red), vesicles (aphthæ), cheilitis, gingivitis, various forms of stomatitis, noma, scorbutus, Ludwig's angina, ulcers (syphilis, carcinoma, decubital, tuberculosis), hyperkeratosis, macrocheilia, thrush, scars, wounds, action of corrosives, lead-line, neoplasms, etc. Note pillars of fauces, size, shape and condition of uvula. If the teeth have not been inspected during the general examination they should receive attention at this time. Note malformations, anomalies, neoplasms (adamantoma, odontoma, dental osteoma, various forms of cysts, epulis, giant-cell sarcoma, papilloma, fibroma, etc.)

2. **Tongue.** Mucosa normally is moist and grayish-red. Note discolorations, coatings, crusts, scabs, exudates, various forms of stomatitis, "geographical tongue," glossitis, abscess, fissures, ulcers (syphilis, carcinoma, decubital), chancre, wounds, action of corrosives, scars (epilepsy, syphilis), tuberculosis, neoplasms (carcinoma, lymphangioma, hæmangioma, papilloma, leukæmic lymphocytoma, adenoma, thyroid adenoma [struma baseos linguæ], and rarely sarcoma, congenital fibroma, lipoma, myxoma, chondroma, osteoma and dermoid cysts), thrush, actinomycosis, leprosy, trichinæ, cysts (lymphangiectatic), hyperkeratosis, leukoplakia, "black hairy tongue," macroglossia, partial or total hypertrophy. All forms of syphilitic lesions may be found upon the tongue (chancre, condyloma, plaques, papules, fissures, rhagades, ulcers, gumma, etc.) "Smooth atrophy" of the base of the tongue is regarded by various authors as pathognomonic of tertiary or congenital syphilis. Cysticercus and echinococcus are very rare.

3. **Pharynx.** Normal mucosa is smooth and gray-red. Note contents, color and character of mucosa, atrophy, congestion, œdema, exudations (mucous, purulent, croupous, diphtheritic, thrush), ulcers, scars, hyperplasia of lymph-follicles, adenoids, various forms of acute and chronic pharyngitis, retropharyngeal abscess, syphilis, tuberculosis, neoplasms (nasal polypi, lymphosarcoma, leukæmic lymphocytoma, aleukæmic lymphocytoma, carcinoma, retropharyngeal dermoids, lipoma, cysts, fibroma, chondroma, etc.), glanders, leprosy, actinomycosis, rhinoscleroma, cysticercus and echinococcus.

4. **Tonsils.** Size (how far do they project?), smooth or showing depressions, color (normally uniformly gray-red), atrophy,

hypertrophy, hyperkeratosis, various forms of inflammation (acute and chronic tonsillitis, diphtheria, angina superficialis, lacunaris, follicularis, pseudomembranosa, purulenta and phlegmonosa, tonsillar ulcers, cysts and abscess), syphilis, tuberculosis, actinomycosis, thrush, concretions, neoplasms (carcinoma, primary is rare, secondary from primary in tongue or larynx more common; lymphosarcoma or lymphocytoma, either aleukæmic or leukæmic, is the most common neoplasm of the tonsil, other forms of sarcoma and connective-tissue tumors are rare), cysticercus and echinococcus are rare.

5. **Nose.** If the brain is not removed and the nasal tract not examined by the method of Harke, as much of the nose as possible should be inspected, and the various conditions noted, as described in Chapter VI.

6. **Oesophagus.** Contents, size (dilatation, stenosis, diverticula), color and character of mucosa (normally smooth, transparent, pale, grayish-white, often hypostatic on posterior surface), inflammation, swelling of mucosa, leukoplakia, œdema, erosions, ulcers, action of corrosive poisons, perforation, foreign bodies, varices (cirrhosis, splenic anæmia), hemorrhage, aneurismal erosion, infective granulomata (tuberculosis, syphilis and actinomycosis are all rare), neoplasms (benign are rare, sarcoma rare; carcinoma most common usually at the lower or middle third), parasites (thrush the most important infection). Postmortem softening of the œsophagus from the regurgitation of stomach-contents must not be mistaken for pathologic conditions. Oesophagomalacia is of the rarest occurrence during life.

7, 8. **Larynx and Trachea.** Nature of contents, character and position of *epiglottis* and *plicæ aryepiglotticæ* (the latter should be thin; greatly thickened in inflammation and œdema), mucosa (normally gray-red and smooth); *vocal cords* (position and relations as viewed from above; should be thin and tendon-like; mucosa thickened in inflammation and œdema; may be atrophic), œdema, inflammation, diphtheritic membranes, ulcers, syphilis, tuberculosis, leprosy, glanders, actinomycosis, rhinoscleroma, neoplasm, foreign-bodies, etc. An extreme œdema of the glottis may disappear after death, and its occurrence be shown only by the wrinkled appearance of the mucous membrane. Anomalies are rare, the most common being a laryngocele. In typhoid fever erosions and ulcers are not rare in the larynx. In smallpox ulcers, diphtheritic inflammations and hemorrhages may occur. The most common tumor is the fibroma or fibro-epithelioma (papilloma), occurring particularly in children and singers ("children's nodule," "singer's nodule"). Angioma, myoma, lipoma and chondroma are rare. Thyroid adenoma, the so-called "amyloid-tumor" and adenoma of the mucous glands are rare. Sarcoma is also rare. Lymphosarcoma and leukæmic infiltrations are not common. Primary carcinoma is more frequent than sarcoma, but is relatively rare. It occurs most frequently in men, arising on the true vocal cords, and is squamous-celled. In trichinosis the laryngeal muscles usually show an early and abundant invasion. The most important pathologic conditions of the trachea are anomalies (diverticula, fistula, tracheocele), inflammation (catarrhal, membranous, pseudomembranous), tuberculosis, syphilis, secondary erosions, ulcers and perforations (tumors of thyroid, cancer of œsophagus, tuberculosis and suppurating lymphnodes, aneurisms), stenosis, compression from enlarged thyroid, thymus or lymphnodes, dilatation, tracheotomy, intubation, and neoplasms (relatively rare). The cartilages of both trachea and larynx should be examined for inflammation, pigmentation, etc.

9. **Thyroid.** *Weight* is 30-60 grms. The *dimensions* of the lateral lobes are: Length 5-7 cm., breadth 3-4 cm., thickness 1.5-2.5 cm. They should be symmetrical. Note variation in *form*, character of *cut-surface* (normally glassy, granular and yellowish-pink). The colloid is transparent, yellow or brown in color, and rises above the cut-surface. Cysts of varying size are very common, likewise encapsulated adenomata. A firm, yellowish, moderately enlarged thyroid is often seen in cases of pulmonary tuberculosis. Increase of the stroma with hyaline change and calcification is common. The most important pathologic conditions of the thyroid are: *goitre* (struma diffusa, nodosa, maligna, benigna, parenchymatosa, hyperplastica, adenomatosa, colloides, gelatinosa, cystica, vasculosa, fibrosa, hæmorrhagica, calculosa, ossea, amyloides, inflammatoria, etc.), *inflammation* (thyreoditis simplex, purulenta, abscess), *neoplasms* (carcinoma the most common form of malignant tumor, sarcoma not rare, adenoma and cystadenoma very common, combinations of sarcoma and carcinoma have been observed; other forms rare), *granulomata* (tubercles and gummata are rare), *parasites* (echinococcus). Especial examination should be made of the thyroid in cretinism, myxœdema, all forms of cachexia of unknown etiology, infantilism, lymphatic constitution, unexplained death, rachitis, chondrodystrophia, acromegaly, giantism, idiocy, etc. In marked constitutional disturbances conditions of athyreosis, thyreoplasia and hyperplasia of the thyroid may play an etiologic

rôle. Accessory thyroids are not uncommon in the neck, in the supraclavicular fossæ and behind the sternum. They usually show the structure of fœtal adenomata, but may become cystic or undergo carcinomatous change.

10. **Parathyroids.** These organs are usually four in number, sometimes more, sometimes only one or two. They are usually paired, and are found near the inner posterior borders of the lobes of the thyroid, near the two terminal branches of the inferior thyroid artery. They vary in size from 3-15 mm. in length, 3-4 mm. broad, by 1-2 mm. in thickness. They are normally brown in color, and soft in consistence. It is often difficult to distinguish them from the hæmolymph nodes that are common in this region. The parathyroids should be examined in all cases of tetany, paralysis agitans, acromegaly, epilepsy, infantile atrophy, myotonia and obscure cachexias. Conditions of supposed hypoparathyreosis have been reported. Hypertrophy of the parathyroids has been observed in acromegaly. Adenoma has been described by several writers. Cysts, fatty degeneration, fatty infiltration, colloid degeneration, cloudy swelling and tuberculosis have been reported as occurring.

11. **Cervical Lymphnodes.** Note *number, size, color, consistence, character of cut-surface.* etc. The most important pathologic conditions are: tuberculosis, secondary carcinoma, Hodgkin's disease, lymphosarcoma (leukæmic and aleukæmic), various forms of inflammation, dermoid and epidermoid cysts, cystic lymphangioma (congenital cystic tumor of the neck), branchiogenic carcinoma, and hyperplasia in syphilis, rachitis and status lymphaticus. In acute inflammation the lymphnodes are red and soft; in chronic inflammation they are usually grayish-white and firm.

12. **Salivary Glands.** The *parotid, submaxillary* and other *salivary glands* are examined as to *size, color, consistence* and *character of cut-surface*. The most important conditions are: parotitis (epidemic and secondary), chronic inflammation, calculi, cystic dilatation of ducts [ranula], Ludwig's angina, salivary fistula, granulomata (tuberculosis, syphilis and actinomycosis), neoplasms (most common forms are the mixed tumors containing cartilage, fibrous connective-tissue and myxomatous tissue and cords or rows of cells regarded by some observers as endothelial, by others as epithelial; other less common tumors are adenoma, fibroma, carcinoma and sarcoma). Symmetrical enlargement of the salivary and lachrymal glands occurs as the result of aleukæmic or leukæmic lymphocytoma ("Mikulicz's disease").

13. **Cervical Vessels and Nerves.** Examine the arteries and veins, noting contents, thickness and character of walls, size of lumen, changes in the intima, sclerosis, atheroma, calcification, thrombosis, embolism, etc. In death from strangulation or hanging the intima of the carotids may be torn. The *aorta* is usually examined after the section of the neck-organs. Note size of lumen. In the adult it usually admits the index-finger or thumb. The circumference of the thoracic aorta is 4.5-6 cm.; that of the abdominal aorta is 3.5-4.5 cm. Note its elasticity, contents, thickness of wall, changes in intima, etc. Fatty degeneration of the intima, sclerosis, atheromatous plaques and ulcers, calcification and thrombosis are the most common conditions. Syphilis is a very common cause of mesaortitis, shown by linear or radiating depressions of the intima. The *carotid gland* (paraganglion intercaroticum) at or near the division of the carotids should be noted. It is about the size of a rice-grain, oval, vascular and of firm consistence, resembling very much the superior cervical ganglion. Alveolar tumors apparently primary in this gland have been observed by a number of writers. Its epithelial nature is denied by some observers who class it with the sympathetic system. The *nerves* and *ganglia* should be examined and any change from the normal noted, such as atrophy, effects of pressure, involvement in scar-tissue, hæmorrhage, inflammatory processes, neoplasms, etc.

14. **Deep Muscles of Neck.** Note same conditions in these muscles as mentioned above for abdominal and thoracic muscles. Retropharyngeal abscesses and hemorrhages resulting from fractures and luxations of the vertebræ are the most common conditions.

15. **Cervical Vertebrae.** Anterior surface should be smooth. Fractures, luxations and tuberculosis are the most common conditions. In caries of the vertebral bodies the surfaces become rough and sharp. In luxations irregular prominences and deviations are found. The prominent portion usually shows sharp edges.

CHAPTER X.
THE EXAMINATION OF THE ABDOMEN.
I. METHODS OF EXAMINATION.

The preliminary general inspection of the peritoneal cavity was made after the main incision. (See Chapter VII.) After the examination of the neck and thoracic organs has been completed, the abdominal organs are removed and examined separately. The method to be followed must be varied to meet the conditions. In the case of extensive carcinomatosis, general peritonitis, peritoneal tuberculosis, pseudomyxoma peritonei, etc., when adhesions are numerous and the abdominal organs matted together, the examination becomes very difficult, and it may be necessary to remove the abdominal organs *en masse* and dissect them on the table. If the œsophagus and aorta have not been removed from the thorax they are stripped down to the diaphragm, which is cut on both sides, so that aorta, œsophagus and the abdominal organs *en masse* can be stripped down to the brim of the pelvis and there cut off to be examined outside the body.

For the ordinary autopsy the following order of examination of the abdominal organs is recommended: The **spleen** is first examined. It is lifted up from beneath the left under-surface of the diaphragm by tearing or stretching the ligamentum phrenico-lienale and the gastrosplenic omentum. In the case of wandering spleen the technique of removal must be modified to suit the conditions. When the spleen is very soft great care must be taken not to tear or rupture it. When adhesions to the diaphragm are present these must be torn or cut. The spleen is then laid upon the left edge of the ribs. In this position it may be sectioned by an incision made from upper to lower pole, and then, after it has been examined, it is allowed to slip back into the abdominal cavity, when its removal from the body is not desired. If it is to be removed and examined outside of the body, its ligaments and vessels are cut with the knife directed against the edge of the ribs, taking care not to cut the stomach or tail of the pancreas. It is then weighed and measured, and examined by means of a chief incision through its convex surface, from upper to lower pole, and reaching to the hilus. Parallel sagittal or transverse cuts may be made as desired. The cut surface is then thoroughly examined. Bacteriologic examinations should

SECTION OF INTESTINES. 141

be made when indicated, before the organ is sectioned. A portion of the capsule is seared and the pipette introduced through the seared area.

The **intestines** are examined next. They may be opened inside the body without separating them from the mesentery, but the best method by far is to remove and open them outside of the body. The middle portion of the transverse colon is lifted up by the left hand and the ligamentum gastrocolicum and the mesocolon transversum cut close to the intestine, toward the left, separating the left half of the transverse colon, then the splenic flexure and the descending colon and the sigmoid flexure to the rectum. After the splenic flexure has been separated the descending colon can usually be stripped down to the sigmoid by the hands without using the knife. When the sigmoid has been freed from its mesocolon two ligatures are put around the upper portion of the rectum, about an inch apart, and the intestine is then cut between the ligatures. The freed portion of the large intestine is then carried over into the right side of the abdomen and as much of the lower portion as is possible is put into a pan or tray resting upon the cadaver's right thigh. The right half of the transverse colon, the hepatic flexure and the ascending colon are now freed down to the beginning of the ileum, care being taken not to cut off the appendix when loosening the cæcum. The entire large intestine is then gathered into the tray resting on the cadaver's thighs, and the intestine is pulled down firmly by the left hand in a line corresponding to the main axis of the right thigh. The coils of small intestine are left in their natural position. The ileum is then severed from the mesentery as follows: The intestine is pulled by the left hand straight down in the middle line of the right thigh, putting the mesentery on a stretch. The long section-knife is used by the right hand to cut the mesentery close to the intestine in a manner resembling the use of the bow in violin-playing. The blade of the knife is held slightly obliquely against the mesenteric insertion of the intestine, and as the left hand pulls up the coils of intestine against the knife, the latter in the bowing or sawing movement severs the mesentery from the intestine as close to its insertion as is possible without cutting the intestine. The freed portions of intestine are caught in the tray resting on the thighs, and the left hand grasps in succession new portions of the small intestine and pulls them against the knife until the entire intestine is freed up to the duodenum and the root of the mesentery. A double ligature is put around the jejunum and the intestine severed between the ligatures, and the freed jejunum, ileum and large intestine are now removed in the tray for examination. The severing of the intestine from the mesentery in this manner can be carried out very quickly after a little practice. Care must be taken to cut the mesentery as close as possible to the intestine without nicking the latter. If too much mesentery is left on the intestine it cannot be laid out straight and its opening is made more difficult. If the coils of the small intestine are left in their natural position, and if the ileum when it is first taken up by the left hand is not twisted, the coils will unroll before the knife without any difficulty. Some prosectors begin with the jejunum, ligating it at the point where it comes out from beneath the mesentery, cutting it between the ligatures and separating it from the mesentery downward until the entire intestine as far as the rectum has been freed. The latter is ligatured and the freed portions removed. When the saving of time is of great importance the large intestine may be freed as described above, a ligature put around the upper end of the jejunum, and the mesentery severed at its root, so that the entire mass of small intestine with its mesentery is removed for further separation from the mesentery outside of the body. When peritoneal adhesions that cannot be easily torn are present it may be necessary to remove the intestines with mesentery attached.

After the removal of the intestines from the body they are opened by the intestinal shears, beginning either with the jejunum or the large intestine, the cut being made in the line of the mesenteric attachment. As the intestine is opened careful attention should be paid to the contents of each portion. It is very poor technique to dilate the intestine with water or to run water through it before it is opened. There is danger of washing away parasites, blood, etc. When the intestine is distended the opening is easy, but when collapsed it can be more easily opened if an assistant straightens it out and holds it on the stretch in advance of the enterotome. It may be opened on the table, in the tray, or in a pail. The latter method is a clean and convenient one. As the intestine is opened it is passed on the flat beneath the handle of the pail as it rests on the rim, so that the intestinal contents are scraped off into the pail and the clean mucosa examined as it is pulled from the pail into a basin or tray. The ileocæcal valve should be carefully examined from above before it is cut through. The appendix may be opened from the intestine by the small probe-pointed shears, the cut being made on the side opposite the mesenteric attachment. Transverse sections can be made, if desired. When the intestines are opened within the body, the enterotome is introduced into an opening made in the ileum just above the ileocæcal valve and the intestine is cut upward to the duodenum, along its mesenteric attachment, the coils being drawn upon the probe-pointed blade of the enterotome with the left hand. After the small intestine is opened the enterotome is introduced through the ileocæcal opening and the large intestine cut in the anterior tænia as far as the rectum. The opening of the intestine within the body should be left until all the other abdominal organs have been examined, because of the disagreeable mess made by the escape of the intestinal contents into the cavity.

The **duodenum** is opened next. The curved scissors, or the enterotome, is introduced into its lower end through an opening made above the ligature, and the inferior and descending portions of the duodenum are cut in the middle line of the anterior wall. The superior portion is then cut up to the pylorus, the cut passing through the inferior wall of this portion, the enterotome being held in the axis of the canal and pylorus, while the duodenum is pulled over to the right by the left hand. Before the pylorus is cut it should be explored, as to its width or constriction, by the index-finger of the left hand. The duodenum may also be opened first in the lower part of the descending portion. The root of the mesentery is pushed over to the left and a fold of the anterior wall is picked up by the thumb and index-finger of left hand and cut with the shears, so that when let free by the left hand there is formed a longitudinal incision in the duodenal wall large enough to admit the long blade of the enterotome. The duodenum is then cut up to the pylorus as described above. The inferior part of the duodenum is then opened from the point where the first incision is begun. The duodenum may also be opened downward, beginning at the pylorus, a small transverse cut being first made in the stomach wall just above the pylorus and the stomach opened along the greater curvature as far as the cardia. The enterotome is then placed through the pylorus and the duodenum cut in the median line of its anterior wall throughout its entire length. When the duodenum is opened, the *papilla*, the *ductus choledochus* and the *ductus Wirsungianus* are to be carefully examined. The papilla can usually be easily found by stretching the duodenal mucosa transversely over the head of the pancreas. It lies below the middle of the head of the pancreas, and about four finger-breadths below the pylorus. Pressure should be made upon the gall-bladder to force bile through the duct and papilla, and thus demonstrate their patency. When this cannot be done a sound should be introduced, and the common duct opened into the hepatic and cystic ducts. If the duodenal mucosa just below the papilla be stretched forcibly downward the duct can usually be opened by the small scissors without the aid of a grooved director. The duct of Wirsung may be explored with the sound from the papilla to the left of the common duct, or from its separate opening when the two ducts do not open in common. Both the bile-duct and the duct of Wirsung may be opened in the opposite direction, from the liver and pancreas respectively.

The **stomach** is opened from the pylorus after the size of the latter has been ascertained. The anterior wall may be cut midway between the greater and lesser curvatures, or the cut may follow the greater curvature, extending through the cardia into the œsophagus. As the stomach is opened its contents are inspected and removed. They should not be allowed to escape into the abdominal cavity. When the organs are removed *en masse* the stomach may be opened from the cardiac end. The organ may also be opened by an incision through its posterior wall or along its lesser curvature, as occasion may demand. If it is desired to save the pyloric ring the incision may stop above or below it and begin again on the other side. The stomach, with the lower portion of the œsophagus and the superior portion of the duodenum, may be separated from their attachments and examined outside of the body.

The **pancreas** is examined by turning the stomach toward the thoracic cavity, cutting or tearing the gastrocolic omentum, and cutting the exposed organ by a longitudinal incision through head, body and tail, or by means of parallel transverse incisions made through the different parts of the organ. The ducts of Wirsung and Santorini should be explored. It must be freed from the duodenum before it is weighed. The pancreas may be removed in connection with stomach, duodenum and liver and examined outside of the body. This is advisable in all cases of perforation of the stomach, ulcer, carcinoma and surgical anastomoses, carcinoma of pancreas, acute pancreatitis, obstruction of common duct, duodenal ulcer, etc.

The **liver** may be examined in the body without removal. The left hand is put between the diaphragm and the convex surface of the right lobe of the organ, and the liver raised up out of the cavity. With the long section-knife a main incision is made deep into the organ, from left to right, about a hand's-breadth above the lower border. Parallel incisions to the main incision may be made. After the examination of the cut surface the organ is dropped back into the abdomen. When the liver is to be weighed and measured it is removed from the body by cutting first the ligamentum hepatoduodenale, examining, as they are cut, the *common duct, hepatic artery* and the *portal vein*. The left lobe of the liver is then taken in the left hand and raised as high as possible. The left triangular ligament, the left half of the coronary ligament, the suspensory ligament, the right half of the coronary ligament and the right triangular ligament are cut from left to right. The inferior vena cava is cut at the same time. In the case of adhesions between liver and diaphragm these must be cut or the diaphragm itself removed in connection with the liver. In such a case the diaphragm must be trimmed off before the liver is weighed. The liver may also be removed in the opposite direction, raising up the right lobe and severing all connections as far as the median line of the spinal column. The right lobe is then pulled upon the right edge of the thorax-wall, and the connections with the left lobe are severed. In separating the under surface of the right lobe care must be taken not to damage the right adrenal. The liver is then weighed and measured, and placed upon the board with the right lobe toward the prosector. A long, deep cut is then made by drawing the long-section-knife across the left and right lobes, extending the cut through to the porta. Additional cuts may be made parallel to this chief-incision. When occasion demands a number of sagittal incisions may be made instead. As mentioned above, it is often best to remove the liver with stomach, pancreas and duodenum and examine on the table.

The **gall-bladder** is opened from its fundus with the fine probe-pointed shears; its contents are caught in a vessel and examined. The cystic, hepatic and common ducts may be explored from the gall-bladder, if they have not been from the intestine. The gall-bladder may be dissected from the liver and removed in connection with the duodenum.

The **portal vein** is opened into its radicles; the examination of the splenic vein is of especial importance. The **portal lymphnodes** are examined at this time.

The **mesentery** and the **mesenteric lymphnodes** are now examined. The former may be cut off at its root and examined outside of the body. The lymphnodes may be opened by longitudinal or transverse incisions.

The **left adrenal** and **kidney** are now examined. If the pancreas and stomach have not been removed from the body they are turned over toward the thoracic cavity, so as to expose completely the left adrenal. The movability of the kidney is then tested.

Beginning above the adrenal an incision is made through the peritoneum and underlying tissue, curving outward around the kidney and downward to its lower pole, taking care not to bring the incision too far around the lower pole of the organ for fear of cutting the ureter. The knife is then laid aside, and the adrenal and kidney are pulled upward toward the median line until they are entirely free save for the blood-vessels and ureter. The loose tissue about the fatty capsule of the kidney is usually easily separated. The blood-vessels are then cut from above downward against the spinal column, the ureter being left uncut. Holding the kidney in the two hands, it is pulled downward toward the pelvis, stripping the ureter free as far as the pelvic brim. At this level the ureter may be cut, or, if it is desired to remove the kidneys in connection with the pelvic organs, the ureter is left uncut and the kidney laid over the pubis until the pelvic organs are removed. When the kidney and adrenal are removed they are placed upon the board and the adrenal separated. The latter organ is then examined by means of parallel transverse incisions, or by an incision in its longest axis in the middle of its flat surface. When the adrenal is left in the body it may be examined by means of the same incisions. The fatty capsule is then stripped from the kidney and the organ weighed and measured. It is then held in the palm of the left hand with the ureter between the middle fingers, the convex border up, the thumb placed on one flat surface, the fingers on the other, holding the organ tightly. The kidney is then opened by means of a long incision made with the long section-knife, beginning at the upper pole, drawing the knife through the convexity, to the lower pole, and extending the cut through the organ to the pelvis. As the knife approaches the hilus the grasp of the left hand upon the organ is loosened and pressure upon the knife lessened so as not to cut through the hilus. The edges of the fibrous capsule are then caught by the fingers or forceps and the capsule stripped from the cortical surfaces. The external surface and the cut surfaces are then examined. When indicated other incisions into the kidney substance may be made. The ureter is sounded from the pelvis, and opened with the fine probe-pointed shears. The renal artery and vein may be examined now, or better when the kidney is being removed.

The **right adrenal** and **kidney** are removed in the same way, by making a curved incision around the outer border of the organs, pulling them up toward the median line and cutting the blood-vessels from above downward against the spine, and then stripping the ureter downward to the pelvis. After removal the adrenal is separated from the kidney and examined as directed above for the left adrenal. The kidney and ureter are then examined in the same way as on the left. When it is desired to remove the right kidney with the pelvic organs the same procedure is carried out as advised above in the case of the left one. In the removal of the right adrenal care should be taken not to injure the vena cava. In the case of displacement of either kidney the incisions for the removal of the organ must be altered to suit the case.

When the kidneys are removed before the examination of the intestines and liver, the removal of the left adrenal and kidney usually follows the examination of the spleen. The small intestines are pulled over to the right; the peritoneum is incised over the left kidney between the descending colon and the spinal column so that the right hand can be worked beneath the peritoneum up above the adrenal and kidney, freeing them, and lifting them toward the median line. The vessels are then cut as directed above, and the ureter stripped down to the pelvis. On the right side the cæcum and ascending colon are raised and a cut made through the peritoneum at the brim of the pelvis. The cæcum, ascending colon and peritoneum are now stripped upward with the left hand until the right hand can be passed up above the right adrenal to loosen it and the kidney toward the median line. When this is accomplished the adrenal and kidney are held in the left hand, while the right cuts the blood-vessels from above downward against the spine, sparing the ureter, which with the two organs is stripped downward to the pelvic brim. The close proximity of the right adrenal to the under surface of the liver makes the removal in this way much more difficult than when the liver is removed first. Usually, when the method of removing the kidney after the spleen is adopted, the adrenal is left in the body until after the removal of the liver.

So many variations in the order of section of the abdominal organs are given by different writers that it is impossible to escape the conclusion that the best order is the one best adapted to the individual case. A very common order is *spleen, left adrenal* and *kidney, right adrenal* and *kidney, duodenum, stomach, pancreas, liver, intestines, pelvic organs* and *genitalia*. **Beneke** advises the removal of spleen, then the removal of the entire intestines, stomach and pancreas, in connection with the gall-bladder, which is stripped from the liver and removed in connection with common duct and duodenum, the whole mass removed from the body and examined outside. Other prosectors begin with the *liver,* then the *spleen, urinary bladder* and *kidneys* and *genital organs,* the *gastro-intestinal tract* being left to the last. It may then be opened inside the body without inconvenience resulting from the escape of its contents into the peritoneal cavity. After surgical operations when permission for autopsy is refused, the abdominal, and also the thoracic organs, may be removed through the laparotomy wound.

After the examination of the abdominal viscera is completed the **abdominal aorta** is opened in the median line of its anterior wall and followed into its branches, the iliacs and hypogastrics. When occasion demands it may be stripped from the spine and opened outside of the body. The **inferior vena cava** is also opened throughout its length and followed into its branches. The abdominal portion of the thoracic duct should receive attention before the aorta is removed. The receptaculum chyli is found by lifting up the right edge of the aorta at the level of the second or third lumbar vertebra and dissecting out the duct up to its thoracic portion. It may then be opened by the fine probe-pointed shears. The **retroperitoneal lymphnodes** and **haemolymphnodes** are examined *in situ,* or removed with the blood-vessels and examined outside of the body. The **sympathetic ganglia,** particularly the *suprarenal* and the *cœliac plexuses,* and the *splanchnic nerves* are to be examined, especially in cases of Addison's disease. The section of the abdomen closes with the examination of the **ileopsoas muscles** and **diaphragm** by means of longitudinal or transverse incisions, and the inspection of the **vertebrae.** Pathologic conditions in the latter are examined according to indications.

II. POINTS TO BE NOTED IN THE EXAMINATION OF THE ABDOMEN.

1. **Peritoneum.** Normally the peritoneum is moist-shining, grayish and translucent. It is cloudy, dry, lustreless, injected, swollen or covered with exudate in acute inflammation; thickened, hyaline ("iced" or "Zuckerguss") in chronic inflammation. Note degree, character and location of adhesions. The most common pathologic conditions are inflammation, tuberculosis, secondary carcinoma and pseudomyxoma peritonei. Lymphomata are found in cases of typhoid fever and in leukæmia. Primary neoplasms (lymphangioma, endothelioma, carcinoma, lymphosarcoma, angiosarcoma, etc.) are rare. Ovarian cysts of the structure of cystadenoma may give rise to implantation-metastases over the peritoneum. The parasites are echinoccocus and cysticercus.

2. **Spleen.** Weight 150-250 grms., length 12 cm.; breadth 8 cm., thickness 3 cm. Varies greatly in size and weight. Describe shape, character of borders, number of notches, etc. Accessory spleens are common in the gastrosplenic omentum. *Capsule* should be delicate, smooth, shining and transparent. Note *tension of capsule* (loose, wrinkled, tense), adhesions, hyaline thickenings, exudates or neoplasms. *Color* of spleen through capsule is bluish-red. Fresh anæmic infarcts appear as yellowish or reddish-yellow areas surrounded by a darker red zone. Cicatricial depressions on the surface of the spleen are usually the result of healed infarcts. *Consistence* of spleen normally is that of muscle. In acute hyperplasias and congestions the spleen is softer and more friable (acute

infections, typhoid fever). In chronic hyperplasias and congestions, atrophy, amyloid degeneration, etc., the consistence is firmer than normal, even to that of a wooden hardness in advanced amyloid disease. (Apply iodin test.) The large, firm spleen is characteristic of leukæmia, splenic anæmia, syphilis and chronic malaria. On section note the *pulp, follicles* and *trabeculæ*. In the normal spleen the cut surface is dark red or bluish-red, smooth, and the trabeculæ and follicles easily seen. In acute hyperplasias the pulp swells up over the trabeculæ as a thick red or grayish-red gruel-like substance. In chronic hyperplasias the pulp is atrophic, grayish-red, and firm. In subacute hyperplasias the cut-surface often presents a shagreened appearance. The *color* of the cut-surface is blood-red in typhoid fever, grayish-red in septicæmias, chocolate-brown in potassium-chlorate poisoning and hemosiderosis due to other causes. In amyloid spleen the amyloid portions are glassy; when confined to the follicles the latter look like grains of boiled sago. The *follicles* are about the size of medium pin-heads, grayish in color, not elevated and cannot be scraped out with the knife. They are more numerous and larger in young individuals than in adults. Note size and number, degenerations, etc. The *trabeculæ* appear as fine gray lines, sharply outlined, increasing in size toward the hilus and capsule. They are more distinct in atrophy and chronic hyperplasias. In anthracosis of the spleen black granules are seen in the pulp, particularly about the trabeculæ. Tubercles appear as grayish-white, semitranslucent nodules, elevated above the surface, and can be scraped out with the knife-point. When caseation has begun their centres are opaque and yellowish. Gummata are grayish-white, with opaque centers, and have a periphery of vascular granulation-tissue or hyaline scar-tissue. The most important pathologic conditions of the spleen are: acute and chronic passive hyperæmia, embolic infarctions, abscess, acute and chronic hyperplasias (typhoid, malaria, plague, pneumonia, septicæmia, leukæmia, pseudoleukæmia, splenic anæmia, hepatic cirrhosis, syphilis, Kala-azar, other forms of tropical splenomegaly, tuberculosis, rachitis, idiopathic splenomegaly of the Gaucher type, etc.), wandering spleen, absence of spleen, amyloid disease, atrophy, syphilis, tuberculosis, actinomycosis, traumatic rupture, cysts (peritoneal), neoplasms (primary are rare [angioma, angiosarcoma, fibroma, chondroma, osteoma, lymphangioma, endothelioma]; secondary sarcoma [chiefly lymphosarcoma and melanosarcoma] and carcinoma are also infrequent; secondaries of malignant syncytioma are more frequently found), parasites (echinococcus, cysticercus and pentastomum).

3. Intestines. In the examination of the *large intestine, appendix* (average length about 9 cms.), *small intestine* and *duodenum* note the *contents* of the various portions with respect to amount, color, odor, consistence, presence or absence of bile, food-remains, parasites, foreign-bodies, blood, pus, concretions, etc. Note *character of wall, size of lumen, color* (normally gray) and *character of mucosa, folds* and *villi, solitary follicles, Peyer's patches, mouths of bile-duct* and *pancreatic ducts, ileocæcal valve* and *opening into appendix*. Postmortem digestion of the mucosa, often leading to perforations, postmortem hypostasis, imbibition of bile, pseudomelanosis, and contractions of portions of the bowel must not be mistaken for pathologic conditions. Redness of a portion of the intestine does not in itself mean inflammation; the latter condition is shown by excess of mucus, swelling of the mucosa, hyperplasia of the follicles, hæmorrhage, etc. The contents of the small intestine are usually gruel-like in consistence, thinner in the upper part, thicker toward the ileocæcal valve. The *hook-worm, ascaris lumbricoides* and *intestinal trichina* occur in the duodenum; *tænia solium, saginata* and the *bothriocephalus latus* in the jejunum and ileum, *tricocephalus dispar* in the cæcum, and *oxyuris vermicularis* in the large intestine and rectum. *Ulcers* of the intestine may be due to typhoid fever, tuberculosis, carcinoma, dysentery, embolism or thrombosis of mesentery vessels, etc. Diphtheritic ulcers are caused by a variety of infections and poisons. They are usually found in the large intestine, but occasionally occur in the small intestine in cases of uræmia. Typhoid ulcers usually have their longest diameter parallel with the longitudinal axis of the intestine; tuberculous and carcinomatous ulcers usually encircle the intestine, forming "ring ulcers;" diphtheritic and dysenteric ulcers are irregular, involving the surfaces of the folds. Solitary round or peptic ulcers occur in the duodenum and jejunum. Decubital ulcers, associated with fecal concretions, gall-stones or foreign-bodies are found in appendix and rectum most commonly, more rarely in other portions of the intestines. *Perforations* of the intestines may be traumatic, or due to infections (typhoid, tuberculous, purulent, dysenteric, etc.), neoplasms (carcinoma), embolic gangrene, ileus, fecal impaction, erosion of calculus or foreign-body, parasites (round-worm?), overdistention, etc.

The most important pathologic conditions of the intestines are: anomalies (atresia, diverticulum, stenosis, dilatation, hernia), acute and chronic passive congestion, hæmorrhage, stasis, embolism and thrombosis, hæmorrhagic infarction, gangrene, traumatic injuries, ileus, volvulus, strangulated hernia, enteritis(catarrhal, follicular, hyperplastica, cystica, purulent, ulcerative, croupous, diphtheritic, dysentery, cholera, typhoid, etc.), appendicitis (catarrhal, ulcerative, perforative, obliterative), tuberculosis, syphilis (chiefly in rectum, ulcers, stenosis and perforations), actinomycosis, anthrax, intestinal sand, concretions, foreign-bodies, and neoplasms (primary carcinoma the most important [adenocarcinoma, colloid, scirrhous, medullary, etc.], most frequent in large intestine and rectum, secondary carcinoma is rare; adenomatous polypi are common, particularly in rectum; primary sarcomata [lymphosarcoma chiefly] are much less common than carcinoma, secondary sarcoma more common than primary [melanotic sarcoma, lymphosarcoma]. Benign connective-tissue tumors [lipoma, fibroma and myoma] are relatively rare. Primary carcinoma and sarcoma occur in the appendix, as well as secondary carcinoma). Leukæmic infiltration is common in leukæmia.

4. **Bile-passages.** Note patency, character of mouth, contents, etc. The most important conditions are inflammation, gall-stones, obstruction, stenosis, dilatation, perforation, carcinoma, and anomalies (in the newborn). Round-worms may obtain entrance and block the duct.

5. **Stomach.** On the external examination the size (dilatation, contractions due to scirrhous carcinoma or scars), shape (hour-glass, etc.), position, color of surface, consistence of wall, presence of adhesions, etc., should be noted. When the stomach is opened note presence of *gas* (odor), *character of contents* (fluid, gruel-like, food-remains, curds, foreign bodies, mucus, pus, blood, parasites, drugs, etc.), *odor* (yeasty, sour, acid, sweetish, foul, H_2S, odor of foods or drugs), *reaction* (acid or alkaline), *color* (yellow, greenish, grayish, brown, black, bloody, etc.) Describe the character of mucus on the mucosa (tough, glassy, difficult to remove in acute catarrh; softer, grayish or grayish-red, often containing small black blood-specks in chronic catarrh). Bile gives a yellow or greenish color. The presence of blood may give to the stomach-contents the appearance of "coffee-grounds;" in hæmorrhage by diapedesis the contents may be brownish. Cloudy swelling of the glands is common in sepsis, chronic anæmia and various poisonings. It affects cells in deepest portion of glands, as shown by excising a bit of the mucosa and examining microscopically. The brownish or black discoloration of the mucosa associated with softening of the latter (gastromalacia, postmortem digestion) must not be taken for a pathologic condition. The mucosa becomes soft, cloudy or jelly-

like and strips easily from the whitish submucosa. Softening of the entire wall leads to perforations that must not be mistaken for pathologic ones. Their edges show no signs of disease. The normal mucosa is grayish in *color*. In chronic passive congestion the color may be dark red. Hypostatic congestion is common in the large veins of the fundus. Hæmorrhages occur chiefly in the fundus and along the greater curvature (caused by vomiting). In potassium cyanide poisoning the mucosa is often rosy-red in color and has a soapy feel. The normal mucosa is nearly smooth when the folds caused by contraction are spread out. Localized hyperplasias occur in chronic gastritis (etat mamelonné) and cannot be smoothed out by stretching. Erosions (common in chronic passive congestion) and ulcers (round or peptic, carcinomatous, due to corrosives, very rarely to tuberculosis and syphilis) are to be carefully examined and described. The different layers of the stomach wall are to be examined with respect to their absolute and relative thickness. Thickening of the submucosa may be caused by œdema, purulent infiltration, increase of connective-tissue, carcinomatous or sarcomatous infiltration. Hyperplasia of the muscular coat occurs chiefly at the pylorus in cases of stenosis.

The most important conditions of the stomach are anomalies (congenital stenosis of pylorus, situs inversus), acute and chronic passive congestion (portal stasis), hæmorrhages, hæmorrhagic erosions (portal stasis), gastritis (acute, chronic, catarrhal, purulent, fibrinous, diphtheritic, phlegmonous, atrophic, hypertrophic), tuberculosis (rare), syphilis (rare), anthrax, action of corrosive poisons (acids, concentrated lye, carbolic acid, mercuric chloride, silver nitrate, oxalic acid, potassium cyanide), round or peptic ulcer, perforation, neoplasms (carcinoma the most common [adenocarcinoma, medullary, scirrhous, colloid]; primary sarcoma rare [lymphosarcoma], secondary are less rare; metastases of malignant syncytioma may occur in the stomach wall; benign tumors are rarely important. The most common are adenomatous polypi, fibroma, myoma and fibromyoma), stenosis, dilatation, contraction, wounds, concretions, foreign bodies and parasites (temporary as gordius, round-worms occasionally enter, intestinal form of trichina).

6. **Pancreas.** Weight 60-100 grms.; measures 17-20 cm. long, 3-4.5 cm. broad, and 2.5-3 cm. thick. *Color* reddish-grayish-yellow; *consistence* firm; *lobules* distinct. Postmortem change occurs quickly. The most common pathologic conditions are: atrophy, fatty infiltration, hyperæmia, hæmorrhage, inflammation (degenerative, parenchymatous, hæmorrhagic, necrotic, gangrenous, purulent, chronic fibroid or interstitial [inter- and intra-acinar], cirrhosis

PATHOLOGIC CONDITIONS OF LIVER. 153

of pancreas), tuberculosis (very rare), syphilis (gumma not common, interstitial pancreatitis most common form), fat-necrosis, cysts, congenital cystic pancreas, concretions in duct, hæmosiderosis, neoplasms (primary carcinoma the most important [scirrhous, medullary, adenocarcinoma]; primary sarcoma rare; secondary melanotic sarcoma and lymphosarcoma occur, secondary carcinoma less frequently; benign tumors rare, cystadenoma being the most common), and parasites (echinococcus, round-worm in duct). In fat-necrosis or acute pancreatitis the pancreatic ducts should be examined for obstruction due to calculi or stenosis. Areas of fat-necrosis appear as opaque, white, yellow or brown, firm nodules. Accessory pancreatic tissue not rare in wall of intestine. May occur more rarely in stomach-wall, omentum or abdominal wall.

7. **Liver.** Weight 1,500 grms.; measures 22 cm. sagittally, 30 cm. transversely and 8 cm. thick. A dimension of over 30 cm. is enlarged; when all dimensions are under 20 cm. the liver is smaller than normal. Note *size* (enlarged in congestion, cloudy swelling, fatty infiltrations, leukæmia, neoplasms; smaller in atrophy, acute yellow atrophy, cirrhosis), *changes of form* (congenital furrows, deep furrows with thickened capsule in syphilis, fine or coarse granulations and contractions in cirrhosis, edge rounded in fatty and amyloid liver, sharper in atrophy, capsule wrinkled in acute yellow atrophy), *capsule* (normally smooth and transparent; thickened, white, and opaque in chronic inflammation, the thickening being usually most pronounced along the ligaments, blood- and lymph-vessels. Small, hyaline nodules or patches may be scattered over the capsule, or the entire capsule may be tendon-like ["iced" or "Zuckerguss-leber"]. Adhesions with diaphragm, stomach, omentum, spleen, intestine and abdominal wall may occur. Fibrinous and purulent exudates may be found on the capsule, particularly on the diaphragmatic surface; when encapsulated by adhesions they form the so-called subdiaphragmatic abscess.), *consistence* (increased in fat-infiltration, cirrhosis, atrophy and amyloid; diminished in acute parenchymatous degenerations, leukæmia, acute yellow atrophy, acute congestion; fluctuation is present over abscesses, echinococcus cysts and softened tumors), *color* (normally brown-red; dark-brown in atrophy, dark red or bluish-red in passive congestion, "nutmeg" appearance in chronic passive congestion, chocolate-brown in hæmosiderosis, greenish in chronic icterus, yellow in acute icterus, fatty liver, leukæmia and anæmia, grayish-white

or yellow in cloudy swelling and fatty degeneration; sharply circumscribed dark bluish-red areas are caused by cavernous angiomata), *cut-surface* (normally smooth and of uniform color, blood-content abundant, before the age of puberty lobules are seen with difficulty; in adults they are recognizable from their yellowish-brown periphery and red central zones. They are about 1-2 mm. long by 1-1.5 mm. broad. Note size of lobule, color of central, intermediate and peripheral zones, distinctness of boundary of lobules, elevation of lobules above surface. Lobules are elevated in fatty infiltration and in cirrhosis, depressed in atrophy. In acute yellow atrophy they cannot be made out. Fatty infiltration begins usually in the peripheral portion of the lobules, fatty degeneration in the central zone, amyloid in the intermediate zone, hæmosiderin is found in the peripheral and hæmatoidin in the central zone. In extreme fatty infiltration affecting the entire lobule the outlines of the lobules cannot be made out. The normally shining surface is dull, cloudy, appearing as if cooked in cloudy swelling and fatty degeneration). Note amount of stroma; it is increased in cirrhosis, so that the lobules may be entirely surrounded by connective-tissue, or the connective tissue may invade the lobules. Note also size and contents of hepatic and portal blood-vessels and bile-ducts.

The most important pathologic conditions of the liver are acute and chronic passive congestion, thrombosis of portal veins, atrophy (simple and brown), fatty infiltration, cloudy swelling, fatty degeneration, acute yellow or red atrophy, amyloid, phosphorus-liver, abscess (metastatic, tropical, purulent cholangitis), cirrhosis (Lænnec's or atrophic, Hanot's or hypertrophic, fatty, biliary, cardiac), pericarditic pseudocirrhosis, tuberculosis, syphilis (very common: gummata, interstitial hepatitis, cirrhosis, hepar lobatum), actinomycosis, leukæmic infiltrations, glycogen infiltration (diabetes), pigmentations (hæmosiderosis in pernicious anæmia, malaria, hæmolytic poisons, etc., hæmatoidin in atrophy, bile-pigment in icterus, anthracosis, argyrosis, malaria pigment, melanin), neoplasms (most common tumor is the cavernous angioma, usually in old people, rarely of clinical significance; primary carcinoma and sarcoma rare; secondary very common [melanotic sarcoma, lymphosarcoma, metastases from carcinoma of gall-bladder and duct, stomach, pancreas and intestine, metastases of malignant syncytioma], adenoma and cystadenoma are rare), cysts, congenital cystic liver, parasites (echinococcus hydatidosus, granulosis and multilocularis, cysticercus, distomum hepaticum, pentastomum denticulatum, coccidium oviforme).

8. **Gall-bladder.** Note *size* (length 8-17 cm., diameter 3 cm., thickness of wall 1-2 cm.), *amount* and *character of contents* (clear and watery in hydrops, seropurulent or purulent in inflammation, excess of mucus in catarrhal inflammation), calculi, bile-sand, thickening and indurations of wall, œdema, character of mucosa, carcinoma (adenocarcinoma, squamous-celled). Note size, contents, thickness of wall and character of mucosa of ducts.

9. **Portal Vein.** Note contents, character of wall, occurrence of stenosis, thrombosis, pylephlebitis, thrombopylephlebitis, syphilitic changes, calcification, pressure from without.

10. **Mesentery.** Amount of fat, color, condition of vessels, blood-content, occurrence of œdema, inflammation, abscesses, hæmorrhages, infarction, gangrene, fat-necrosis, aneurism, embolism, thrombosis, cysts, parasites (bilharzia hæmatobia), tumor-infiltrations and primary tumors (lipoma).

11. **Mesenteric Glands.** Size, appearance on section (rose-red in acute inflammation, grayish-white in chronic), occurrence of tubercles, secondary tumors, calcification, abscesses, pigmentation, typhoid necrosis, primary lymphosarcoma, leukæmic hyperplasia, Hodgkin's, etc.

12. **Adrenals.** Weight 4-7.5 grms. measurements are 5-6 cm. long, 2.5-3.5 cm. broad, 0.5-1 cm. thick. Normally the consistence is firm; it is increased in amyloid degeneration, tuberculosis, syphilis, fibroid induration and atrophy; diminished in hæmorrhage, soft caseating tubercles, degenerating tumors. Postmortem autolysis of the medulla takes place very quickly, the cortical portion remaining as a hollow capsule. On section note the relations of the grayish-white cortex (more yellow and opaque in adults from the amount of fat contained in the cells), the intermediate brown zone and the central grayish, translucent portion of the medulla. The most important pathologic conditions are tuberculosis, syphilis, atrophy, compensatory hypertrophy, hæmorrhage, infarction, thrombosis of adrenal vessels, secondary tumors (melanotic sarcoma, carcinoma), primary neoplasms (hypernephroma, accessory adrenals typical and atypical, lipoma, glioma, neuroma, sarcoma), parasites (echinococcus).

13. **Kidneys.** Right kidney weighs 110-145 grms., and measures 10-12 cm. long, 4.5-5.0 cm. broad, and 3-4.5 cm. thick. Left kidney weighs 150-180 grms. and measures 12 cm. long, 5-6 cm. broad, 3-4.5 cm. thick. The left kidney is usually larger and heavier than the right. Note position and movability of kidneys, thickness and color

of fatty capsule (increased in lipomatosis, atrophy of kidney), purulent infiltrations and fibroid thickenings of the perirenal fat. Normally the fibrous capsule is thin and translucent, easily stripped off, the inner layer remaining attached around the blood-vessels passing from capsule into cortex. The capsule is adherent in chronic inflammations and over healed infarcts and localized inflammatory processes, tubercles, tumor-nodules, etc. Note alterations in *shape* and *size* ("horse-shoe kidney," "hog-back," round, fœtal lobulations, fissures; enlarged in acute parenchymatous nephritis, pyelonephritis, hydronephrosis, chronic passive congestion, etc.; diminished in atrophy, chronic interstitial nephritis, etc.). *Character of cortical surface* (normally smooth, grayish-brown in color; a fine or coarse, regular or irregular granulation of the surface occurs in chronic nephritis, the elevations corresponding to the preserved portions of the parenchyma, the depressed portions to the areas of connective-tissue increase; localized depressions or fissures may be caused by old or recent scars of infarcts, abscesses, rupture, etc. Distinguish fœtal furrows from pathologic depressions. Flat, puckered or radiating scars point to syphilis. Elevations of the surface may be due to fresh infarcts, tubercles, abscesses, neoplasms, etc. Accessory adrenal tissue (resembles adipose tissue) and small papillary adenomata are very common on the cortical surface. Retention- and degeneration-cysts are also very common, particularly in the kidneys of adults). In atrophic kidneys the glomeruli can be seen through the cortical surface. Note condition of superficial vessels (stellate veins). The *color* of the cortical surface depends essentially upon the blood-content and the condition of the parenchyma. In acute or chronic parenchymatous nephritis the color is whitish or grayish-white. Localized fatty degeneration and cloudy swelling cause pale, grayish-yellow, opaque spots or streaks. Hæmorrhages appear as red or brown-red spots. In extreme passive congestion the kidney may be a dark purplish-blue (cyanotic kidney). In hæmorrhagic nephritis the surface may be covered with pin-point or pin-head hæmorrhages. In pyæmia or acute ascending pyelonephritis the surface may be dotted with gray or yellowish pin-head abscesses. Metastatic abscesses are uniformly distributed; others are arranged in groups. In miliary tuberculosis the surface may contain numbers of grayish translucent miliary tubercles, with opaque centers when caseation has taken place. They cannot be so easily scraped out with the knife as the abscesses. Calcified glomeruli may also appear as white spots. Proliferations of the interstitial tissue cause large, red kidneys. Anæmic infarcts are yellow, brick-red or rusty, with a deeper red zone about them. Pseudomelanosis (usually postmortem) gives a gray-green color to the kidney. In icterus the color may vary from brownish-yellow to deep bronze. The *consistence* of the kidney is increased in chronic passive congestion, atrophy, interstitial nephritis and amyloid degeneration; decreased in acute degenerations and inflammations.

On section note *color, blood-content* and *consistence of cut-surface, relations of cortex and medulla*. The cortex is normally 0.5-1.0 cm. broad (increased in acute degenerations and inflammations, diminished in chronic inflammation and atrophy). Note number, size and color of the *glomeruli*. They appear as red pin-head points in congestion; in anæmia as small colorless granules; in the normal kidney as small reddish points against the lighter color of the labyrinths. In amyloid disease they are enlarged and glassy. Calcified glomeruli are white and opaque. In venous congestion the interlobular veins appear as bluish-red stripes; hæmorrhages appear as red points in the glomeruli and convoluted tubules, as red stripes in the collecting tubules. The blood-content is increased in chronic passive congestion and chronic alcoholism. On the cut-surface anæmic infarcts are usually wedge-shaped, with the base toward the cortical surface. The color of the kidney-parenchyma is usually gray; in fatty degeneration and cloudy swelling it becomes yellow or grayish-yellow. The areas of greatest degeneration appear as cloudy, opaque, yellowish points and stripes. Slight degenerations are shown by slight cloudiness of the cortex. The contrast between the grayish-white cortex and the dark-red medulla is often very striking in severe parenchymatous nephritis. In uric-acid infarction of the new-born ochre-yellow or vermilion-red stripes or lines are seen in the medullary pyramids; white lines indicate chalk-infarction; golden-yellow lines a bilirubin infarction. In gout whitish deposits of urates occur in the kidney; they are usually surrounded by scar-tissue. In purulent pyelonephritis yellow stripes of pus surrounded by hæmorrhage occur in the pyramids. Tuberculosis begins usually in the papillæ, destroying the pyramids first and then the cortex, forming a multilocular sac lined with caseating tissue. In hydronephrosis due to obstruction of the ureter the kidney becomes converted into a multilocular sac without ulceration or caseation of its papillæ. Note size of *pelvis* and calices, contents, character of mucosa, concretions, etc. The normal mucosa is grayish-red and delicate; it is rose-red in inflammation and often shows petechiæ. In severe inflammations grayish-white sloughs encrusted with urates are often found. Concretions of urates, phosphates or oxalates may be present, often associated with decubital ulcers of the mucosa. Tuberculous ulcers of the pelvic mucosa are common. The *ureters* are straight and about 4 mm. thick. Note size, contents, thickness of wall, changes in the mucosa, obstruction, dilatation, concretions, etc.

The most important pathologic conditions of the kidneys are anomalies (horse-shoe kidney, dystopia, double ureters, congenital lobulation), floating kidney, congestion, anæmia, infarction, thrombosis and embolism of renal vessels, atrophy (simple, arteriosclerotic), hydronephrosis, nephrolithiasis, nephritis (parenchymatous, hæmorrhagic, secondary contracted, primary contracted), rupture, amyloid degeneration, abscess, pyelonephritis, tuberculosis, syphilis, actinomycosis, uric-acid infarct, hæmatoidin- and hæmosiderin-infarct, bilirubin-infarct, chalk-infarct, argyrosis, retention- and degeneration-cysts, congenital cystic kidney, neoplasms (hypernephroma and adenoma the most common; carcinoma infrequent, sarcoma more common, particularly the congenital adenosarcoma or rhabdomyosarcoma; fibroma, leiomyoma, lipoma and angioma are relatively rare. Secondary carcinoma and sarcoma are common), pyelitis, ureteritis (cystica, polyposa, diphtheritica, purulenta), pyonephrosis, parasites (distomum hæmotobium, echinococcus, filaria, cysticercus, pentastomum and dioctophyme renale).

14. **Abdominal Aorta, Iliacs** and **Vena Cava.** Note size of lumen, thickness of wall, character of endothelium and contents. Sclerosis, fatty degeneration of intima, atheroma, calcification, aneurism, inflammation, thrombosis, stenosis, dilatation, compression, and infiltrations with pus or neoplasm are the most important conditions.

15. **Lymphatic Vessels.** Inflammation, obstruction, rupture, tuberculosis and invasion by malignant neoplasms are the most important conditions. (See also Thoracic Duct, Chapter VIII, Page 130.)

16. **Lymphnodes.** The retroperitoneal *lymphnodes* and *hæmolymph nodes* are described as to their number, size, color, consistence, occurrence of hyperplasia, lymphadenitis, atrophy, congestion, œdema, hæmorrhage, pigmentation, tuberculosis, metastatic tumors, primary tumors (lymphosarcoma), leukæmic hyperplasias and Hodgkin's disease.

17. **Sympathetic.** The solar plexus, semilunar ganglia and adrenal plexus should be examined, particularly in Addison's disease, for atrophy, degenerations, involvement in inflammatory processes, hæmorrhages, tumor-infiltrations, etc.

18. **Psoas Muscles and Diaphragm.** Examine for purulent, phlegmonous or gangrenous inflammations, tuberculosis, atinomycosis, trichinosis, atrophy and scar-tissue. Pus from carious processes in the thoracic and lumbar vertebræ burrows downward along the psoas muscle.

19. **Vertebrae.** Fractures, dislocations, curvatures, deviations, tuberculosis, caries, actinomycosis, etc.

CHAPTER XI.
THE EXAMINATION OF THE PELVIC ORGANS.
I. METHODS OF EXAMINATION.

1. **Male Pelvis.** When the removal of the external genitals is permitted the fundus of the bladder is taken in the left hand and pulled toward the head of the cadaver while the anterior wall is separated from the pubis. This can be done with the fingers of the right hand or the point of the knife. The loose connective-tissue is torn on both sides around the urethra and rectum until the hand can be passed beneath the rectum, completely encircling it and the prostate which must be freed as far as its anterior border. The legs of the cadaver are then separated, and an incision is made with the large section-knife, through the skin, beginning above at the root of the penis, at the termination of the main incision, and following the arch of the pubis around the external genitals down to the left, passing around the anus to the coccyx. A similar incision is then made on the right side of the external genitals to meet the first incision behind the anus. The outer genitals are then held in the left hand and pulled downward between the legs while they are dissected from the pubis, cutting the suspensory ligament of the penis, to the level of the posterior border of the symphysis. The knife is then run through into the pelvis just beneath the symphysis, and while traction is made upon the external genitals toward the right, a sweeping cut is made downward to the left along the pubic arch, severing the insertion of the cavernous portion of the penis on that side. A similar cut is then made on the right side. The penis thus freed is then pushed up beneath the symphysis into the pelvis and the scrotum pulled up after it, putting the perineum on the stretch and pulling up the anus so that it can be seen. While the external genitals are forcibly pulled upward in the pelvic cavity toward the head, the encircling incision behind the anus is deepened, cutting the fat-tissue, connective-tissue, and muscle around and behind the rectum, until the whole mass of genital organs and rectum is so loosened that it strips up easily to the brim of the pelvis, where any remaining attachments of peritoneum or blood-vessels are severed and the entire mass removed for examination on the board.

The mass is laid upon the board with *rectum* uppermost. The latter is then opened from the anus, using the intestinal shears, and scraping off the contents into a pail so as not to contaminate the other tissues. The rectum is then separated from the base of the bladder and prostate, guiding the incision along the outer muscular layer of the rectum, and stripping off the latter until the *seminal vesicles* are wholly exposed. These are then examined by means of transverse cuts, or are opened longitudinally with the knife or fine probe-pointed scissors. The *prostate* may also be sectioned from its posterior surface, if it is desired to preserve the urethral side intact. *Cowper's glands* are also accessible from this incision. The organs are then turned over, the penis put on a stretch and the anterior wall of the urethra cut in the median line from the meatus to the bladder. A pair of strong, medium-sized probe-pointed scissors should be used. The incision is extended through the anterior wall of the bladder. The mouth of the *ureters, ejaculatory ducts* and ducts of *Cowper's glands* are examined. If the prostate has not been examined from the rectal side it may now be examined by means of transverse incisions across the urethra and extending entirely through the gland. The section of the genitalia is then finished by the examination of the *testicles.* The latter are removed by enlarging the inguinal canal on each side, slipping the testicles up through them, and bisecting each gland so that the incision falls through the head of the epididymis. The testicles may also be examined by means of incisions made in the scrotum over the glands, which are forced through the incisions and then bisected. If the vasa deferentia are to be preserved they should be dissected out before the semicircular cuts on each side of the external genitals are made.

When the kidneys have been removed, and the ureters left uncut, to be examined in connection with bladder and external genitals, they are usually left lying on the thighs until the abdominal examination is finished. They are then laid in the abdomen until the pelvic organs have been separated up to the brim of the pelvis. At this point care should be taken to see that the ureters are not cut when the whole mass of pelvic organs, ureters and kidneys is removed. When placed upon the board the ureters are laid straight and the kidneys placed in their respective positions. The *ureters* are sounded from the bladder and when desired opened upward from the bladder to the kidneys. The section of the kidneys may then proceed according to the directions given in the last chapter.

When the external genitals cannot be removed, the *testicles* can be examined by enlarging the inguinal rings and canal, and

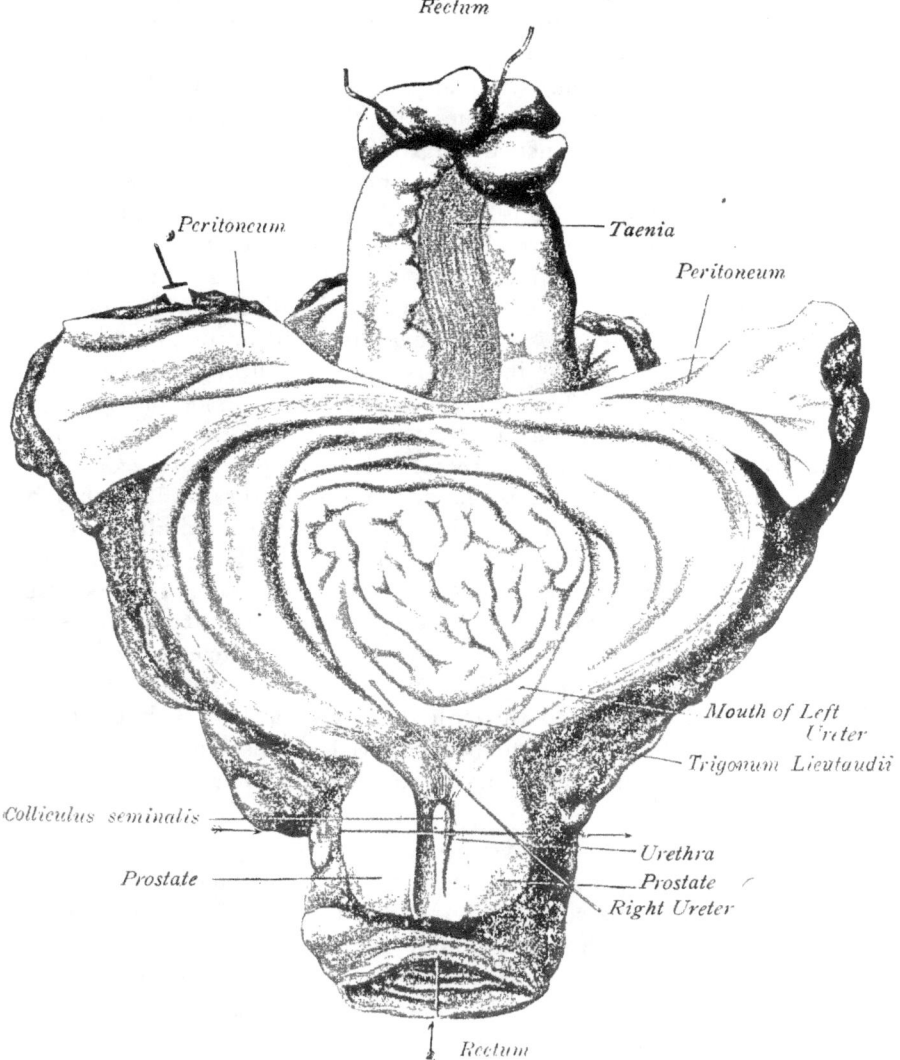

Fig. 45.—Section of male pelvic organs. Arrows mark line of incisions through prostate and rectum. (After Nauwerck.)

forcing each testicle up from below, through the ring. The gland is then sectioned and, after examination, returned to the scrotum.

The anterior wall of the bladder is then separated from the pubis and the tissues about rectum and prostate loosened until the hand can completely encircle the rectum and prostate. These organs and the bladder are then pulled up firmly toward the head of the cadaver, and with the cartilage-knife hugging the pubic bone the rectum is cut just above the internal sphincter, and the urethra just anteriorly to the prostate. When it is desired to get as much of the penis as possible, its attachments to the pubis are cut from the pelvic side, and the body of the penis pulled up into the pelvis, while the skin of the organ is loosened as far as the glans. The body of the penis may be severed from the glans or the glans may be freed from the prepuce and removed with the entire organ, leaving only the skin to be used for the restoration of the part. After the rectum and urethra are severed, the mass of pelvic organs is stripped up to the brim of the pelvis and removed, as given above. They are examined upon the board, opening first the *rectum*, then the *seminal vesicles, prostatic urethra, bladder* and *prostate*. The prostatic urethra and anterior bladder-wall are cut with the small probe-pointed shears, while the prostate is cut transversely with the long section-knife.

The *bladder, prostate* and *seminal vesicles* may be examined *in situ*, or separated from the rectum and examined outside of the body. The anterior wall of the bladder is freed from the pubis, and the lateral connections of the prostate separated. The bladder is then opened in its anterior wall by an incision from its fundus into the prostatic portion of the urethra. The prostate is then cut transversely at about its middle, the cut extending entirely through the organ. The fore-finger of the left hand is then hooked underneath the prostate, and the bladder stripped forcibly from the rectum, upward toward the pelvic brim. The base of the bladder is thus brought up into view, exposing the seminal vesicles, which are examined by transverse incisions.

In the employment of any one of these methods, the urine, if it is to be saved for examination, should first be drawn through a catheter. This is also the cleanest way of emptying the bladder, particularly when it is greatly distended. The employment of force to squeeze the urine out of the bladder through the urethra is not advisable when there is any disease of bladder or urethra present.

2. **Female Pelvis.** The contents of the pelvis and the external genitalia are removed from the female cadaver in the same way as in the male. The anterior wall of the bladder is first freed from the pubis and the tissues separated around and behind the rectum so

164   THE EXAMINATION OF THE PELVIC ORGANS.

that the hand can be carried around the vagina and rectum. When the external genitalia are to be removed with the internal organs, an encircling incision is made on both sides of the external genitals,

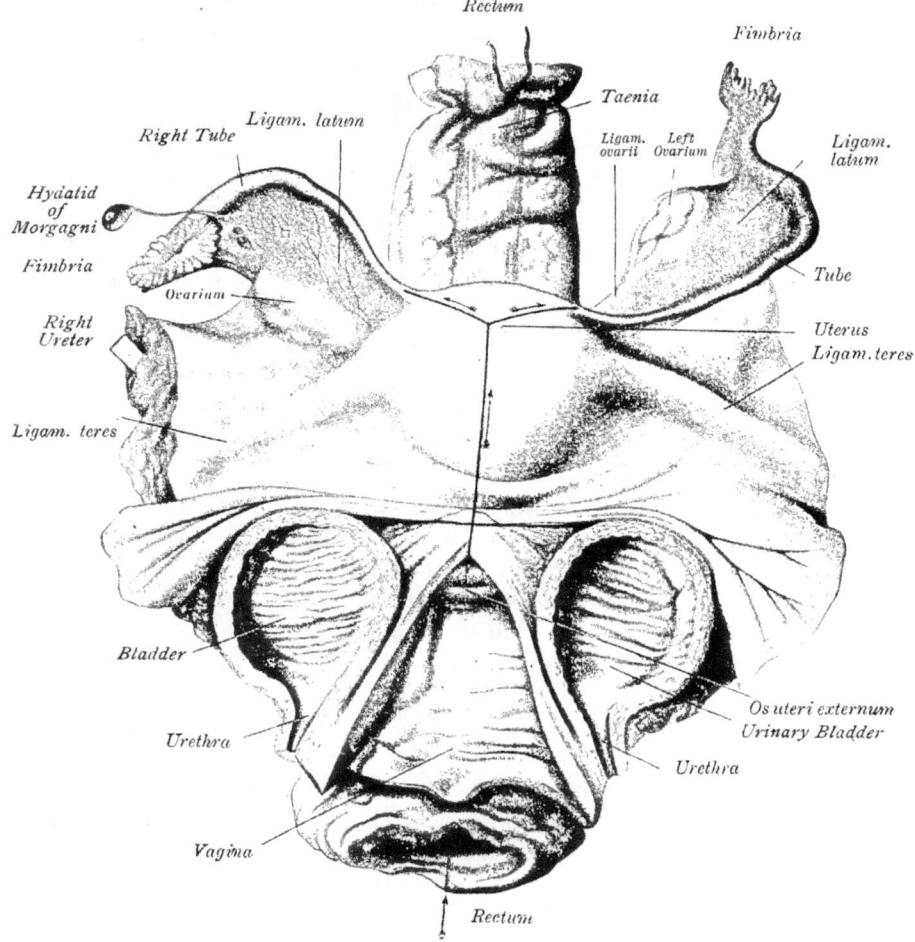

Fig. 46.—Section of female pelvic organs. Urinary bladder bisected and vagina opened in anterior median line. Arrows show direction of incisions. (After Nauwerck.)

beginning above at the termination of the main incision at the beginning of the anterior commissure, and meeting behind the anus. The external genitals are then dissected away from the arch of the pubis until the knife can be passed up beneath the symphysis and the attachments to the posterior border of the arch cut on both sides, so that the vulva can be pulled up beneath the pelvic arch, putting the perineum on the stretch. The posterior portion of the encircling incision is then deepened until the entire mass of external genitals and anus can be stripped up with the internal organs to the brim of the pelvis, where they are held up perpendicularly and any remaining attachments of peritoneum and blood-vessels cut, care being taken to cut outside of the ovaries and tubes. The mass thus removed is laid on the board with *rectum* uppermost and the latter opened first. The organs are then turned over, and the *urethra* and *bladder* opened in the anterior median line with the probe-pointed shears. The *vagina* and *uterus* are then opened in the anterior median line, bisecting the urethra and bladder. A heavy pair of shears having one blunt-pointed blade should be used. If it is desired to save the bladder and urethra, they can be dissected over to the right, or the vaginal wall can be cut on its left side. When the cervical canal will not admit the scissors the *uterus* may be cut in the median line with a knife. The horns may then be opened with the scissors. Additional cuts may be made into the uterine wall as desired (tumors, placental site, etc.). The *tubes* may be sounded from the abdominal extremity and then opened for their entire length with the fine probe-pointed shears, or they may be examined by means of transverse cuts. The *ovaries* are held with their flat surfaces between thumb and index-finger and then sectioned in the plane of greatest dimension from the convex border to the hilus. The *broad ligaments, parametrium, parovarium* and *lymphnodes* are examined by means of cuts made parallel with the sides of the uterus.

When the external genitals cannot be removed, the vagina and rectum, after they have been freed from the surrounding tissues, are put on the stretch toward the head of the body and cut through as close to the pubic outlet as possible. When this is carefully done it is possible to secure the inner labia and the urethra intact. The rectum is cut as close to the anus as possible. The organs are then stripped up to the brim of the pelvis, then held up perpendicularly while the remaining connections are severed. The organs thus removed are examined on the board in the same manner as given above. When the organs cannot be removed from the body, the bladder and urethra are examined by an anterior median incision after they have been freed from the symphysis. The uterus and vagina are then cut with the knife in the anterior median line, either through the bladder or after the latter has been dissected away. The ovaries, tubes and broad ligaments are then examined as directed above. The uterus and vagina may also be dissected from the rectum and opened by a posterior median incision. This method is used in medicolegal examinations.

To facilitate the removal of the genital organs in either sex a symphysiotomy may be performed and the pubic arch pulled apart, or a portion of the pubis may be cut out with the saw.

When permission to open the body by means of the usual main-incision cannot be obtained, it is possible to remove the thoracic and abdominal organs through the vagina or rectum. The cadaver is placed on its back, with buttocks near the end of the table, the thighs separated as widely as possible and flexed upon the body. In the male the scrotum is drawn up out of the way. A circular perineal incision is then made, beginning anteriorly at the perineoscrotal junction and extending around the anus. The arm may be introduced through this opening after the removal of the rectum and the abdominal and thoracic organs pulled downward and removed. In the female the uterus and vagina are removed through the vaginal opening; the arm is then introduced and the abdominal and thoracic organs removed.

II. POINTS TO BE NOTED IN THE EXAMINATION OF THE PELVIS.

I. MALE PELVIS. 1. **Penis.** Size, anomalies, condition, character of prepuce, evidence of circumcision, presence of smegma, character of meatus, discharge, wounds, scars (on and back of corona), evidence of syphilis, neoplasms, etc. Postmortem priapism occurs particularly in leukæmia. It may be caused also by traumatic or infective thrombosis and hæmorrhage, tumor-metastases, inflammatory infiltrations, and in death from hanging. The most important pathologic conditions of the penis are: inflammations (balanitis, posthitis, cavernitis, gonorrhœa, etc.), gangrene, phimosis, paraphimosis, præputial concretions, soft chancre, hard chancre, secondary syphilides, traumatic lesions (fracture, hæmorrhage, urine-infiltrations, etc.), anomalies (hypospadias, epispadias, etc.), tuberculosis (rare), condylomata, elephantiasis, cornu cutaneum, carcinoma, sarcoma (rare; melanotic sarcoma the most common form), secondary carcinoma (primary in prostate), lipoma, angioma and teratoma.

2. **Scrotum.** The most important pathologic conditions of the scrotum are: œdema, inflammation, gangrene, trauma, burns, elephantiasis, carcinoma, melanotic sarcoma, lipoma, fibroma, myofibroma, lymphangioma and teratoma.

3. **Testis and Epididymis.** Testis and epididymis weigh 15-30 grms. Note *size, form* and *consistence.* Normal color of cut-surface is grayish yellow; becomes brown in atrophy. Note character of tunics (color, lustre, smoothness, consistence, etc.), and contents of sacs (hydrocele, hæmatocele, empyema, etc.). The most important conditions affecting the testes are: inflammation (orchitis, epididymitis, vaginitis, abscess, hæmatogenous inflammations in pyemia, mumps, scarlet fever, typhoid fever, variola, chronic fibroid orchitis in syphilis, gonorrhœal epididymitis), tuberculosis, gonorrhœa, syphilis, actinomycosis, leprosy, leukæmic infiltrations, atrophy, compensatory hypertrophy, cryptorchidism, hydrocele, varicocele, spermatocele, cysts, malignant teratomata (syncytioma, cysts, cystocarcinoma, adenocarcinoma, adenoma, adenosarcoma, cystosarcoma, rhabdomyosarcoma, chondroma, osteoma, myxoma, etc.), carcinoma, sarcoma, lipoma, fibroma, etc., metastatic sarcoma and carcinoma, dermoid cysts, benign teratoma, parasites (echinococcus is rare). Tuberculosis is most common in the epididymis; syphilis more frequently affects the body of the testis. Torsion of the vas deferens may occur; atrophy of the testis may result. Twisting or thrombosis of the spermatic vessels may cause gangrene of the testicle.

4. **Rectum.** Note *contents* (amount, color, consistence, odor, etc.), *color* and *character of mucosa* (normally grayish red or reddish gray, smooth and translucent, solitary follicles just visible). Normally the rectum should contain formed brownish féces; in catarrh the contents are fluid and not formed, while the mucosa is covered with a thick glassy mucus. In obstruction of the gall-ducts the féces are gray ("clay-color"). In catarrhs and chronic passive congestion the mucosa is red. Decubital ulcers are often green from the imbibition of bile, and are surrounded by hæmorrhages. They are circular or correspond in shape to the fécal mass pressing upon them. Traumatic ulcers, hæmorrhages, diphtheritic inflammation, follicular ulcers, foreign bodies, stricture, fécal impaction, hæmorrhoids, fissures, fistulous tracts, tuberculosis, syphilis, adenomatous polyps and carcinoma are the most common pathologic conditions. The oxyuris vermicularis is the most common animal parasite. Gonorrhœa of the rectum is not uncommon. Stricture is most commonly caused by syphilis.

5. **Prostate.** Normal size is about that of a walnut or horse-chestnut. Weighs 19-25 grm. Average dimensions are 2.7 cm. long, 4.0 cm. broad, 2.0 cm. thick. Note form, consistence, color of cut-surface (smooth or granular), amount of secretion, corpora amylacea (color brown to black), size of gland-spaces, cysts, abscesses, tubercles, neoplasms. The most common pathologic conditions are: hyperplasia (usually inflammatory, the result of old gonorrhœal infection, less commonly due to chronic pyogenic infection), neoplasms (carcinoma is relatively common, usually developed in a prostate showing chronic inflammatory hyperplasia, adenoma, myoma, fibroma, myofibroma), cysts, acute inflammation (usually gonorrhœal), typhoid prostatitis, abscesses, tuberculosis, syphilis (rare) and atrophy. Thrombosis and the formation of phleboliths are very common in the prostatic veins; they are usually associated with gonorrhœal infection. The inflammatory hyperplasia may involve one or all three lobes of the prostate. In old men showing no evidences of prostatic inflammation the prostate may be atrophic.

6. **Seminal Vesicles and Duct.** Should be symmetrical. Note size, contents, character of wall, and appearance of lining membrane. They measure 3-5 cm. long, 1-2 cm. broad and 0.7-1.5 cm. thick. Gonorrhœal inflammations and tuberculosis are the most common conditions. In old men the vesicles contain a brownish-yellow mucoid substance. As a result of chronic inflammation the walls of the vesicles are thickened, often hyaline; the lumen is sometimes wholly obliterated. Calcification of the wall is not uncommon. Concretions are found in the vesicles following obstruction. Cystic dilatation may occur. Primary neoplasms (carcinoma and sarcoma) are rare.

7. **Urethra.** Mucosa should be grayish-red, smooth, shining and transparent. The most common and important pathologic condition is gonorrhœa (acute, chronic, anterior, posterior, erosions, ulcers, abscesses, perforation, stricture, periurethral abscess, cavernitis, etc.). Non-gonorrhœal urethritis is rare (colon- and influenza-bacillus, streptococcus, pneumococcus, etc.). Trauma (crushing, laceration, perforation, urine-infiltration, hæmorrhage, periurethral abscess, phlegmon, gangrene, stricture, urinary fistula, etc.), soft chancre, hard chancre, secondary and tertiary syphilitic lesions (gumma), tuberculosis (lupus), leprosy and neoplasms (rare: adenoma, carcinoma, melanotic and round-cell sarcomata [lymphosarcoma], fibroma, angioma) may occur. The most common anomalies are hypospadias and epispadias.

8. **Bladder.** *Size, degree of distention, amount* and *character of contents, character* and *color of mucosa* (normally gray-red, smooth and transparent), *muscle-coats* (hypertrophic, atrophic). The most common pathologic conditions are: anomalies (ectopia, ecstrophia, vesica bipartita, vesica bilocularis, diverticula), congestion, œdema, cystitis (acute and chronic catarrh, cystitis granulosa, cystica, purulent, phlegmonous, diphtheritic, emphysematous, interstitial, peri- and paracystitis, erosions, ulcers, gangrene, malakoplakia), tuberculosis, dilatation, trauma (rupture, perforation, fistula), neoplasms (papillary fibro-epithelioma, carcinoma, adenoma, myxoma, myoma, rhabdomyoma, angioma cavernosum, sarcoma, dermoids, secondary carcinoma [usually from prostate], and sarcoma [melanotic sarcoma]), concretions (urates, uric acid, oxalates, phosphates, carbonates, cystin and xanthin), and parasites (filaria sanguinis, distomum hæmatobium, echinococcus, trichomonas, ascaris and oxyuris).

II. **FEMALE PELVIS.** 1. **Rectum.** Note same things as given above for the examination of the rectum in the male. Gonorrhœa, stricture due to syphilis and traumatic fistula (due to childbirth) are more common in the female.

2. **Vulva.** The most important pathologic conditions are: congestion, œdema, hæmorrhage, hæmatoma, trauma (laceration), vulvitis (catarrhal, gonorrhœal, chronic, diphtheritic, gangrenous, phlegmonous, ulcerative, abscess), erythema, eczema, herpes, acne, furunculosis, pruritus, kraurosis vulvæ, leukoplakia, Bartholinitis, retention-cysts, cysts of the glands of Bartholin, hydrocele muliebris, syphilis (primary, secondary and tertiary lesions), tuberculosis (lupus), elephantiasis, condylomata, neoplasms (lipoma, fibroma, lymphangioma, papilloma, fibromyxoma, fibromyoma, chondroma, neuroma, carcinoma [usually very malignant in type], sarcoma [rare] and metastatic tumors [very rare]).

3. **Urethra.** Same conditions as noted above for the male. Small polypoid granulomata (caruncles) are very common; usually gonorrhœal in origin. Primary carcinoma is more common in the male.

4. **Bladder.** Note same conditions as given above. Rectovesical and vesicovaginal fistulas are not rare as the result of childbirth. Secondary carcinoma is more common than in the male (from uterus and cervix), primary carcinoma more rare. Ascaris and oxyuris may enter bladder from vagina through a rectal fistula.

5. **Vagina.** Note size (about 5-8 cm. long), contents (foreign bodies, pus, blood, etc.), color of membrane, condition of rugæ,

hymen, etc. The color of the mucosa varies from a delicate rosy red to a bluish purple in the late stages of pregnancy. The most important conditions are: colpitis (acute and chronic, catarrhal, diphtheritic, gangrenous, emphysematous, granular, nodular, adhæsiva, exfoliativa, vetularum, ulcerative; gonorrhœa the chief cause; also caused by mercuric chloride and other poisons; occurs also in cholera, typhoid fever, variola, scarlatina, diphtheria and other infections), ulcers, abscesses, erosions, strictures, varices, prolapse, atresia, trauma (lacerations, rupture, hæmatoma, fistula), tuberculosis (rare), syphilis (primary less common than on vulva, secondary lesions common, gumma rare), thrush, cysts (retention, remains of Müllerian and Wolffian ducts, gas-cysts), neoplasms (papillary fibro-epithelioma, fibroma, myxoma, myoma, rhabdomyoma, rhabdomyosarcoma, myxosarcoma, carcinoma (primary rare, secondary relatively common, particularly of malignant chorio-epithelioma; primary ectopic chorio-epithelial tumors occur in vagina also), and parasites (trichomonas vaginalis, oxyuris vermicularis). Note particularly condition of hymen.

6. **Uterus.** The developed uterus weighs 33-41 grms. In women who have not borne children the dimensions are 7-8 cm. long, 4 cm. broad, 2.5 cm. thick; in women who have borne children the dimensions are 8-9 cm. long, 5-6 cm. broad, and 3 cm. thick. The dimensions of the postpartum uterus vary greatly, where normal contraction has taken place the length is 8-9 cm., breadth 5-6.1 cm., thickness 3.2-3.6 cm., and weight 102-120 grms. Note *size, shape, character of peritoneal coat, consistence, character of cut-surface, size* and *contents of cavity.* Length of uterine cavity 5.2-5.7 cm. Note relations between body of uterus and cervix. In adults the circumference of the body of the uterus is greater than that of the cervix; before the age of puberty it is less than that of the neck. In old age the entire organ contracts, but the body more than the cervix, so that the organ again assumes an infantile form. The external os in the virgin uterus is round or oval; in women who have borne children it appears as a transverse cleft. The most common conditions of the cervix are the so-called erosion and ectropion, cystic glands (ovula Nabothi), cervical catarrh, hyperplasia, ulcers, polypi, myofibroma and carcinoma. Note contents of cervical canal (normally glassy, tough mucus; in catarrh becomes thin, cloudy or purulent); length and shape of canal (elongations, dilatations, stenosis, etc.). Color of mucosa should be grayish-red; the folds should be distinct and symmetrical. Purulent and diphtheritic inflammations, lacerations, polypi, cysts, fibromyoma, carcinoma

and tuberculosis are the most common conditions affecting the cervical canal.

The uterine cavity is normally empty; during menstruation or as the result of inflammation it may contain blood and bloody mucus; and the mucosa may be deep-red. The normal mucosa is gray-red and 0.5-1.0 mm. thick. In the puerperal uterus portions of the placenta, fœtal membrane, purulent or bloody lochial discharges are present. The placental site is shown by its uneven surface and presence of blood-clots. Gangrenous and purulent areas are greenish, gray, brownish-green, and black, with opaque and ragged surface. Gas-bubbles may be present. The normal consistence of the uterus is firm, diminished in the puerperal uterus, increased in chronic metritis. The cut-surface is smooth in the virgin uterus, rough in the uteri of women who have borne children and in chronic metritis. The most common pathologic conditions of the uterus are: abortion, hæmorrhage, apoplexia uteri, hæmatometra, hydrometra, pyometra, rupture, perforation, traumatic lesions, endometritis (acute, chronic, hæmorrhagic, interstitialis, glandularis, hyperplastica, cystica, polyposa, adenomatosa, infective, decidual, atrophic, etc.), foreign bodies, tuberculosis, syphilis, actinomycosis, hyperplasia, metritis (acute, chronic, hyperplastic, atrophic), perimetritis, parametritis, atrophy, neoplasms (myoma and myofibroma the most common; adenoma, adenomyoma, adenomatous polypi are very common; carcinoma [adenocarcinoma, cystocarcinoma, medullary, papillary, colloid, scirrhous, squamous-celled, malignant chorio-epithelioma] very common; sarcoma less common but it is not rare [myosarcoma the most common form; often represents a sarcomatous transformation of a myofibroma]; metastatic carcinoma and sarcoma are rare). and parasites (echinococcus).

7. **Tubes.** Note *length, thickness, shape, character of peritoneum, patency, fimbriated extremities* (swelling, redness, exudate, tubercles, hæmorrhage), *contents, color* and *thickness of mucous membrane, thickness* and *consistence of entire wall.* Tubes should be straight, not tortuous; in inflammation they are usually twisted, tortuous or bent. Hæmatosalpinx is usually caused by a tubal gestation. The most common pathologic conditions are: salpingitis (usually gonorrhœal, acute, chronic, catarrhal, purulent, pyosalpinx, hydrosalpinx, interstitial, perisalpingitis, tubo-ovarian abscesses and cysts), tuberculosis. actinomycosis (rare), syphilis (very rare), hæmatoma (ectopic gestation relatively frequent), neoplasms (rare: adenomyoma, fibromyoma, fibroma, myosarcoma, sarcoma,

carcinoma, chorio-epithelioma and teratoma; secondary carcinoma from uterus, ovary and intestine).

8. **Ovaries.** Note *size, form, consistence, color, character of cut-surface,* number of Graafian follicles, corpus luteum, etc. Ovary at puberty weighs about 10 grm., measures 4-5.2 cm. long, 2-2.7 cm. broad, 1.0-1.1 cm. thick. The adult ovary weighs about 7 grm., and measures 2-4 cm. long, 1.4-1.6 cm. broad, 0.7-0.9 cm. thick. A corpus luteum is 1.0-2.0 cm. in diameter. Ovary is compared to an almond in size and shape. In young individuals the surface is grayish-white and smooth; with age the surface becomes more and more irregular, the organ smaller and its consistence firmer. The cut-surface in young individuals is normally very moist (this should not be regarded as œdema). The most important conditions are: inflammation (acute and chronic, hæmorrhagic, purulent, etc., oöphoritis, abscess), tuberculosis, cystic follicles, lutein-cysts, cystadenoma (multilocular, monolocular, surface papilloma, simplex, papillary), parovarian cysts, carcinoma, fibroma, sarcoma, dermoid cysts, teratomata, malignant teratomata, embryoma, parasites (echinococcus is very rare).

9. **Uterine Ligaments, Vessels and Lymphatics.** Peritoneum over the broad ligament should be moist-shining, delicate and transparent. Inflammatory processes are very common in the parametrium, particularly in puerperal cases. The peritoneum is cloudy, opaque, injected, or covered with fibrinous or purulent exudate. Great numbers of small cysts containing clear fluid are often found in the peritoneum of the broad ligament as the sequelæ of inflammation. Note contents of blood-vessels (thrombi, concretions, neoplasms), and character of walls. Parovarian cysts, myomata, adenomyomata (round ligament), secondary carcinoma, chronic inflammations, hæmatoma and tubercles are the most common pathologic conditions.

CHAPTER XII.
SPECIAL REGIONAL EXAMINATION.
I. METHODS OF EXAMINATION.

1. **Bones and Bone-Marrow.** The methods employed will depend wholly upon the indications in any given case, the anatomic relations and the aim of the examination. Anatomic knowledge should be applied in the removal of any bone. In the case of the extremities adequate incisions should be made in the skin extending the entire length of the bone which is to be removed, and the soft parts dissected from the bone before the latter is disarticulated or cut out. When the bone is examined *in situ* it may be opened with hammer and chisel or cut with a saw, either transversely or longitudinally, so as to give the most instructive picture of the condition present. The spinal column may be cut longitudinally. The symphysis pubis is first cut through, a block of wood is placed beneath the lumbar vertebræ, and the vertebral bodies are sawed through in the median line, from below upward, moving the block toward the head as the sawing proceeds. The cut-surfaces of the vertebræ are then inspected. The *pelvis* may be removed whole in connection with the lumbar vertebræ and the upper halves of the femurs. The *spinal column* and the *pelvis* may also be removed entire by sawing the ribs on each side of the spine, cutting the occipito-atloid ligaments above, and disarticulating the femurs or sawing them at their upper half or third and removing them with the pelvis. Of the long bones the *femur* is the one most frequently examined. An incision is made in the skin from the groin in the direction of the large vessels extending to the middle of the leg. The ligamentum patellæ is cut through and the skin and muscles turned back at the knee until the joint is laid bare; the capsule of the joint is opened and the femur disarticulated. The skin and muscles are then separated from the upper part of the femur, the hip-joint opened, and the femur disarticulated and removed. When held in a vise it may be opened longitudinally by sawing. Other bones are removed as indicated; the chief points to be observed in their removal are the anatomic considerations and the making of the incisions in such a way as to cause the least possible disfigurement. For the examination of the *bone-marrow*

the tibia or femur, sternum, a rib and the body of one of the vertebræ are usually opened by means of the saw or chisel.

2. **Joints.** The joints are opened for examination with attention to the same considerations given above for the examination of the bones. Approved surgical incisions may be used. If fistulous openings into the joint are present these should not be cut until the joint is open. When bacteriologic examinations are to be made the joint should be opened with a sterile knife, or the capsule seared and punctured with a sterile pipette through which the contents of the joint-cavity are secured. The articular surfaces, epiphyses and diaphyses should be examined by transverse or vertical incisions.

3. **Lymph-glands.** The cervical, axillary and inguinal lymph-nodes can be secured for examination by carrying the skin-flaps of the main-incision far enough back to make these regions accessible. For the examination of other glands, such as the cubital, popliteal, interscapular, posterior cervical, etc., the cadaver should be placed in a convenient position, and the skin-incisions should be made so as to expose sufficiently the part to be examined, without unnecessary mutilation.

4. **Peripheral Blood-vessels and Nerves.** Skin-incisions are made along the course of the vessels and nerves, and these are then exposed by careful dissection. In the case of the upper extremity the clavicle is removed when the entire course of the nerves and vessels of the arm is to be exposed.

5. **Sympathetic System.** The cervical, thoracic and abdominal sympathetic systems are examined either at the close of the examination of each one of these regions or at the end of the autopsy. Careful anatomic dissections are necessary for the demonstration of the sympathetic ganglia and nerves.

6. **Organs of Special Sense.** These may be examined at the close of the autopsy, according to the methods given above, if they have not been examined at the close of the section of the brain.

II. POINTS TO BE NOTED IN SPECIAL REGIONAL EXAMINATION.

1. **Bones and Bone-marrow.** Note size, form, color of surface, consistence (diminished in necrosis, osteomalacia, rachitis, senile osteoporosis, etc.; increased in sclerosis), fragility, fractures, separation of epiphyses, fissures, dislocations, elevation or separation of periosteum, periosteal defects, changes in periosteum (thickened, indurated, and showing hard white elevations in chronic

inflammation; swollen and easily stripped from the bone in acute inflammation; hæmorrhages and collections of pus beneath periosteum cause separation of periosteum; in chronic inflammation the periosteum may become more firmly adherent to the bone and contain spongy, compact, cartilaginous or osteoid osteophytes that vary in color according to the degree of calcification [bluish-red, yellowish, dirty-white, shining-white]; the normal periosteum is grayish-white in color; it is reddened in hyperæmia and hæmorrhage). The surface of bones normally is smooth and grayish-yellow in color; it becomes red with an increase in the number and size of the medullary spaces, and paler, grayish-white or white in necrosis; a dull, rough, uneven surface indicates lacunar absorption. Note localized or general thickening (exostoses, hyperostosis). On section note thickening of the bone (osteomyelitis ossificans), thinning (osteoporosis, excentric atrophy), enlargement of medullary spaces, obliteration of spaces by newly-formed bone (osteosclerosis; bone becomes heavy and solid like ivory), and caries (pyogenic infection, tuberculosis, syphilis, actinomycosis, neoplasm). Caries occurs in both spongy and compact bone, but more often in the former. The necrotic bone appears as soft, friable granules (molecular necrosis) or sequestra, between which living bone or granulation-tissue may be found. The necrotic granules feel like fine grains of sand when the finger is rubbed over the cut-surface. The color depends essentially upon the amount of granulation-tissue present (gray, grayish-red or deep bluish-red). Purulent areas are cloudy, opaque and yellowish. Tubercles appear as round, grayish, semitranslucent areas, with opaque yellowish centers when calcification has occurred. In young subjects the developing portions of the bone (epiphyses, cartilages) should receive especial examination. Note *amount, color* and *consistence* of bone-marrow. In the young individual the marrow is red; after puberty the red marrow gradually becomes restricted to the flat bones and the short spongy bones, while in the long bones there develops a yellow, fatty marrow. In old age the marrow of the long bones may become brownish, transparent, myxomatous or soft like colloid, or contain large cystoid spaces filled with a thin mucoid fluid or liquid fat. Red lymphoid marrow is found in the long bones in severe anæmias; it is grayish-red or deep red according to its blood-content. In leukæmia the marrow may be red, violet, pink, grayish or grayish-yellow (pyoid); in chloroma the marrow may be greenish. In cachexias the marrow may become gelatinous as in old age. A hyperæmic fatty marrow should not be mistaken for lymphoid marrow; the fatty shine serves to distinguish the former. Cloudy yellowish areas in the marrow point to purulent infiltration. Firm sulphur-yellow masses are gummata.

The most important pathologic conditions of the bones are: atrophy, osteomalacia, rachitis, fractures, dislocations, periostitis, osteomyelitis, ostitis, acromegaly, necrosis, syphilis, tuberculosis, actinomycosis, leprosy, exostosis, hyperostosis, hyperplasia, defects, hypoplasia, dwarfism, giantism, neoplasms (primary sarcoma the most common malignant tumor [periosteal, myelogenous, myeloma, lymphosarcoma, chloroma, leukæmia]; secondary carcinoma [primary in mamma, thyroid, prostate, adrenal] also relatively common; osteoma, lipoma, exostosis cartilaginea, fibrosa and ossificans, fibroma, myxoma, lipoma, angioma, chondroma, etc.), cysts, and parasites (echinococcus, cysticercus).

2. **Joints.** *Capsule* (thickness, tension, defects, tears, perforations, adhesions), *cavity* (contents [normally a few drops of light-yellow, clear fluid, more in knee-joint than in other joints; may be serous, purulent, hæmorrhagic or fibrinous], adhesions, granulation-tissue, rice-bodies, free bodies, joint-mice, obliteration of cavity, osseous, fibrinous or cartilaginous ankylosis, changes in internal articular ligaments), *synovial membrane* (a delicate pale grayish, smooth membrane; rough from exudate or formation of granulation-tissue; red in hyperæmia or hæmorrhage. Note folds and villi; subserous fat-tissue), *articular surfaces* (loss or increase of cartilage, separation of cartilage, newly-formed bone, granulation-tissue, deposits of lime-salts or urates, necrosis or purulent infiltration of the cartilage, erosions, eburnations, defects or enlargement of ends of bones; in degeneration and necrosis the bluish-white, transparent cartilage becomes opaque, cloudy and yellowish). The most important pathologic conditions of the joints are: arthritis (acute, chronic, serous, purulent, gangrenous, primary, secondary, gonococcal, pneumococcal, streptococcal, tuberculous, syphilitic, deformans, villosa, prolifera cartilaginea, adhæsiva, ulcerosa, sicca, neuropathic), dislocations, deformities, abnormal position, congenital anomalies, chondritis, spondylitis, gout, necrosis, ankylosis, tuberculosis, syphilis, free bodies, neoplasms (rare: angioma, sarcoma, chondroma, lipoma; secondary more common from an extension of sarcoma of neighboring structures; metastatic tumors rare), and parasites (echinoccocus very rare).

3. **Lymphnodes, Peripheral Vessels and Nerves, Sympathetic and Organs of Special Sense.** The pathologic conditions of these structures have been given above.

CHAPTER XIII
THE AUTOPSY OF THE NEW-BORN.
I. METHODS OF EXAMINATION.

The **Section of the New-Born** differs from that of the adult in several particulars, as follows:—

a. Spinal Cord. The spinal canal may be opened with the scissors alone, as the soft, bony structures of the spinal column are easily cut.

b. Skull. The cranium is opened, after the removal of the scalp, in the usual way, by cutting with the scissors into the posterior angle of the anterior fontanel and then introducing the shears into the longitudinal sinus, and cutting the latter posteriorly in the line of the sagittal suture. The sinus is then opened anteriorly. The sutures between the frontal and parietal bones, and between the parietal and occipital bones, are now cut with the shears down to the level of the greatest circumference of the cranium. The cranial bones with the adherent dura are then pressed outward from the brain, and are either held in this position or cut through with the bone-shears so that sufficient room for the removal of the brain is afforded. The anterior falx is then cut and the brain removed as in the adult, using great care because of its very soft consistence. When too soft to be removed the brain may be opened within the skull; or a horizontal section may be made with the large, flat brain knife at the level of greatest circumference. Some prosectors freeze the brain before removal, or remove it while the cadaver is immersed in a strong solution of brine.

c. Section of Thorax, Neck-organs and Abdomen. A small block of wood is placed beneath the lumbar vertebræ, and the main-incision reaching from thyroid cartilage to the pelvic crest is made, the incision passing to the left of the umbilicus, and diverging outward below it so as not to cut the left umbilical artery. The incision is now extended through the abdominal wall into the peritoneal cavity, the right half of the abdominal wall turned up so as to expose the umbilical vein, which is cut loose from the abdominal wall, so that a second diverging incision can be made through the abdominal wall, beginning just above the umbilicus and passing down to the right of the right umbilical artery, without cutting the umbilical vein. There is left between the two diverging cuts a triangular flap of abdominal wall (see Fig. 47) containing the umbilicus, urachus and umbilical arteries, and connected with the liver by the umbilical vein. The umbilical vessels are then probed and examined by transverse sections; and the triangular flap of abdominal wall turned down over the pubis. After the height of the diaphragm has been noted the thorax is opened by cut-

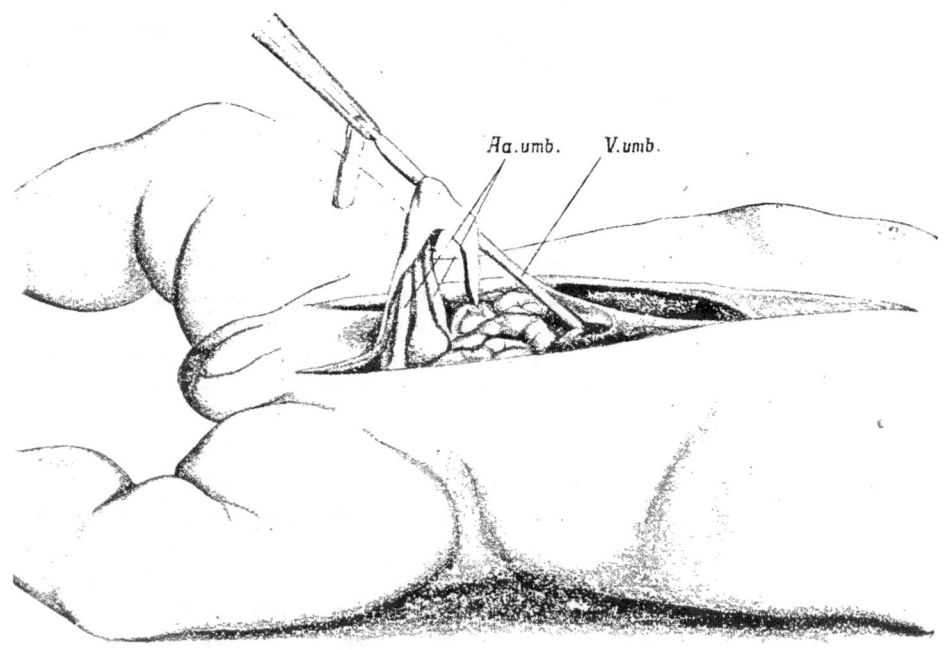

Fig. 47.—Method of opening the abdomen in the new-born, with especial reference to the examination of the umbilical vessels. Note triangular flap, including umbilicus, urachus and umbilical arteries, and attached to umbilical vein. (After Nauwerck.)

ting the ribs outside of the costochondral articulations so as to give more room. The thymus gland is then examined and removed. The heart may be opened in the same way as in the adult, extending the cut into the pulmonary artery up to the ductus arteriosus, which is examined by the probe. The ductus arteriosus is easily found by cutting the pulmonary artery in the middle of its anterior wall. In the median line beyond the right and left branches of the pulmonary artery is the opening of the duct, which can be probed into the descending aorta. (See Fig. 48.) The heart may then be removed, and the foramen ovale carefully examined.

THE AUTOPSY OF THE NEW-BORN. 179

It is usually better to take out the neck and thoracic organs *en masse* and examine on the table. This must always be done in cases of suspected thymic death and when the question of the child having been born alive or dead is to be settled. The position of the

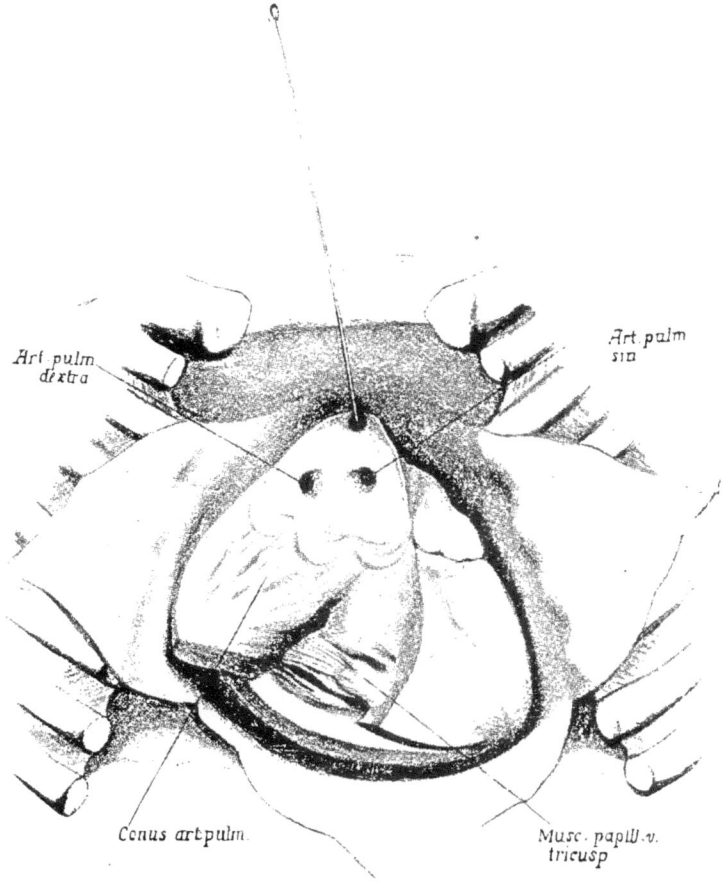

FIG. 48.—Section of pulmonary artery and pulmonary ring in the new-born, showing openings of right and left pulmonary arteries and ductus arteriosus (containing probe). (After Nauwerck.)

diaphragm must be taken before the thorax is opened. The upper air passages are then ligated. The thoracic cavity is then opened; the pericardium and heart opened and examined. The larynx and trachea are opened above the ligature, and the whole respiratory tract with the ligature in position is removed from the thorax and placed in a vessel of clean water. The air passages below the ligature are then opened, and the lungs, after their floating power has been tested, are cut beneath the water in order to see if air-bubbles

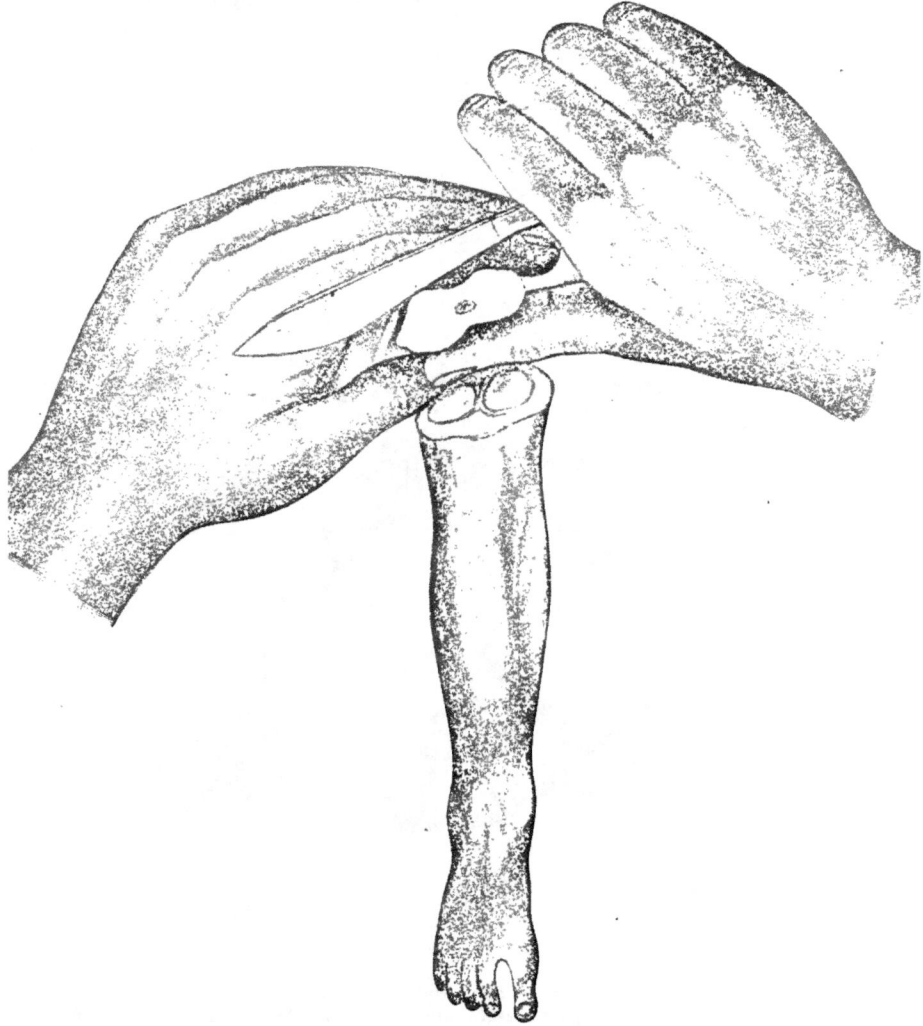

Fig. 49.—Method of demonstrating the Béclard center of ossification in the lower epiphysis of the femur. (After Nauwerck.)

arise from the cut-surface or from the bronchioles. The lungs are examined piece by piece for air-containing portions, noting their floating power, crepitation, occurrence of bubbles, etc. In the case of suspected thymic enlargement the trachea should be explored from above for a stenosis, before the thorax is opened. If evidences of pressure upon the trachea cannot be demonstrated in this way the body of the child can be fixed in formalin and then opened. The thymus and trachea are then examined by means of transverse sections. The stomach should be ligated at both ends and then removed, and opened under water. The presence of air points to extra-uterine "swallowing" movements. This test is worthless if decomposition has set in. When the thoracic organs are taken out *en masse* the ductus arteriosus can be examined from the aorta. The removal of neck, thoracic and abdominal organs *en masse* is often of advantage in the examination of the infant cadaver, as the organs can be much more easily examined on the table than in the body. The neck organs are first removed after ligating trachea and œsophagus, and with the thoracic organs are stripped down to the diaphragm and then lifted up out of the body and laid over the left side of the body. The diaphragm is then cut laterally and posteriorly. The rectum is ligated and cut between ligatures. The crura of the diaphragm, the cœliac vessels and root of mesentery are then cut, and the viscera, including the kidneys, are stripped down to the brim of the pelvis, where the peritoneum and blood-vessels are cut.

The *ear-test* (the demonstration of the opening-up of the Eustachian tube and middle ear by the establishment of respiration) may be shown by the examination of the middle-ear from the cranium. The ear-drum must be examined to see if it is intact.

The *Béclard center of ossification* in the lower epiphysis of the femur is examined by opening the knee-joint, flexing the leg, and then making parallel transverse cuts perpendicularly to the long axis of the bone, until the greatest diameter of the center of ossification is cut.

The eye-ball may be removed and examined for the pupillary membrane. The eye is cut through a few millimetres back of the cornea, the anterior segment is fixed in dilute chromic acid or alcohol and then examined microscopically; or it can be examined in the fresh state, the membrane being visible even to the naked eye.

Bacteriologic examinations should be made in the usual way, the material being secured by sterile pipette, sterilized knife or platinum loop, smears, etc. In the examination of a very fresh cadaver the possibility of danger from infection with syphilis must always be borne in mind.

II. POINTS TO BE NOTED IN THE SECTION OF THE NEW-BORN.

Aside from establishing the cause of death, the autopsy of the new-born has for its aim the determination of the age of the infant, its viability and whether it was born living or dead. Special attention must therefore be paid to all points that may be of value in settling these questions.

The *average length* of a full-term new-born child is 50 cm. (42-58 cm.), boys being somewhat longer than girls; 58 cm. may be taken as the maximal length, 48 cm. the minimal. Both length and weight vary within wide limits. The length of the fetus in the first five months of intra-uterine life corresponds approximately to the square of the month. In the last five months the age of the fetus equals approximately the length in centimetres divided by five. Viability is usually regarded as beginning in the eighth month and with a body-length of over 32 cm. The *average weight* of the full-term new-born is 3,200 grms., for boys 3,310 grms., girls 3,230 grms.; maximum weight 5,500 grms., minimal 2,500. The weights for the different months are: second month, 4 grms., third month 5-20 grms., fourth 120 grms., fifth 284 grms., sixth 434 grms., seventh 1,218 grms., eighth 1,549 grms., ninth 1,971 grms., tenth 2,334 grms.

Look for traces of *vernix caseosa*. The *skin* of the well-nourished, full-term, new-born is smooth, not wrinkled, white or grayish-red rather than red in color (a slight icteric tint is so common as to be regarded as normal), and showing the fine *lanugo hair* only on the shoulders. The *hair* of the scalp averages 2-3 cm. in length. The *finger-nails* are firm, horny and extend beyond the finger-tips. The subcutaneous panniculus should be abundant. The average length of the *umbilical cord* is about 50 cm., and it is inserted about the middle of the body or just below it. As a rule it is thrown off on about the 5-6th day. The *cartilages of the nose and ears* are firm. In male infants the *testicles* lie in the firm and wrinkled scrotum (they begin to descend in the seventh month); in the female the outer *labia* usually meet, but occasionally the inner ones are visible. In the seventh and eighth months the *clitoris* rises above the greater labia. A small amount of blood-stained discharge is often present in the vagina of the new-born. From the *mammæ* of both male and female new-born a whitish turbid fluid ("Hexenmilch") can usually be expressed. The *great fontanel* is 2-2.5 cm. broad, while the posterior one is nearly closed. The *pupillary membrane* is absent after the eighth month. The *ductus arteriosus* remains open 4-5 days after birth; the *foramen ovale* is not completely closed until the second or third month of extra-uterine life, although by the tenth day the opening is nearly obliterated. The *center of ossification* in the lower epiphysis of the femur should be present and measure 2-9 mm. It is not present in the eighth month and in a large proportion of cases begins to develop in the ninth month. Only rarely is it absent in normal full-term infants. It appears in the bluish-white cartilage as a lenticular mass of red or reddish-brown color in which the blood-vessels can be easily seen. It may be absent in congenital rachitis or syphilis, or in the latter disease it may show the characteristic appearance of osteochondritis syphilitica.

The head should be examined for the presence of the *"head-tumor"* or *"caput succedaneum,"* the œdematous swelling of the scalp over the parietal eminences. Minute hæmorrhages may be present in the tissues. The tumor usually grows smaller or disappears within 12-48 hours. In difficult labors a *hæmatoma neonatorum* may be produced between the periosteum and bone, usually over the right parietal eminence. It appears as a circumscribed tumor which may increase after birth and persists for a long time. As the result of a periostitis ossificans a wall of bone may be formed about the extravasate, or it may be encapsulated with small bony plates. After the absorption of the extravasate the newly-formed bone may persist throughout life in the form of a "crater-like" or "coral island" elevated circle of bone. Infection of the hæmatoma not infrequently leads to the formation of a subperiosteal abscess, purulent infiltration of the cranial bone and purulent meningitis. The cranium should also be carefully examined for other evidences of conditions due to the mechanism of birth, such as the general shape of the head, condition of sutures, movability of the cranial bones, depressions, over-lapping, etc.; of the cranial bones. Wounds of the scalp and face should be carefully noted. The circumference of the *cranium* is 34.5 cm., sagittal diameter 10-13.5 cm., transverse 8-9.5 cm., diagonal 12-14 cm. The *brain* of the infant is normally rosy-red in color, rather translucent, soft, almost jelly-like, and moist. Tearing of the pial veins or meningeal arteries during delivery may produce fatal meningeal hæmorrhages.

The *weights* of the internal organs are: brain 380 grms., thymus 7-10 grms., heart 20.6 grms., lungs 58 grms., spleen 11.1 grms., kidneys together 23.6 grms., testicle 0.8 grm., liver 118 grms. The *mature placenta* weighs about 500 grms., and measures 15-20 cm. in diameter, 3 cm. thick in the middle and 0.5-1 cm. thick at the edge.

In the examination of the abdomen the *color and appearance of the peritoneum, position of abdominal organs* and *height of diaphragm* should be noted. Before respiration is established the diaphragm is at the fourth rib; after respiration is begun it is about one rib lower on both sides, usually a little lower on the left side than on the right. The condition of the *umbilicus* and *umbilical* vessels is of great importance (umbilical hæmorrhage, infection, insertion of cord, line of demarcation, etc.). Note contents, size of lumen, thickness and character of walls, appearance and moistness of intima. In umbilical infection the process spreads through the sheaths of the umbilical arteries rather than of the vein. The infected arteries contain yellowish-brown purulent thrombi; and the tissues about them show œdema, hæmorrhages, purulent infiltration or small abscesses. The perpendicular position of the stomach, the relatively large size of appendix to that of kidney and spleen, the lobulation of the kidneys, and the relatively large size of liver and adrenals must be borne in mind and not be regarded as pathologic. Examine *adrenals* especially for occurrence of hæmorrhage, infarction and thrombosis. Look for accessory adrenals ("adrenals of Marchand") in broad ligament and along the spermatic cords. Thrombi in the renal and spermatic vessels are not rare in the new-born. Note occurrence and degree of *uric-acid infarction of the kidneys* (formerly supposed to indicate that child was born alive). Meconium is present in the large intestine of the child born at term; when prematurely born it is found only in the small intestine. It is greenish in color and contains cholesterin, crystals of calcium sulphate, bile-pigment, desquamated epithelium and granular detritus.

In the examination of the thorax especial attention should be paid to the *thymus,* noting its size, color, consistence and evidences of pressure upon underlying structures, particularly upon the trachea. In death from suffocation small petechiæ are often found in the thymus and in the serous membranes. The *lungs* rise up over the edges of the pericardium and thymus when respiration has occurred, and their color is a light rose. Areas of atelectasis are bluish. The unexpanded lungs are brownish-red, firm in consistence and distinctly lobulated. Air-containing lung floats in water and crepitates, and gives off bubbles when cut beneath the water. Attempts at artificial respiration may draw some air into the lungs. Gas-bubbles may be produced by decomposition. In *white pneumonia* the lung is pale, grayish-white and airless. The *larynx, trachea* and *bronchi* are to be examined for presence of mucus, amniotic fluid, meconium, foreign substances, etc. The ligated stomach should also be tested as to its floating power, and should be opened under water to determine the presence of air or gas.

The determination of the exact cause of death in the new-born is often very difficult or impossible. In many cases no adequate lesions can be found to explain the occurrence of sudden death in the first days or weeks after birth. Among the more frequent causes of such deaths are congenital syphilis, asphyxia neonatorum (cardiac syphilis, presence of amniotic fluid, etc., in respiratory passages, congenital cardiac lesions, injury to brain, meningeal or cerebral hæmorrhage, congenital marasmus, intra-uterine infections, umbilical infections, enlarged thymus, "overlying," poisoning, congenital hæmophilia, melaena neonatorum, etc.), adrenal hæmorrhage, malformations of gastro-intestinal tract, absence of common duct, nephritis, pneumonia, etc. The most important congenital infections are syphilis, gonorrhœa, tuberculosis, variola, typhoid, pyogenic infection, tetanus, measles, scarlatina, influenza, meningitis, malaria, recurrent fever, pneumococcus, colon bacillus and others, mostly very rare. Congenital leukæmia has been observed. Numerous cases of congenital neoplasm have been reported (hæmangioma, lymphangioma, fibroma, lipoma, neurofibroma, papilloma of the larynx, adenoma, carcinoma [liver, kidneys, stomach, intestine], cystic tumors of liver, pancreas, kidneys and ovary, rhabdomyoma or rhabdomyosarcoma of kidney, heart, etc., adenosarcoma of kidney, dermoid cysts and various forms of teratomata).

Congenital syphilis is so common and such an important condition in the new-born that especial search should always be made for evidence of its presence. Smears of all the organs should be made in the cases examined soon after death, and either stained or examined at once by the dark-field method for the presence of the spirochæte. The most common anatomic manifestations of congenital syphilis are pemphigus, macules, papules, or maceration of the skin, white pneumonia, cardiac dilatation due to interstitial myocarditis, interstitial hepatitis, splenic enlargement and osteochondritis syphilitica. The long bones should always be examined for the last-named condition; they should be removed and cut longitudinally. In the boundary between epiphysis and diaphysis the presence of a yellow, hard zone points to this condition. The area of ossification is increased, irregular, and is separated from the bone by the yellowish zone, which in its earliest stages is soft and cellular, later sclerotic. The area of proliferating cartilage is also increased and may contain medullary spaces, showing as red lines. In rachitis the ossification-zone is wholly or partly wanting, while the zone of proliferating cartilage is broader and rich in red medullary spaces. In place of the ossification-zone there may be present a layer of soft, grayish-white osteoid tissue containing medullary spaces. No sharp line exists between the different zones.

CHAPTER XIV.
THE MEDICOLEGAL AUTOPSY.

As has been stated above, every autopsy should be conducted as if it were a medicolegal case, and autopsy-protocols should be so complete and accurate that they may be accepted as evidence in any case in which such testimony can be introduced. While the ordinary autopsy may give satisfactory evidence as to the nature of the pathologic processes found and the cause of death, the scope of a medicolegal autopsy includes not only the cause and manner of death, but also the identification of the body, the determination of the commission of a crime, the manner in which the crime was performed, its motive and the detection of the criminal. Under such conditions the prosector must extend the field of his observations and conclusions to meet the possibilities of the witness-stand. The general technique of the medicolegal autopsy will vary but little from that of the ordinary, and these variations will be given here, as follows:—

The medicolegal autopsy should always be performed in the presence of two witnesses, one of whom should be a physician competent to judge of the methods employed in the autopsy. The autopsy findings should be dictated during the progress of the autopsy, and at its close should be verified and signed in the presence of the witnesses. No other spectators should be permitted in the room. The examination should be made by daylight, and not until positive signs of death appear. If the cadaver has been frozen it must first be allowed to thaw out at room-temperature. The prosector should, if possible, see and examine the body before it is removed from the place where it is found, and he should carefully examine the surroundings, clothes and external surface of the body for possible clues. All known information concerning the circumstances of the case, the personal history of the deceased, the occurrence of any injury, previous illness, etc., should be in the hands of the prosector. Undertaker's manipulations, such as the injection of embalming fluids, puncture of intestines, aspiration of fluid-contents, etc., must not be permitted before the autopsy.

Especial attention should be given to the **identification** of the body (measurements, weight, build, shape of head, deformities or defects, color of hair and eyes, teeth, dental work, thumb-markings, tattoo marks, birth-marks, scars, evidences of previous diseases, occupation, clothing, etc.). In doubtful cases the body should be photographed. Roentgen-ray pictures may also be made. When only portions of a body are found the microscopic examination alone may be able to throw light upon the case and give positive evidence as to the sex, age, existence of certain physical characteristics, birth-marks, scars, disease, etc. When no conclusions can be reached a minute description of the remains should be placed in the protocol. The approximate **time of death** is to be determined with greater care in the medicolegal case (temperature of body, rigor mortis, putrefaction, dissolution, mummification, character of stomach-contents, changes in eye-balls, etc.).

In the performance of the autopsy the greatest care should be taken to avoid the production of artefacts. Hammer, chisel or wedge should not be used; bones should be sawed through completely, particularly in the case of the skull and spine. Especial care should be exercised in the removal of brain and cord. Examine vertebræ in all cases when cause of death is unknown. The main-incision may begin at the chin. The mouth and pharynx should be examined for foreign-bodies before the mouth- and neck-organs are removed. These should be taken out *en masse*. Particularly in young infants is the examination of the larynx of great importance. Examine thoracic organs *in situ* before removing them; then remove in connection with neck-organs and examine on table. Ligate cardiac end of œsophagus to prevent escape of stomach-contents. Cut œsophagus above ligature. Open pulmonary artery before lungs are sectioned. Examine abdominal organs *in situ* before removing them. Bullet- and stab-wounds should be accurately located, traced, measured and course described. Recover missiles for use as evidence. The origin and cause of hæmorrhage must be accurately determined. Remove genital organs *en masse* after examination *in situ*. Examine particularly contents of vagina and anus; make microscopic examination of same (semen, blood, foreign-bodies, etc.). Do not put probe, knife or shears into cavity of uterus, but open with a clean cut in the median posterior line. Examine ovaries for presence of corpus luteum.

In cases of **suspected poisoning** especial attention should be paid to the condition of the gastro-intestinal tract (position, distention, odor, consistence, condition of blood-vessels, etc.). A ligature should be placed about the cardiac end of the stomach and another around the duodenum below the mouth of the common duct, and both organs removed. They should then be opened outside the body and the contents examined (amount, consistence, color, composition, reaction, odor), and the latter then placed in clean, sterilized glass or porcelain jars, which are sealed and labeled. The mucosa of the organ is then carefully examined and described, and the organ itself finally preserved in a sealed and labeled jar. The small and large intestines and the œsophagus are similarly ligatured, removed and examined, and with their contents are preserved for chemic reaction by sealing them in separate sterilized jars properly labeled. Blood from the heart and large veins should be saved for spectroscopic and chemic examination. The contents of the urinary bladder likewise are saved for chemic analysis. Finally, portions of the brain, liver, kidney, intestine, spleen and other organs and tissues are preserved in separate vessels for chemic and microscopic examination. When possible an expert chemist should be present at the autopsy and receive the organs and contents directly from the pathologist. Especial care must be taken that no contamination of the material can occur. The manner of removal of the organs, the character and condition of the instruments used, nature and condition of receptacles for material, manner of sealing, use of preservatives, method of transportation to the chemist, and other fine points of detail will all be threshed over in court in the endeavor to discredit the testimony, and the pathologist and chemist must be thoroughly prepared to meet all questions of this nature. In certain cases the presence of a poison may be told by the finding of a granular or crystalline substance in the stomach or intestines (arsenic-poisoning), by the color (green from aceto-arsenite of copper, yellow from potassium chromate or iodin, purple from iodin, red from bromin) or by the odor (bitter almonds, phosphorus, alcohol, chloroform, laudanum, carbolic acid, lysol, garlic in arsenic poisoning). Excessive acidity or alkalinity of the stomach contents is found in poisoning with acids, alkalies or potassium cyanide. Portions of poisonous plants, mushrooms, matchheads, etc., may be found in the stomach.

Certain pathologic conditions, as fatty degeneration of the liver, cloudy swelling of the kidney, nephritis, malignant jaundice, acute yellow atrophy of the liver, dysentery, and others may be caused by such poisons as phosphorus, arsenic, mercuric chloride, potassium chlorate, chloroform, etc. When such changes are found at autopsy the pathologist must always carefully differentiate between disease and poisoning. He must decide as to the actual occurrence of poisoning, the source and nature of the poison, how and when administered, amount of poison, number of poisons, primary and secondary effects, attendant circumstances, accidental, suicidal or criminal administration, motive, etc. Some poisons produce no characteristic gross or microscopic changes in the organs or tissues. In such cases no pathologic conditions sufficient to cause death may be found, and when there is doubt a chemical examination should be made. Other poisons produce more or less characteristic changes, either by their local action, by selective action upon certain organs, by excretion, or by acting upon the blood. The effects will vary according to the amount of the poison, its concentration, length of action, condition of gastrointestinal tract, rapidity of excretion, etc. The most important and common poisons producing recognizable autopsy conditions are as follows:—

Acids. In *carbolic-acid* poisoning there may be dry, brown, leathery spots on the face about the lips; grayish-white eschars on mucosa of lips, mouth, tongue, pharynx and œsophagus; œdema of the glottis and pharyngeal submucosa; white or gray longitudinal eschars in stomach and duodenum; leathery appearance of stomach wall; cloudy swelling of kidneys, odor of phenol in urine, which is dark in color; general passive hyperæmia. In *sulphuric-acid* poisoning there may be brown, leathery and dry eschars on lips and skin, grayish-white to black eschars in mucosa of mouth, stomach and œsophagus; black, dry and brittle clots in the blood-vessels; perforation of stomach; sloughing of mucosa; parenchymatous nephritis. *Hydrochloric acid* has little or no action on the skin; on mucous membranes the action is similar to that of sulphuric acid except that the drying of the eschars and blood-clots is less marked. In *nitric-acid* poisoning the eschars are yellowish; hæmatin is not separated and dissolved, so that the brown black eschars seen in sulphuric- and hydrochloric-acid poisoning are not formed. *Oxalic acid* causes a white or grayish escharotic condition of the mouth, œsophagus and stomach; crystals of calcium oxalate may be found in the blood-clots and in the kidney-tubules. *Glacial acetic acid* may produce a grayish-white escharotic condition of the mucosa of the upper respiratory tract, and pneumonia, when inhaled.

Alcohol. In concentrated solutions coagulates albumin and has a corrosive action on mucous membranes. The ingestion of large amounts causes asphyxia, gastro-enteritis, cloudy swelling of ganglion cells of brain, and parenchymatous degeneration of kidney and liver. Lungs, liver, brain and stomach may give an alcoholic odor. In chronic alcoholism there may be chronic atrophic or hypertrophic gastritis, atrophic cirrhosis, sclerosis of arteries, miliary aneurisms of pial vessels, fatty degeneration of heart and liver, and "hog-back kidney."

Alkalies. Mucosa of mouth and œsophagus swollen and red, with desquamation of epithelium; mucosa of stomach swollen, dark brown and ecchymotic, with diphtheritic patches; croupous bronchitis may result from aspiration of caustic soda or potash, and bronchopneumonia from inhalation of ammonia. Stricture of the œsophagus, due to contraction of scar-tissue, may occur when the patient survives the immediate effects of the poison.

Antimony. In acute cases the mucosa of mouth, œsophagus and stomach is inflamed, with erosions and ulcerations; in chronic cases there is marked emaciation.

Arsenic. Mucosa of stomach œdematous, hyperæmic and ecchymotic; over the hæmorrhages there may be grayish-white sloughs or erosions. In these there may be found granules or crystals of the poison. The glands of the mucosa show cloudy swelling and fatty degeneration. Yellow sulphide of arsenic may be seen on the gastric mucosa. The small intestine is filled with a rice-water-like fluid, as in cholera, and the mucosa is congested, swollen and hæmorrhagic; the lymphoid tissue may be swollen. There is slight icterus, cloudy swelling of all organs and ecchymoses in pericardium and pleura. In chronic poisoning with dilute solutions characteristic gastrointestinal changes are wanting. In cases of suspected arsenic poisoning it is important to take portions of all organs and tissues for chemical examination.

Atropine. Death from asphyxia, resembles heat-exhaustion.

Chloral-hydrate. Hyperæmia of lungs, brain and cord. Examine urine.

Chloroform. Fatty degeneration of liver and heart. In delayed poisoning the liver shows picture of acute yellow atrophy, with marked icterus, widespread ecchymoses, cloudy swelling of kidneys and fatty degeneration of heart. Lungs, brain and liver may or may not give odor of chloroform.

Ergot. Sclerosis and contraction of arteries; gangrene of endometrium; in chronic cases sclerosis of the posterior columns of the cord.

Formalin. Corrosive action on mucosa of stomach; formic-acid in urine.

Hydrocyanic Acid and Potassium Cyanide. The mucosa of stomach is deep red, swollen, softened and sometimes translucent; soapy to the touch; odor of bitter almonds or ammonia; blood is fluid, dark or light cherry-red; red hypostasis.

Illuminating-gas and Carbon-monoxide. Blood fluid and cherry-red; cadaver life-like; pink hypostasis; carbon-monoxide-hæmòglobin in blood demonstrated by spectroscope. In poisoning by coal-gas the changes are less marked because of the greater amount of carbon dioxide present. Inhalation of smoke is shown by black, sooty deposits upon the mucosa of the respiratory tract.

Lead. In acute cases severe gastro-enteritis; black fluid in intestines; cloudy swelling of kidneys. In chronic cases arteriosclerosis, fatty degeneration of muscles, liver, kidneys and spleen; cirrhosis; blue line on gums.

Mercury. Mucosæ congested, ecchymotic or showing grayish-white eschars; diphtheritic inflammation of pharynx, colon and vagina; decalcification of bone;

cloudy swelling and calcification of kidney. In chronic cases ulcerative stomatitis.

Nitrobenzol. Cadaver cyanosed; blood and muscles brown; mucosa of stomach hyperæmic and ecchymotic; odor of bitter almonds; brownish methæmoglobin in collecting tubules of kidney.

Opium and Morphine. No characteristic findings. Condition of pupils not conclusive.

Phosphorus. In very acute cases there may be few changes; odor of phosphorus; cloudy swelling of heart, liver, kidneys and gastric mucosa. In subacute cases there is icterus, hæmorrhage, marked fatty degeneration of all organs; in chronic poisoning there is universal fatty degeneration, and not rarely a necrosis of the jaw-bone.

Potassium Chlorate. Hypostatic spots and blood are of chocolate color; methæmoglobinæmia; hæmorrhagic nephritis.

Ptomaines. Gastro-enteritis, fatty degeneration; icterus, cloudy swelling of kidneys.

Strychnine. Intense and persistent rigor mortis; blood fluid and dark as in asphyxia. Urine should be saved for the frog-test.

Other causes of death requiring especial consideration in a medicolegal examination are:—

Abortion. Determined by the finding of fœtal tissues, chorionic villi, decidua, enlargement of uterus, formation of sinuses at placental site, curetted surface, corpus luteum of pregnancy in ovary, punctures or lacerations of uterus and cervix, effects of corrosive fluids, infective endometritis, evidences of poisoning.

Asphyxia. Death due to lack of oxygen and excess of carbon dioxide, produced by interference with respiration, choking, drowning, hanging, paralysis of muscles of respiration, intoxication, etc. When respiration is suddenly checked ecchymoses are usually found in the pericardium, pleura, meninges, thymus, and rarely in peritoneum. Lips, skin of face and neck, and finger-nails may be deeply cyanotic; the blood is dark and fluid; passive congestion of lung is usually present. In death caused by hanging or strangling there may be fracture of the hyoid bone, thyroid cartilage or tracheal rings, marks upon the skin, hæmorrhage, laceration of the intima of the arteries, fracture or dislocation of the cervical vertebræ and injury to the cord. In death from drowning the bronchi, lungs and stomach may contain fluid, there is watery fluid in the pleural cavities, maceration of skin, greater water-content in blood of right heart than of left, with consequent raising of freezing point.

Infanticide. The points to be considered in determining the age and viability of the child are given in Chapter XIII. The most important causes of death in the new-born are also given in the same chapter.

Electric Shock. Burns of skin, "lightning figures," signs of asphyxia, laceration of internal organs.

Burns and Scalds. Extent of burn more important than depth of the burn; death usually ensues if one-third of the surface is burned. Burns show scorching, singeing or marks of the hot object; scalds usually show some action of the hot fluid on the skin or mucous membranes. Demonstration of carbon-monoxide in blood of internal organs proves the inhalation of carbon monoxide. When exposed to intense heat the soft parts of the body show marked shrinking.

Heat or Cold. No characteristic lesions in death from these causes. Diagnosis must be made by exclusion and history of case.

Starvation. Marked disappearance of fat and atrophy of all organs, stomach and small intestines empty, marked emaciation, blood anæmic, concentrated when subject was deprived of water.

Violence. Wounds must be minutely described as to character, degree of laceration, contusion, extravasation, damage to tissues, direction of force, character of instrument, means and method of infliction, path of projectile or stab-wound, etc. Postmortem changes and injuries must be differentiated, as must be also antemortem and postmortem lesions, primary and secondary effects of the injury, effects of injury and pre-existing diseases. Intracranial hæmorrhages must be carefully differentiated with respect to causation by violence or disease. Effects of *contrecoup* must be borne in mind. The presence of other marks of trauma, the exclusion of disease, the location of the clot, the age of the clot, the age of the patient, etc., are some of the factors to be considered. In young people without alcoholic history or syphilis intracerebral hæmorrhages without signs of violence are rare. When associated with fractured skull they are usually regarded as due to the trauma.

CHAPTER XV.
THE RESTORATION OF THE BODY.

When the autopsy is finished the body-cavities are cleansed and then thoroughly dried. No blood, stomach- or intestinal-contents should be left in the cadaver. All bleeding or dripping parts should be tightly secured; the anus and vulva should be tightly stitched, and the penis ligated. If necessary, the organs are then cleansed and returned to the body, as nearly as possible to their normal positions, although the brain, because of the difficulty of getting it back into the skull-cap, is usually put into the thoracic cavity. When several autopsies are done at the same time, care should be taken not to mix the organs. The undertaker should always be aided in his work; and, if he so desires, an embalming powder or fluid may now be sprinkled or poured into the cavities.

The skull-cap must be securely fastened in its normal position, so that no slipping can occur. If the body is not to be shipped any distance the posterior interlocking joint will usually hold it firmly in place if the scalp is drawn tightly together and closely stitched. When the body is to be moved some distance, the skull-cap must be more firmly fastened. This can be accomplished by drilling holes at the sides of the saw-cut and fastening the skull-cap to the cranium by means of copper wire, which must be tightly twisted and pressed flat against the bone. When this is done in the temporal region the wire is completely concealed by the temporal muscles when these are drawn up with the scalp, or if these have been cut away pads of cotton can be put in their place. The cranial fossæ and the skull-cap may be filled with plaster-of-Paris; while this is still soft a piece of wood may be pushed through into the foramen magnum and allowed to project high enough above the saw-cut to hold the skull-cap on, when it, filled with plaster, is put in position. With the setting of the plaster the skull-cap is firmly held. A little ingenunity will suffice to improvise various other methods of securing the skull-cap, by the use of bandages, metal pins, etc. After the employment of Harke's method the halves of the skull must be brought together and securely fastened at the base or in the occipital region. After resection of the temporal bone for the examination of the auditory apparatus the defect must be filled in with cotton or other substance, and the lower jaw and external ear restored to their normal positions. After examination of the orbit and the removal of the posterior half of the eye-ball a wad of red- or black-stained cotton should be used to fill out the eye so that it will have the same degree of fullness that the other eye has. When the eye is enucleated a glass-eye may be substituted and the lids fastened together by fine stitches made on the conjunctival side. If it is desired to save the skull-cap an artificial skull-cap may be molded from a square piece of pulp-board of the thickness of 0.5 cm. in the case of the adult, somewhat thinner for children. The pasteboard is soaked in warm water for about fifteen minutes, and is then molded over the skull-cap. It is then cut parallel with the edges of the saw-cuts so that the edge of the board will extend about 1 to 1.5 centimetres over the edges of the skull-cap to overlap the bones below the saw-cut. The cranial cavity is then filled with plaster or cotton. The pasteboard is removed from the skull-cap before it becomes too dry for its lower edge to be adapted easily to the lower border of the saw-cut. Ridges or folds are trimmed off with the knife and the surface made smooth. It is then adjusted and firmly fastened in position by passing several turns of strong twine around the lower border overlapping the cranial bones. The temporal muscles and the scalp-flaps are then drawn up and tightly stitched. A close base-ball stitch should be used to fasten the scalp-flaps, and a black thread should be used. If the scalp has been stretched so that it is loose and baggy, a portion of it may be cut out, so that when sewed together the flaps will fit tightly. The hair must be freed from all bone-dust and blood-clots, washed if necessary, then dried, and arranged in its former position in such a manner as to hide the sutures.

The place of any bone that has been removed may be filled by a piece of wood cut to the required proportions, and securely fastened by wire or bolts, or plaster-of-Paris may be poured about it and allowed to set. After removal of the spinal column or of portions of it, there may be substituted a block of wood or an iron pipe of suitable size, which may either be securely fastened above and below by means of wire or bolts, or it may be held in place by imbedding it in plaster-of-Paris. These expedients are not necessary after the removal of the cord alone, but only when entire sections of the spinal column are removed. When the cord is removed posteriorly the skin-incision is tightly closed with a base-ball stitch, and then covered with a strip of surgeon's plaster or collodion to prevent leakage of blood and serum after the body is turned over.

The thoracic and abdominal cavities are filled with dry bran, sawdust or finely-cut excelsior to fill out the normal contour, a piece of old cloth or paper is laid over the whole, and the sternum replaced. It is usually not necessary to fasten the latter, but if desired the costal cartilages may be stitched together, or wired when the needle cannot be pushed through the cartilage. When the tongue and neck-organs have been removed, the lower jaw must be held in position by fine stitches in the mucous membrane of the lips to prevent the jaw from dropping and leaving the mouth open. The contour of the neck may be restored by a pad of cotton.

The main-incision is then closed by a continuous base-ball stitch, using a stout linen pack-thread and a rather large, slightly curved needle. The first stitch begins in the middle-line about 1 cm. above the beginning of the main-incision, the needle being introduced from below through the incision, and the thread secured at its end by a knot. The stitches are then made about 5-7 mm. apart, the needle each time being pushed through the skin from the inside, so that it comes through the skin about 5 mm. on either side of the incision, alternately to the left and right. The thread is kept tightly pulled, and as perfect coaptation as possible is secured. At the end of the incision the thread is secured by a knot before it is cut. Collodion or surgeon's plaster may then be used to cover the entire incision. All other skin-incisions are sewed up in the same manner. When the testes and the body of the penis have been removed, it may be necessary under certain conditions to restore the form of these parts before the main-incision is closed. Cotton wads may be used for this purpose.

When all incisions are finally closed the cadaver is carefully washed and all blood-stains and discolorations removed. When formalin has been used as an injection-fluid blood spilled upon the skin may produce a brownish stain that is removed with difficulty. Corn-meal or hand-sapolio may be used to remove such stains. After the cadaver has been thoroughly washed, it is dried, and can then be turned over to the undertaker.

CHAPTER XVI.
OTHER SOURCES OF PATHOLOGIC MATERIAL.

1. **Autopsies on Animals.** In the case of the small animals used ordinarily for laboratory purposes, such as the mouse, rat, guinea-pig, rabbit, cat and dog, the animal is put upon its back and fastened to the autopsy-board either by small nails driven through the extremities or by slip-knots of string or rope passed over the latter. Autopsy board and holders designed especially for the purpose can be obtained from makers of laboratory apparatus. A main-incision is made in the anterior or median line from the chin to the genitalia, and the skin stripped back from the thorax on each side to expose the ribs. The thoracic cavity is then opened by cutting the ribs with the bone-shears or bone-forceps, and the sternum and cartilages are removed. The neck, thoracic and abdominal organs may then be removed *en masse* and examined outside the body, or the organs may be removed singly and examined in succession, following in general the same methods of procedure as in the autopsy on the human body, adapting the methods given above to differences in anatomic structure and size. For the opening of the skull and spinal canal the bone-forceps alone may be used, or in the case of larger animals the saw may be needed. Anatomic considerations should govern the method of opening the skull. Directions for the performance of autopsies on inoculated animals will be found in text-books on bacteriology; and veterinary methods of autopsies on the larger domestic animals are given in text-books on veterinary pathology. In all cases of autopsies on animals full protocols should be kept, following the general order of the autopsy, altered to suit the individual case.

2. **Surgical Operation.** A very large part of the material obtained for pathologic examination is removed by the surgeon for diagnostic purposes. The question of the surgical technique employed may be left to the surgeon, but as far as the pathologic aim is concerned certain principles should be followed, if the object of the examination is to be secured. Unfortunately these principles are not recognized by the great majority of practitioners, and pieces of tissue to be examined are taken at haphazard from the surface or from necrotic areas, to be run through by the pathologist, only

to find that no diagnosis is possible, either because the portion of tissue removed did not extend deeply enough or is wholly necrotic. Great care and judgment should be exercised in the choice of the portions to be removed for diagnosis. The part removed must be characteristic of the condition present. It is necessary not only to ascertain the character of the pathologic change but also the nature of the reaction in the surrounding tissue. A neoplasm may show the histologic structure of an adenoma, but at its periphery may be found infiltrating the neighboring tissues as an adenocarcinoma. If the piece of tissue for examination is removed from the central part or surface of the tumor, an incorrect diagnosis may be given. This is especially true in the case of rectal and uterine polypi, papillomata of the mouth and penis, horny warts, etc. The rule to be followed in all cases is that the excised portion must be at the boundary-line of the neoplasm or morbid process, and extending across it so as to include both pathologic and surrounding normal tissues. The cut must be deep enough to extend into living tissue, and in the case of epithelial surfaces to go below the basement membrane. It should be made at right angles to the surface. Necrotic, softened, or degenerating portions should be avoided, unless a portion of this is removed in addition for the purpose of ascertaining the nature of the degenerative changes present. The scraping away of superficial scabs, exudates, etc., should never be practiced for purposes of diagnosis. Time is saved if a satisfactory excision be made the first time, and to secure this the tissue must be living, the cut must be deep enough, and the portion removed must fully represent the nature of the condition present. When organs are removed, as in the case of the appendix, uterus, tubes, ovaries, mamma, etc., several portions of tissue representing different structures of the organ should be secured for the examination.

Tumors and other pathologic specimens received from the surgeon should be fully described as to *size, form, weight, consistence, color, relation to surrounding tissues* (encapsulated, well-defined borders, growth by infiltration or expansion, zone of inflammation, etc.), *character of cut-surface* (color, moisture, translucency, smooth or elevated, homogeneous, character of cell-scraping, evidences of structure, etc.). Accompanying all pathologic material sent to the pathologist should be concise and accurate notes giving the name, sex, age, nationality, occupation and status of the patient, anything in the individual or family history bearing upon the condition, the source of the specimen, its exact location and relations, manner of growth and character of operation. The pathologist should have full data upon which to construct his diagnosis. A very common idea among surgeons is that the specimen alone should be sufficient for the pathologist, and that other data are not necessary for the formation of his opinion. Many other considerations than the mere histologic picture presented by a specimen enter into the formulation of a pathologic diagnosis, if it is to bring to the aid of the surgeon all that a pathologist's knowledge and experience can give. This is particularly true when the pathologist, as is usually the case, is asked to give a prognosis. Both in hospital service and in private surgical practice it is best to have printed history forms to be filled out and to be sent to the pathologist with each specimen.

Another factor seriously interfering with the efficiency of the pathologist's work is the failure of the surgeon to see that the material removed for diagnosis is properly taken care of before it reaches the pathologist. Tissues removed for examination should never be allowed to dry. They should not be exposed to the air, but should either be placed at once in a fixing fluid or covered with damp cloth. Curettings should be placed for a moment upon a pad of gauze to remove the excess of blood, and the fragments of tissue are then picked up and put into the fixing solution. When sent by mail or express fresh tissues should be wrapped in damp cloth and then in rubber cloth; or if the distance is great they should be put into fixing fluids. A sufficient quantity of the latter should be used, or decomposition may take place before the specimen reaches the pathologist. All material for bacteriologic examination should be removed under proper precautions, put into sterilized vessels, properly sealed and sent to the pathologist under proper precautions.

PART II.

THE TREATMENT OF THE MATERIAL.

INTRODUCTION. The material obtained by autopsy, surgical operation, currettage, excision, spontaneous discharge, animal experimentation, etc., may be examined microscopically in the fresh state, or prepared for microscopic examination by methods of fixation, hardening and imbedding. The methods necessary for such histologic studies of pathologic material are given in the following pages, arranged as far as possible in their logical order. Only those methods are given that, in the light of the writer's experience, yield the best results, from the standpoints of economy of time, labor, and expense, and perfection of result. The number of histologic methods contained in the literature is so great that it is out of the question for the student or practical worker to try out all of them. To give all of these methods would create confusion. I have attempted to avoid this by giving in full detail only those which in our laboratory experience have yielded the best results. So many methods represent but slight variations of some original method, and in the great majority of cases these variations add so little or nothing of value to the original method that in such cases the latter alone is given in full, with references only to the variations of the method. The individual equation plays such a large part in the judgment of laboratory methods that allowance has been made for this when certain variations or alterations in original methods have been strongly recommended by expert laboratory workers.

The purpose of the microscopic examination is the revealment of pathologic changes too small to be recognized by the naked eye, and the securing of a diagnosis that cannot be made macroscopically, as well as the confirmation of diagnoses based upon the gross appearances. Aside from these more immediate practical considerations, the microscopic examination of tissues is concerned with the solution of etiologic and pathologic problems, and the extension of our knowledge of disease. The aim of pathologic technique is the fixation of tissues for microscopic examination in such a manner that all of the morphologic and chemical elements and constituents of the tissue are perfectly preserved, so that with differential staining methods they are all brought out with sufficient contrast to be readily and correctly identified. In a certain number of methods this ideal is attained, and to Weigert, more than to any other worker in the field of pathologic technique, are we indebted for such ideal methods.

The choice of methods will depend upon the source and nature of the material, the object of the examination, the time-element and the degree of responsibility involved. The cellular elements of all pathologic fluids, secretions and excretions should be examined in the fresh state as well as in fixed preparations. For the demonstration of various chemical and morphologic features that are lost or altered by processes of fixation and imbedding, and when a rapid diagnosis is required, the examination of the material in its fresh state or by the freezing method is indicated. When the freezing method cannot be employed because of the changes in cells and tissue produced by it, when very thin or serial sections are desired, when a rapid diagnosis is not required, and when a very careful and minute study is desired, with the application of various staining methods, then the material should be fixed, hardened and imbedded and cut upon a microtome. Whatever method is chosen, it must be borne in mind, particularly in practical diagnostic work, that the portions chosen for microscopic examination must represent the characteristic anatomic structures of the tissue or organ, that living tissue be included, that the pathologic condition be represented both in its fully-developed state and at the transition-border between it and the healthy tissue, and that when sections are cut the block or tissue must be so oriented as to give the most comprehensive view of the tissue and the pathologic process. To accomplish this fully it is often necessary to make a number of blocks representing different areas of the material, and to cut these in different planes.

CHAPTER XVII.
THE LABORATORY OUTFIT.

For practical diagnostic work or for pathologic research various instruments and utensils are necessary, although the expense of fitting up a working pathologic laboratory is not as great as it is often thought to be. The most expensive item, as well as the most important, is the **microscope.** This should be of the best make, and should be carefully selected and tested before the final purchase. As a rule the German makes, Zeiss, Leitz, and others, are to be preferred to the American instruments, in spite of the higher cost due to the duty imposed. I have found the German microscopes uniformly good and standing the wear and tear of a teaching laboratory much better than the American-made stands. I have never seen a poor Zeiss or Leitz objective, but cannot say the same thing of other makes. On the other hand, I have seen some American objectives that were as good as any German ones, but there are not many such. If one is going to buy an American microscope it should be bought on the same principle that one would buy a violin or a piano, wholly on its individual merits; and these can be ascertained only by having the instrument carefully examined and tested by an expert. Most laboratory workers will agree that the Zeiss instruments are the best; they are also the most expensive. For all practical purposes a Leitz stand costing ninety to one hundred dollars is quite good enough. A medium-sized continental stand, with rack and pinion and micrometer screw for coarse and fine adjustment, a triple nose-piece with dust-protector, Abbé condenser, iris diaphragm, plane and concave mirrors, three objectives (low, high and 1-12 oil-immersion), and two eye-pieces, a low and a high, form a complete outfit that answers all practical requirements. The new type of stand with curved arm and large stage, permitting the examination of all parts of a Petri dish or glass plate, and with the mechanism of the fine adjustment protected from any strain when the instrument is lifted by the arm is especially recommended. I have also found the black-finish very practical. The entire outfit need not be purchased at once; the stand with its accessories and a low power may first be purchased, and the higher-power objectives obtained later. One of the first luxuries is a movable adjustable stage. A very good and relatively cheap one is made by the Spencer Lens Co., of Buffalo. If a Zeiss stand is purchased the objectives A, D, and 1/12 oil-immersion, and oculars 2 and 4 best meet the requirements. Of the Zeiss apochromatic series, the objectives 16.0, 8.0, 4.0, and oil-immersion 2.0 mm., apert. 1.30, and oculars 4, 6 and 8 are most serviceable. The apochromatic objectives and the compensation-oculars are expensive, and need not be used for ordinary work, but are indispensable for photographic work. The Leitz

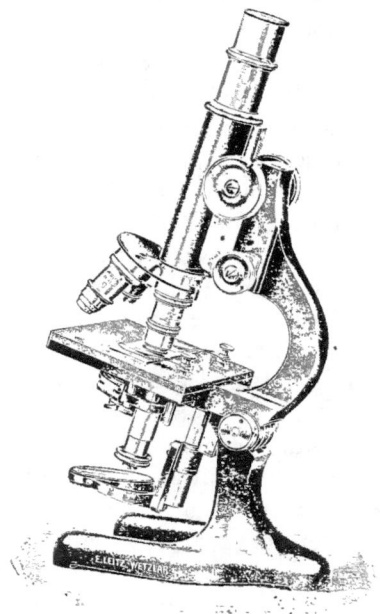

FIG. 50.—A satisfactory outfit for the working laboratory. Continental stand, medium-sized, with large stage, three objectives, etc.

objectives, 3, 6, or 7, and 1/12 oil-immersion, with oculars 2 and 4, and the equivalent objectives of the Spencer Lens Co. or Bausch and Lomb will answer all ordinary needs. For the purpose of microscopic measurements an ocular micrometer is necessary. This may be obtained as a separate eye-piece, or as a round piece of glass with measured divisions marked upon it that may be put into an ocular. The value of the scale must be determined for every lens and tube-length by estimating the number of its parts covering one part of a stage-micrometer marked in hundredths of a millimetre.

An instrument of any one of the above-mentioned makes, carefully selected and tested, should last its owner a life-time if proper care is taken of it. It should receive the same careful attention accorded a good violin or piano. It should be protected from dust, action of chemicals, heat, sunlight, and rough usage. When carried it should be supported in such a way that its weight is not thrown upon the thread of the adjusting screws. The adjustment, draw-tube and iris diaphragm should be carefully oiled at intervals, using the least possible amount of the best microtome oil. It is not necessary here to enter into the construction and theory of the microscope, as this knowledge has usually been obtained before the pathologic laboratory is reached. Experience has shown me, however, that it is always necessary to remind students, even those experienced for some time in the use of the microscope, of certain fundamental principles in the adaptation of microscopic technique to pathologic work. The following rules are of value:—

1. Use a *low-power* objective for all work except for the study of bacteria, microparasites and finer cell-structures. The aim should be to obtain as much of a bird's-eye view of the "geography" of the section as possible. Contrast plays a very important part in pathologic diagnosis; and it is lost in high-power work, so far as the relations of cells and tissue-elements and pathologic products are concerned. The student almost invariably enters the pathologic laboratory with a fixed "high-power habit," and he is usually greatly surprised to learn how much he misses with the high-power and how much he can see with the low-power. A motto used many years in my laboratory, "Low-power objective and high-power cortex," is of greater educational value than may appear at first sight. A slide should be examined first with the naked-eye, as it is held against a window or light; then it should be examined under the low power. Rarely will it be necessary to use a high-power except for the purposes mentioned above.

2. Weak eye-pieces should be used; strong ones darken the field and tire the eyes. Only in the case of apochromatic lenses and compensation oculars can the strong ones be used without darkening the field too much.

3. In the use of higher powers see that the tube is drawn out to the proper length, as indicated in the directions sent with the instrument.

4. For pathologic work an Abbé condenser is essential. It should be pushed up to its proper position beneath the stage, and the plane mirror should be used with it, reflecting the light from a cloud if possible. Daylight is always the best light. When this

cannot be obtained an incandescent or Welsbach lamp with ground-glass globe can be used. The concave mirror should then be used. The yellowish tint of artificial light may be avoided by the use of a piece of blue glass placed beneath the condenser, or a vessel of copper sulphate solution may be interposed. Especial lamps designed to meet the requirements are offered by the trade.

5. The iris-diaphragm should be adjusted by the same hand that moves the slide, usually the left one. With unstained preparations the diaphragm should be nearly closed; when using the oil-immersion it should be fully opened, as is also the case when stained preparations are studied with the lower power. With higher magnification the aperture is diminished somewhat, although color-effects are best shown with open diaphragm. In the study of pigments the diaphragm should be fully closed for a few moments to see if the pigment shows any color by reflected light. It is then examined by open diaphragm. In the study of sections the mirror and diaphragm should be manipulated in various ways to bring out all of the detail of the preparation, and should be adjusted to suit each preparation.

6. Objectives must never be screwed down until they strike the slide or stage. The higher-powers are frequently ruined in this way. When running the objective down always examine from the side to see that there is no danger of its striking the stage. In the use of the oil-immersion place the drop of oil upon the slide or cover-glass, and lower the objective by turning the coarse adjustment until the oil spreads out between the lens and the glass; then focus with the fine adjustment until a well-defined field is obtained. The oil-immersion lens should not be allowed to stand many consecutive hours in the oil. The oil should be cleaned from the lens by wiping the latter with lens-paper or a soft cloth; if the lens is sticky the paper or cloth may be moistened with benzol. The lens itself should never be *wet* with benzol, xylol, alcohol or any cleaning-fluid, because of the danger of softening the balsam in which the lenses are imbedded.

7. Use the mechanical stage only for differential blood-counting, or when the entire section is to be gone over carefully, or when certain details are found with difficulty and it is desirable to mark them for future reference. An immense amount of time is lost in the use of the mechanical stage for ordinary work. By moving the slide with the fingers of the left hand resting upon the stage an entire section may be gone over in a few seconds without missing

any part of it; to accomplish the same thing with the mechanical stage requires much more time.

It is an excellent plan for the student to purchase his microscope when entering the medical school and to use his own instrument throughout his course. It is the one instrument without which no physician can afford to enter practice; and the student who uses his own microscope before graduation will continue to use it afterward. The microscope obtained, the remaining expenditure necessary for the fitting-up of a practical working laboratory of clinical and pathologic diagnosis need not be very great if one's financial condition does not warrant spending with a free hand. It is possible with a little labor and ingenuity to make at home, or to show the local tinsmith how to make, a large part of the necessary apparatus, such as sterilizers, paraffin-ovens, drying ovens, thermo-regulators, etc., at a slight cost. Students of mine have made these things out of old tin cans and glass tubing; one student at a cost of less than three dollars constructed a microtome on which practical working sections could be cut. For the celloidin method no apparatus except the microtome is necessary, as the process of imbedding is carried on in bottles or dishes. These points are mentioned to offset the prevalent idea that a large expenditure is a necessity in installing a practical working laboratory.

In a large diagnostic laboratory, or in one intended for teaching and investigation, there are numerous accessories necessary to modern microscopic technique. For the observation of living objects a *warm stage* is needed. The simple electrical apparatus devised by Ross is the most convenient form, as it can be slipped on and off the slide without changing the focus. It can be attached to any electric light circuit and requires no attention.

For drawing from the microscope the improved form of the *camera lucida*, or the latest model of the *Edinger drawing-apparatus* are recommended. Both of these instruments have recently been greatly improved. The *Zeiss microphotographic apparatus* is by far the best for microphotographic work. For the *polarization-microscope, microspectroscope,* and the complicated and expensive *ultra-violet* and *dark-field* apparatus the worker is referred to the Zeiss catalogues. A simple and practical *dark-field* method for the illumination of bacteria, spirochætes and ultramicroscopic particles suspended in fluids requires only a strong illumination and the use of a *Zeiss, Leitz,* or *Reichert dark-field condenser;* or the very simple "India-ink" method may be used for the demonstration of spirochætes.

(See Staining of Spirochætes.) Especial instruments for easily finding a certain field are obtainable, and are of great convenience in marking slides for photographic purposes.

Next to the microscope the most important instrument in pathologic work is the **microtome.** One that can be used for either celloidin or paraffin work, and that can also be utilized as a freezing microtome, should be selected in private work, when economy is desired. The majority can be used for either paraffin or celloidin, and one of the Becker models can be easily attached to the carbonic

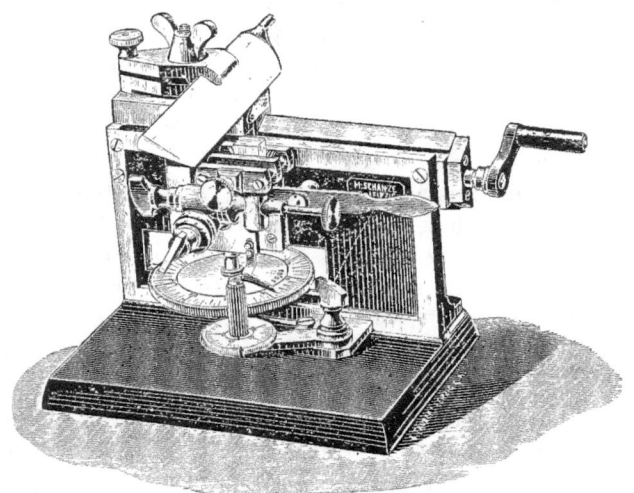

FIG. 51.—A good practical microtome for paraffin and celloidin work. Well-adapted to needs of students and beginners.

acid holder for the cutting of frozen material. The Bardeen freezing microtome is relatively inexpensive, very satisfactory, and can be easily attached to the carbonic acid tanks. It can be recommended for freezing work. The "slide" type, either that in which the knife-holder is moved by the hand directly or by a crank turned by the hand, is advised for ordinary diagnostic work. For students and beginners the crank is of great advantage, as the knife is securely held and cannot jump. The best microtomes are made by Schanze of Leipzig, Jung of Heidelberg, Becker of Göttingen, the Cambridge Scientific Co., the International Instrument Co., and the Bausch & Lomb Co. For either celloidin or paraffin work the medium or large Schanze slide-microtome or the Minot's precision microtome are recommended; for cutting serial sections in paraffin the latest modification of the Minot automatic rotary microtome is especially adapted. The best **microtome knives** are made by Walb of Heidelberg. A long, heavy knife is to be preferred to a light one. For the freezing microtome a knife of the type of the blade of a carpenter's plane set in a wooden handle should be used. Hones and strops of the best quality are necessary.

Paraffin-ovens and **drying-ovens** of suitable size, and constructed preferably of copper, are necessary for paraffin work. The water-space about the oven should be sufficiently large, and the temperature should be controlled by a thermo-regulator. Various models are offered in the trade, but they can be made more cheaply by the local tinsmith. The thermo-regulator can also be home-made by anyone who has the necessary training in glass-blowing usually given in courses in bacteriology.

Various instruments and **utensils**, such as *razors, double-bladed knives, forceps, spatulas, section-lifters, needles, scalpels, scissors, glass rods* and *tubing, test-tubes, graduates, flasks, funnels, bottles, staining dishes, reagent bottles, rubber tubing, water-bath, tripods, centrifuge, Bunsen burners, asbestos pads, gauze, filter-papers, absorbent paper, labels, oil* and *wax colored pencils, slides, cover-glasses, slide-boxes, camel's-hair brushes, glass droppers, platinum wire*, etc., are required for the pathologic laboratory, and can be chosen to suit the individual needs. The solid watch glasses make very good small staining dishes; the enamelled trays and glass dishes used in photographic work are especially adapted to the plate-method, particularly the size used for the 4 x 5 plate. Tea-strainers or small sieves can be used for staining a large number of celloidin sections; and there are different types of staining-dishes designed for the staining of slide- and cover-glass preparations in number. Slides should be of the best quality, colorless and with ground edges, and of medium thickness. Cover-glasses should be square or oblong, round covers having but little use in pathology. For ordinary work the No. 2 square, ¾ inch, is recommended; for work with the higher-power dry objectives a thinner cover must be used. Slides and covers may be cleaned by placing them in a solution of equal parts of one per cent sulphuric and chromic acids and then rinsing in distilled water. A good cleaning fluid is also made of one part acetic acid to three of 80 per cent alcohol. To clean old mounts melt the balsam by heat or dissolve in turpentine, separate slides and covers, boil in ten per cent lysol for half an hour, or for ten minutes in the sulphuric-chromic-acid mixture, rinse thoroughly, dry with cloth having no lint.

The laboratory should be supplied with running water, a sink large enough for washing out specimens, numerous stop-cocks, and a drip-board. Distilled water in abundance must be available. The laboratory-table should have an alcohol- and xylol-proof finish, black on the whole being the most practical color. A portion of the table should be covered with glass beneath which there is laid a sheet of white paper.

CHAPTER XVIII.
THE EXAMINATION OF FRESH MATERIAL.
I. METHODS OF EXAMINATION.

Pathologic material is examined in the fresh state when it is desired to make a diagnosis in the shortest time possible, or when the processes of fixation and hardening produce such alterations in the morphology and chemic constitution of the cells that these features can be recognized only in the unfixed, fresh state. So far as the saving of time is concerned it is possible to take material removed during an operation, examine it in the fresh state, and return a diagnosis to the surgeon, while the patient is still on the table under the influence of the anæsthetic. It is not possible to do this with all tissues or with all pathologic conditions; but, when it can be done, the advantages of such a rapid diagnosis, in the saving of time, labor, expense and danger to the patient, are obvious. The best idea of the cell is also gained by its study in a fresh condition. Vital phenomena and certain morphologic features, as cilia, can be observed only in fresh material. Many of the chemic constituents of cells (glycogen, fat, mucin, pseudomucin, albumin-granules, cholesterin, etc.) are either lost, or are so changed by processes of fixation or hardening that they can no longer be recognized. The majority of specific chemic tests can be made in fresh tissues only. Moderate and slight degrees of fatty degeneration and cloudy swelling are easily recognized in the fresh state; in fixed and hardened preparations they may not be recognized at all. Particularly in the case of the heart-muscle is it necessary to make an examination of the fresh material when the diagnosis of these conditions is concerned. Further, a greater or less degree of shrinking is caused by many of the agents used in fixing and hardening, and this is avoided by the examination of the fresh material. In the case of pathologic fluids (sputum, urine, féces, etc.) an examination of the sediment in the fresh state should always be made as a matter of routine. The formed elements of these fluids are best determined by this means. In the case of tissues, a diagnosis made by means of scrapings, smears, teased bits of tissue, frozen sections, etc., should always be controlled by the examination of fixed and hardened material.

In the examination of fresh material the following methods are employed: *Sedimentation, smears, scraping, crushing, teasing, maceration, sections, shaking or penciling, digestion, intravital staining, injection, the warm stage and "cultivation."*

1. **Sedimentation.** The formed elements of pathologic fluids (urine, sputum, pus, blood, exudates, transudates, cyst-contents, etc.) are examined by collecting the sediment of such fluids from the bottom of a sedimenting glass or bottle, by means of a capillary pipette controlled by the finger. While the sediment is passing up into the tube the pipette should be moved about the bottom of the vessel so as to get some of the sediment from all parts. When the fluid is rich in cellular elements sedimentation is not necessary; a drop of the fluid is placed upon the slide; if too thick it is diluted with physiologic salt-solution or serum. If poor in cellular elements the fluid must be centrifugalized by means of a water- or electric-centrifuge; and a drop of the sediment in the centrifuge tube is then removed by the pipette and placed upon the slide, and covered with a cover-glass. To facilitate the low-power examination of such sediments parallel streaks upon the slide may be made across its entire length, and examined without the use of cover-glasses. To apply the various reagents mentioned below it becomes necessary to use a cover-glass as directed.

2. **Smears.** A clean fresh cut is made into the organ or tissue, and a clean slide or cover-glass is drawn across the surface. Without permitting the smear to dry a drop of salt-solution or any desired reagent is put upon it, and it is then examined. This method is especially applicable to the study of the cells of the spleen, bone-marrow, lymphnodes, etc. Permanent balsam-mounts may be made of such smears by fixing with heat or alcohol and ether, staining, drying and mounting.

3. **Scraping.** A fresh cut is made into the organ or tissue, and the excess of blood absorbed by a pad of absorbent paper devoid of lint. A clean scalpel held at an angle of 45° is then drawn with some force back and forth over the cut-surface until its blade collects a sufficient amount of "tissue-juice" made up of the cells of the tissue. This is then put upon a slide, and covered with salt-solution or any desired reagent, and is then examined. This method is used especially for cellular infiltrations, soft tumors, and parenchymatous organs (spleen, lymphnodes, bone-marrow, liver, etc.), and for the inner wall of cysts (echinococcus-cysts, cysts lined with ciliated epithelium).

4. **Crushing.** A small bit of the tissue is cut out with the scissors or scalpel, and placed upon the slide. A cover-glass is then placed upon it and pressed down so firmly that the bit of tissue is spread out in a thin film or layer beneath the cover-glass. Reagents are introduced beneath the cover-glass, as desired. (See below.) This method is used in the examination of the lung, kidneys and brain for fatty embolism, and of the brain and spinal-cord for "fat-granule" cells, pigment, calcified ganglion-cells, Negri bodies, etc. It is also frequently used in the bacteriologic examination of tissues (crushing of tubercles, etc.).

5. **Teasing.** A small bit of the tissue is cut out and placed upon the slide or in a staining-dish and covered with physiologic salt-solution. It is then teased with fine needles until divided into its ultimate elements. Hard tumors (mature connective-tissue tumors, fibrosarcomata, etc.), muscle (examination for trichina), nerve-trunks, etc., are best examined in this way.

6. **Maceration.** In the case of some tissues the ultimate histologic elements are so firmly held together that they cannot be separated without the aid of a *macerating-* or *dissociation-fluid*. (See below.) **Digestion** is also used for the same end. The tissue should be as fresh as possible and cut into small bits, which are placed in the maceration-fluid in watch-glasses or staining-dishes for twenty-four hours or longer. The macerated bits are then teased until the finest elements are separated. In the case of very minute elements the teasing may be carried on under a hand-lens or the stereoscopic binocular microscope. During the process of maceration all parts of the macerating tissue must be kept covered with the macerating-fluid, or the uncovered portions will become hardened.

7. **Section-cutting.** Sections of fresh tissue may be made with the *curved shears, simple razor, double-bladed razor* and the *freezing-microtome*.

a. *Curved Shears.* The tissue is put upon a stretch, and from the surface a thin, flat section is cut out with the scissors. With care a fairly thin section may be obtained in this way. It may be examined by pressing it upon a slide beneath a cover-glass, or it may be treated as a frozen section.

b. *Simple Razor.* As a part of their required laboratory training medical students should learn how to make working sections with a simple razor. Such a technical knowledge is sure to be of practical use at some time or other. With a little practice sections sufficiently thin for ordinary diagnostic work can be cut. If the piece of tissue is large it may be held in the hand; but when small or soft it may be placed in a matrix of hardened liver, pith, potato, apple, firm lard or butter, paraffin, etc., and cut at the same time with the latter. Both blade and tissue should be wet with physiologic salt-solution. The blade, which must be very sharp, should be *drawn* through the tissue by a shoulder movement, with the wrist-joint fixed. As the sections are cut they are floated off of the razor-blade into physiologic salt-solution, and thence treated as desired.

c. Double-bladed Knife. This consists of two parallel blades arranged so that the space between them can be changed by means of screws. For firm material the blades should be close together; for soft material farther apart. The blades should be dipped into physiologic salt-solution to fill up the space between the blades. The instrument is then drawn through the tissue, and the section between the blades floated out in salt-solution. Some workers use this double-bladed knife to make a perpendicular cut into the tissue, then turning it to either side to cut the lower edge of the section and removing the blades with the section between them. Both the single- and the double-bladed razors require practice for successful section-cutting. Further, it must be borne in mind that sections of fresh tissue obtained by these methods are unsuited for complicated staining methods and can be used only for the simplest staining processes. Nevertheless, in a fairly large proportion of pathologic conditions it is possible to secure a diagnosis by these methods.

d. Freezing Microtome. Much more satisfactory sections can be obtained by freezing the fresh tissue and cutting it upon the **freezing microtome.** Various types of these instruments are in the market. The freezing is accomplished by the use of *ether, ethyl-chloride* or *fluid carbonic acid gas.* The ether and ethyl-chloride freezing-microtomes consist essentially of a metal plate or hollow box on which the tissue rests and against the under-surface of which a spray of ether or ethyl-chloride is forced by means of a rubber bulb connected with a supply of the freezing agent in a bottle. Such freezing attachments can be attached to any microtome, but special instruments as Jung's "student's freezing microtome," Cathcart's, Bausch and Lomb's or Becker's ether-freezing microtome can be recommended for this purpose. (See Fig. 52.) The tissue to be frozen must be of small size and not more than 3-4 mm.

thick. It is placed upon the freezing plate in a drop of water, white of egg or thick gum-arabic, and pressed firmly against the plate. The spray must not be too constant or strong, but should be given with regular pauses of about a second to allow the ether to evap-

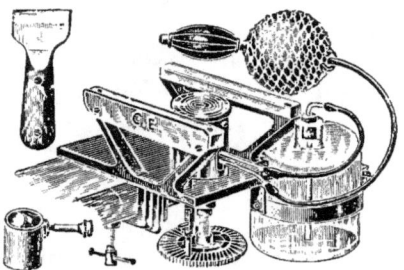

Fig. 52.—Type of freezing-microtome, for the use of ether or ethyl-chloride. Cathcart model.

orate. The tissue must be firmly frozen, but not so hard that it crumbles. It is usually difficult to freeze the upper part of the tissue hard enough to give good sections, and this half-frozen tissue must be trimmed off with the knife until good sections are secured. As the sections are cut they are removed from the knife-blade with the finger and put into physiologic salt-solution that has been recently boiled to drive off the air, so that, in thawing, there may be no formation of air-bubbles in the tissue to cause artefacts. If put into strong alcohol diffusion-currents may damage the tissue; a succession of graded solutions should, therefore, be used if the sections are to be fixed and hardened. The further treatment of frozen sections is given below. The relative slowness of the method of freezing, its greater cost, the necessity of the frequent replacement of the rubber bulbs and tubing, and the greater amount of trouble required by the use of ether or ethyl-chloride are disadvantages that can be avoided by the use of the carbonic acid freezing microtome. Where much work is done by the freezing method the use of the latter is advised.

The *carbonic acid outfit* consists of a microtome arranged so that it can be connected with a cylinder of compressed carbonic acid gas, as shown in the Aschoff-Becker or Bardeen models. (Figs 53 and 54.) The cylinders or drums containing a charge of 15-30 lbs. of the liquid carbonic-acid are furnished by the trade at reasonable rates. It is not necessary to buy the drums, as they are replaced by full ones as needed. They are provided with valves and can be fastened in an upright position or laid flat upon a table, in any way convenient for the attachment to the microtome. Connection is made between the valve of the cylinder and the object-holder of the microtome by means of strong rubber tubing which should be securely wired at

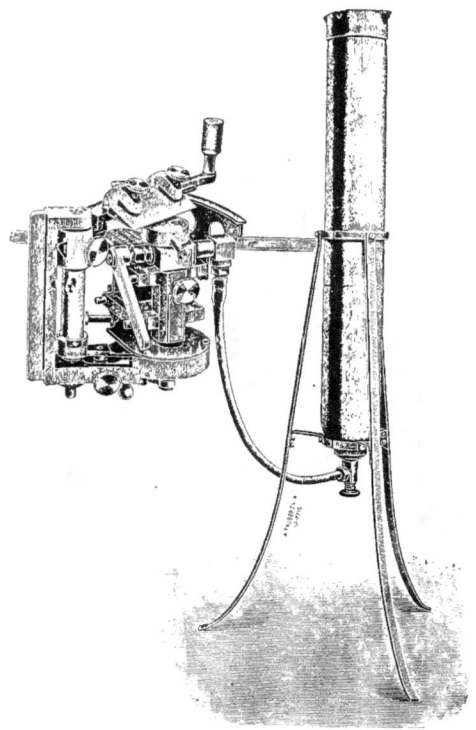

FIG. 53.—Carbonic-acid freezing-microtome. Becker model.

both ends, or by a flexible metallic tube. The latter is preferable, as the rubber-tubing often bursts, or is so stretched by the pressure of the gas that it must be frequently replaced. Object-holders with flexible metallic tube attachment for use in an ordinary microtome are supplied by Bausch and Lomb and other firms. My personal experience makes me prefer the Bardeen freezing microtome (see Fig. 54) to all others. It is cheap and can be easily attached to the valve of the gas-cylinder, which is fastened horizontally to the tabletop, as it has a screw-thread fitted to the uniform thread of the drum-valve. The object-holder can be raised or lowered between the glass-tracks on which the knife runs, so that sections of a definite thickness can be obtained. The most satisfactory knife is that of the type of a plane-bit set in a wooden handle. (See Fig. 55.) It must be well honed and stropped. The tissue, which should not be more than 5 mm. thick, is placed upon the object-holder in a drop of water, albumin fixative, or saturated solution of gum-arabic, and pressed firmly against the plate as the gas is turned on slowly and evenly. Freezing is usually accomplished in one-half to one minute.

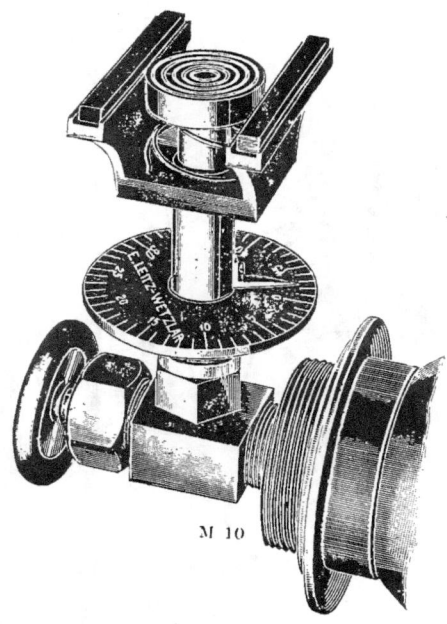

Fig. 54.—Bardeen freezing-microtome attached to carbonic-acid gas-cylinder.

The best results are obtained by turning the gas on for about 15-20 seconds, then turning it off for several seconds; the tissue will continue to freeze; if not hard enough the gas is turned on again for 15 seconds and then turned off. If necessary this may be repeated until the tissue is properly frozen. The interruption of the gas-flow prevents over-freezing and thereby lessens the amount of change in the cells. When sufficiently frozen the gas is then turned off; the knife, with bevel-edge down, is held in the right hand with its handle between the palm and the ball of the thumb with the back of the hand uppermost; and the edge of the knife set at an angle of 45° to the tracks, along which it is rapidly pushed back and forth, shaving the sections from the frozen tissue as the latter is pushed up above the level of the tracks by means of the micrometer screw turned with the left hand. The screw should have been adjusted at the proper height before freezing, so that no time is lost in getting the object-holder up to the height for cutting. By holding the elbow and fore-arm closely against the body and pushing from the elbow with wrist-joint fixed the shaving of sections can be accomplished very quickly, so that with one freezing several hundred sections can be obtained. The microtome-screw should not be turned by the left hand until the knife on its return has cleared the tissue. A little practice in co-ordinating movements is necessary for expert work. The sections should be allowed to collect upon the knife-blade until a large number have been cut; they are then swept off the blade by the finger into cold freshly-boiled phys-

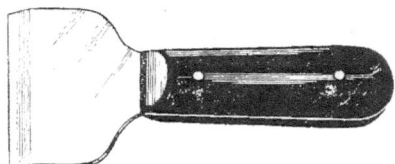

FIG. 55.—Knife for Bardeen freezing-microtome.

iologic salt-solution. Sections of tissue that have been previously fixed can be put into 60 per cent alcohol, where the sections will unroll and straighten out perfectly flat. When the method of freezing by alternately turning on and off the gas, as given above, is followed, and the amount of freezing in the interval noted, there is no danger of over-freezing, and the breaking and crumbling of sections, with the production of marked artefacts, is avoided. When over-freezing has occurred the block may be partly thawed out by the finger. But *over-freezing,* as well as *repeated freezing and thawing,* may cause so much damage to fresh tissue that a diagnosis cannot be obtained from the frozen sections. After thawing out in the physiologic salt-solution the sections of fresh tissue obtained by freezing are treated according to the methods given in the next section of this chapter.

It must be emphasized here that the process of freezing is an active one, and alters the relation of cell-structures. With many fresh tissues the changes resulting from the freezing are so great that no diagnosis can be made. It seems necessary here to warn against the routine employment of the rapid method of freezing and staining fresh tissues in the diagnosis of material obtained by surgical operation. It has become a fad with some surgeons to make a pathologic diagnosis by the freezing method while the patient is on the table. Consequently, as the result of diagnoses made by the rapid freezing and staining method, many mistakes are made, even by supposed experts in this line. Particularly in the diagnosis of sarcoma is it easy to make mistakes because of the altered aspect of the cells caused by freezing. Normal lymphnodes, tonsils and inflammatory infiltrations may look like spindle-cell sarcoma in the sections prepared by the rapid freezing and staining method; and the exact nature of many other pathologic conditions cannot be accurately determined from such sections. On the other hand, a certain number of pathologic conditions can always be recognized in sections obtained in this way, and this fact justifies the employment of the method when properly controlled. *In all cases in which the pathologic condition is not clearly evident in sections obtained by the rapid freezing and staining method no diagnosis should be given.* In such cases the tissue should be fixed and then cut upon the freezing-microtome, or imbedded in celloidin or paraffin and then cut. Even when the patient is upon the table the tissue removed can be put into a 10 per cent formol solution for a few minutes and then frozen directly in gum without washing out the formalin. The longer the time that can be used for this short preliminary fixation the better the sections will be and the less the production of artefacts by the freezing. The process of fixation can be hastened by warming the fixing-fluid. I advise this short fixation before freezing in all cases of operative diagnostic work when the diagnosis is wanted as soon as possible. For all other work with the freezing microtome, when the question of time is not so important, fixation with formol for 12-24 hours should be carried out. This combination of formol-fixation and the freezing method permits the early diagnosis of autopsy and operation material, makes possible the demonstration of fat and other substances altered or dissolved out by the imbedding methods, and is a convenient way of selecting tissues requiring more complicated staining processes. (See also Page 239.) The further treatment of sections of fresh tissue obtained by freezing will be found in the second section of this chapter.

8. **Penciling or Shaking.** For the demonstration of the stroma or reticulum either fresh or fixed sections may be placed upon a slide in an abundance of fluid and gently penciled with a fine, blunt camel's hair brush until the fluid becomes cloudy. The cloudy fluid is washed away and replaced by fresh as long as cells are given off. The same results may be obtained by shaking the sections in a test-tube until the cells are shaken out of the stroma. The removal of the cells from the section is shown by its greater

transparency. One of the practical applications of these methods in diagnostic work is the differentiation between alveolar round-cell sarcomata and carcinomata.

9. **Digestion.** For the demonstration of stroma, parasites, etc., the tissues may be digested with gastric or pancreatic ferments until the required elements are freed. A freshly prepared pepsin in 0.2 per cent HCl in the incubator for 3-5 hours will digest fibrin in fresh clots. Sections of fixed tissues may be imbedded in paraffin, cut, and digested on the slide with Grübler's pancreatin according to the method of Flint.

10. **Intravital and Supravital Staining.** Various methods have been advised for the intravital staining of cell-granules. Intravenous or intraperitoneal injections of methylene blue, alum carmine, neutral red and other stains will produce intracellular granule-staining in various organs of experimental animals. In the study of low forms of animal life staining solutions may be injected, or the animal or its parts may be examined in staining fluids. Human material can be examined by this method immediately after being removed from the body by operation or within 1-2 hours after death. (For details of these methods see article on *"Färbungen, intravitale," Encyklopädie der mikroskopischen Technik.*)

11. **Injection.** Injections for the demonstration of blood-vessels, lymphatics, ducts of glands, etc., are rarely used in pathologic work. The organs to be injected must be fresh, warm from the body, if possible. The vessels should be washed out by a freshly filtered 8 per cent sodium nitrate or sodium sulphate solution, followed by physiologic salt-solution. A cannula is introduced into a main vessel, tightly secured, and then connected with a syringe or a gravity injection-apparatus giving a constant pressure. The injection-mass is then injected under a low pressure. In the case of injections into lymphatic vessels the cannula should be introduced into the largest lymphatics at the periphery of the blood-vessels where larger lymph-vessels are more easily found. Injections are made with either cold or warm solutions; the latter are preferable but require that the organ to be injected be warmed by immersing it in water at a temperature of 40°C. The injection fluid must be of the same temperature. After the warm injection is given the organ is put into ice-cold 10 per cent formol solution until fixed and then after-hardened, imbedded and stained as desired. After the use of cold injections the tissues are fixed in 10 per cent formol, alcohol, or any other desired solution, and treated according to the end sought.

Nuclear and diffuse stains contrasting with the color of the injection mass should be used. The process of injection requires great care; the pressure must be carefully regulated to prevent extravasations, and the injection-fluid must be free from air-bubbles. The injection is continued until the organ appears diffusely stained. Blood-vessels are fixed in their natural blood-injection by such agents as formol and chromic acid, so that stains acting upon the red blood cells cause the veins and capillaries to appear as if they had been injected.

The following injection masses are advised:—

1. **Cold Injection Mass (Beale's Glycerin Carmine):—**
Dissolve 0.3 grm. of carmine in a small quantity of water containing 5 drops of ammonia; add 15 cc. of glycerin and shake; add drop by drop 15 cc. of glycerin containing 8-10 drops of glacial acetic acid. Then add further glycerin 15 cc., alcohol 8 cc., and water 24 cc.

2. **Warm Injection Mass (Thiersch's Berlin-blue Gelatin):—**
   (*a*) Dissolve 1 part of gelatin in 2 parts of water by allowing it to soak 24 hours, and then warming. Filter through flannel.
   (*b*) Saturated water solution of ferrous sulphate.
   (*c*) Saturated water solution of red ferricyanide of potassium.
   (*d*) Saturated water solution of oxalic acid.

Make a solution (*1*) by adding 30 cc. of *a* to 12 cc. of *b*, and a solution (*2*) by adding 24 cc. of *c* to 60 cc. of *a*; both mixtures to be made at a temperature of 30°C. At same temperature add 24 cc. of *d* to solution *2*, and then solution *1*, stirring constantly so that Berlin blue is precipitated. Heat on a water-bath to 90°C.; filter through flannel.

3. **Fischer's Milk-Method.** The vessels are flushed with 8 per cent sodium nitrate or sulphate solution, and then injected with milk. When sufficiently injected the tissue is hardened for 24 hours in a solution of water, 1,000 cc., formalin (40 per cent formaldehyde) 75 cc., and glacial acetic acid 15 cc. Freeze, cut and stain with Sudan III or Scharlach R.; the course of the vessels is outlined by the fat-globules.

4. **Silbermann's** method of injecting indigo-carmine, eosin or phlosin-red into the circulating blood has been used for the demonstration of capillary thrombi, the latter remaining free from the pigment.

12. **Warm Stage.** For the study of vital phenomena in the living cell *Ross's electrical warmer* is recommended. It can be slipped on and off the slide without changing the focus, and is managed without any difficulty. It keeps the centre of the slide at a temperature of 37°C. Reagents can be applied as desired. Deetjen's agar may be used as a medium for the preservation of living cells. (See Methods of Blood-Examination.) Various forms of warm and moist chambers used in experimental embryological work can also be utilized in experimental pathology.

13. **Tissue-cultivation.** The embryologic methods of growing tissues in lymph and blood-plasma as developed by Harrison, Burrows and Carrel have been applied in pathologic work to the experimental study of repair and regeneration, grafting, transplantation and tumor-transplantation. (For methods see *Harrison,* Journal of Exper. Zoology, 1910; *Burrows,* Jour. of Amer. Med. Assoc., 1910; *Carrel,* Jour. of Amer. Med. Assoc., 1910.)

II. REAGENTS USED IN THE EXAMINATION OF FRESH TISSUES.

In the examination of fresh tissue it is often desirable to use certain reagents for the purpose of making chemical tests or to bring out some structures more prominently than others. To introduce these reagents beneath the cover-glass in such a way as to get the desired effect without disturbing given fields requires some practice with a very simple technical method. The preparation is first examined in salt-solution, and the cover-glass adjusted so that it has a slight rim of fluid about its edge, but not enough to make it float. The reagent to be applied is dropped with a glass-dropper at one side of the cover-glass, while at the other the salt-solution is removed slowly by a piece of absorbent paper. The changes produced in the tissue-elements during the progress of the reagent can be observed under low or high powers. Care must be taken to change the fluids so slowly that isolated cells will not be washed away.

1. **Physiologic or Indifferent Fluids.** Serous exudates, blood-serum, hydrocele fluid, etc.; artificial serum made by a mixture of 9 parts physiologic salt-solution with 1 part white of egg; or physiologic salt-solution (0.9 per cent for warm-blooded animals, 0.6 per cent for cold-blooded).

2. **Maceration Fluids.** 33 per cent alcohol (24 hours); chromic acid 1:5000 (24 hours); potassium bichromate 0.1-0.2 per cent solution (2-4 days for nervous tissue); 0.1 per cent osmic acid (12-24 hours); 33 per cent potassium hydroxide ($\frac{1}{4}$-1 hour, for muscle, tissue must be examined in the solution, as the cells dissolve when water is added); Arnold's iodine solution (10 parts of a 10 per cent potassium iodide solution to which are added 5-10 drops of a solution containing 5 grms. of iodine and 10 grms. of potassium iodide in 100 cc. of water. Macerate one or more days. If solution becomes discolored add more of the second solution); very dilute formol solutions (1 cc. to 500 cc. physiologic salt-solution); Müller's fluid (2-3 days, good for nervous tissue).

3. **Glycerin.** Used without diluting as a *clearing agent,* particularly when pigment is present; and as a *mounting medium* for stained preparations that cannot be put into alcohol.

4. **Potassium Acetate.** Saturated water solution for clearing and mounting fresh preparations. Does not clear as strongly as glycerin, hence is better adapted for the examination of fresh tissues.

5. **Acetic Acid.** 1-2-5 per cent solutions are usually employed. Clears the protoplasm and causes the nucleus to shrink slightly and to stand out more distinctly. It differentiates fatty and albuminous granules, dissolving the latter; and is useful in the demonstration of elastic tissue fibres, sharply outlining these against the connective-tissue which swells and becomes clear.

6. **Acetic Acid Fuchsin.** A few drops of fuchsin are added to a 2 per cent solution of acetic acid. With this solution the nuclei are not only brought out more sharply but they are stained red.

7. **Lugol's Solution.** Dilute Lugol's solution to a pale yellow color. It brings out the contours of cell and nucleus, and has a specific reaction with glycogen and amyloid, giving both a brown color. Since glycogen is dissolved out in water-solutions tests for glycogen in fresh tissues should be made with iodine-glycerin or iodine-gum (Lugol's one part, gum arabic 100 parts). Smears or cover-glass preparations may be placed in covered dishes containing a few crystals of iodine.

8. **Potassium and Sodium Hydroxides.** In solutions of 1-3 per cent all tissue-structures swell and dissolve or become unrecognizable except elastic fibres, fat, pigment, amyloid, bacteria, yeasts and moulds. Used especially for examination of skin-scrapings or pus for presence of blastomyces and various forms of parasitic moulds (barber's itch, ringworm, tinea, etc.). Solutions of 33 per cent clear the tissues but do not destroy the cells. Useful for maceration. When diluted the cells are destroyed.

9. **Mineral Acids.** HCl or H_2SO_4 (3-5 per cent). Used to dissolve areas of calcification. Calcium dissolves with liberation of CO_2; the phosphates dissolve without gas-formation, but with H_2SO_4 form crystals of calcium sulphate. Sulphuric acid is also used as a test for cholesterin (red or violet coloration), and with iodine as a test for amyloid.

10. **Osmic Acid.** In a 1 per cent solution this is used to test for the presence of fat (oleates), the fat-droplets become black or brown.

11. **Sudan III or Scharlach R.** Alcoholic solutions of these dyes are used for the demonstration of fat in fresh tissues. They stain fat orange to scarlet. (For method see Staining of Fat.)

12. **Alcohol and Ether.** Used to dissolve fat-granules and to differentiate between these and albuminous granules.

13. **Stains.** Fuchsin, methylene blue, methylene green in 1 per cent solutions in physiologic salt-solution and acetic-acid-fuchsin are the best stains used for the examination of fresh-tissues beneath the cover-glass. They are drawn under the cover-glass according to the method given above.

For the rapid staining of sections of fresh tissue cut by freezing a section is floated from the salt-solution onto a slide, which is then carefully lifted from the salt-solution and the excess of the latter removed. Several drops of methylene blue, carbol-thionin or carbol-kresyl-echt-violett are run upon the section with the glass-dropper, and allowed to remain for 15-30 seconds. The stain is then washed off with salt-solution, a cover-slip put on and the section examined in the salt-solution. Thionin has been especially recommended (Wood, Strouse and others) for the rapid staining of frozen sections; but I prefer to use carbol-kresyl-echt-violett (kresylechtviolett 1 grm., 5 per cent aqueous solution of phenol 80 cc., 95 per cent alcohol 20 cc.). This gives a very good differentiation in the section examined in water, and the picture is clearer than with thionin; the specific staining-reactions with mucin, amyloid, mast-cells, etc., are also more marked than with the latter stain. Such sections are not as clear as dehydrated and cleared sections and their possibilities of diagnosis are correspondingly limited, even in the hands of an expert with sections of this kind.

To make permanent balsam-mounts of the frozen unfixed sections the latter must be fixed in formol or alcohol, or by heat (hot water). The sections may be placed in 4 per cent formol for several minutes, then into 80 per cent alcohol, then stained, washed, dehydrated in absolute alcohol, cleared in carbol-xylol and finally mounted in balsam. Hæmatoxylin and eosin may be used for the staining. Fresh sections may also be fixed in hot water, stained in hæmatoxylin, dehydrated in alcohol and cleared in xylol. To save time the sections may be fixed on the slide for a few minutes in alcohol, care being taken to prevent the sections from rolling up by dropping the alcohol onto the middle of the section after it has been carefully flattened out on the slide. The section may then be stained with hæmatoxylin, borax-carmine or other stains, dehydrated, cleared and mounted in balsam. After fixing with alcohol on the slide the section may be attached to the slide by blotting it with absorbent paper, then covering section with absolute alcohol, draining this off after a few seconds and then running over the section a thin solution of celloidin, which is allowed to drain off, leaving a very thin film over the section and slide. The latter is then immersed in water for a few seconds, and the celloidin-film on setting holds the section to the slide, provided the celloidin has been of proper consistence. The section can now be stained, washed, dehydrated, cleared in origanum and mounted in balsam. When mounted the thin film of celloidin is invisible (Wright's method).

I have originated a much better method which is in use in my laboratory, and can be applied to the staining of frozen sections of fresh tissues in large numbers for class use. The sections are floated from the salt-solution on to a warm solution of New Orleans baking molasses diluted ten times, or a dilute sugar-dextrin solution, and thence are floated on to a clean glass plate and arranged in rows. The plate is drained, and then without drying is immersed in absolute alcohol for 15-30 seconds; it is then flooded with a thin celloidin, drained, the celloidin film allowed to set, and the plate then put into warm water, where the celloidin sheet floats off, carrying the sections, which can now be cut out and treated as single celloidin sections, or the whole sheet can be carried through the staining, dehydrating and clearing solutions to be cut up into single sections before mounting.

CHAPTER XIX.
THE PRESERVATION OF MACROSCOPIC PREPARATIONS.

For preserving gross objects for museum specimens alcohol or formol may be employed. The former bleaches the tissues so that ultimately they are almost destitute of color. Formol in a 5 per cent solution gives better color-effects than alcohol, as the blood-containing parts remain darker. The fluid also remains clear and the tissues are firm. When alcohol is used the fluid must be frequently changed, as it becomes turbid and yellowish, and the tissues finally become soft and lose their form. The best methods of preserving the natural color are found in the various modifications of the **Kaiserling method.** The organs or tissues are placed first in a formol solution until they are just hardened, the formol changing the oxyhæmoglobin into acid hæmatin. They are then transferred to alcohol to bring back the natural color, which is accomplished by the change of the acid hæmatin to an alkali hæmatin, which has a color very closely resembling that of oxyhæmoglobin, so that the natural color is approximately reproduced. The method is carried out as follows:—

Sol. I.—Formalin .... 200 cc.
Water .... 1,000 cc.
Potassium nitrate .... 15 grms.
Potassium acetate .... 30 grms.

The tissues are left in this solution, in the dark, for one to several days, being watched carefully to see that they are not over-hardened.

Sol. II.—80 per cent alcohol for 1-6 hours and then 95 per cent until the color is fully restored (2-24 hours). Watch carefully and remove as soon as best color effect is reached, and preserve in—

Sol. III.—Glycerin .... 400 cc.
Water .... 2,000 cc.
Potassium acetate .... 200 grms.

The specimens must be kept in air-tight jars, and crystals of thymol added to prevent growth of moulds. This is sometimes very difficult, and it becomes necessary to change the discolored fluid for clear. I have found the rectangular museum jars best adapted for the preservation of Kaiserling specimens. I use a wooden top which fits over a thick piece of felt cut just the size of the jar, which in turn fits over a piece of dental rubber cut to fit the jar. The jar is placed upon a wooden bottom which has upright steel rods at the corners, that pass through holes in the wooden top, and have a screw-thread so that they can be fitted with screws, which when screwed down hold the wooden top, felt and rubber sheeting tightly in place, making the jar air-tight, but giving a top easily removable. Very beautiful specimens can be secured by the Kaiserling method, and they can be kept for several years, but sooner or later the color-effect is lost. Light, heat and exposure to the air cause a loss of color.

Some workers prefer the following in place of Sol. I:—

    Hot water .... 2,000 cc.
    Sodium sulphate .... 40 grms.
    Magnesium sulphate .... 40 grms.
    Sodium chloride .... 20 grms.

When salts are dissolved and solution cool add 200 cc. of formalin.

Melnikow-Raswedenkow Method:—

Sol. I—Water .... 100 parts
     Formol .... 10 parts
     Sodium acetate .... 3 parts
     Potassium chlorate .... 0.5 part

Leave in this 1-2-3-4-5 days, according to size of specimen. Large organs must have solution injected into vessels.

Sol. II.—95 per cent alcohol, until color is restored.
Sol. III.—Preserve in: Water .... 100 parts
                        Glycerin .... 60 parts
                        Potassium acetate .... 30 parts

Pick's Method:—

Sol. I.—Water .... 1,000 cc.
      Formol .... 50 cc.
      Carlsbad salts .... 50 grms.

Then transfer to 80 and 95 per cent alcohols, as for Kaiserling, and preserve in water 9,000 cc., glycerin 5,400 cc., sodium acetate 2,700 grms.

Westenhoeffer's method of preserving uric-acid: formol vapor 4-24 hours, then 80-90 per cent alcohol containing mercuric oxide, and preserve in glycerin to which some mercuric oxide covered by cotton or absorbent paper has been added.

Claudius's Method. The specimen is placed on a grating in a closed vessel containing a concentrated solution of ammonium sulphate, an abundance of the crystals being left on the bottom of the vessel. Carbonic acid or illuminating gas is passed through the ammonium sulphate solution for 48-72 hours, and the specimens are then preserved in the same solution. My experience with this method has not been satisfactory.

Gelatin method of mounting Kaiserling preparations: Soak washed Gold Label gelatin in distilled water for 12-24 hours. Take equal parts of water-logged gelatin and glycerin and dissolve by heating in a double boiler, stirring, for 15-20 minutes. Cool to 40°C. Then clarify with white of egg (well-whipped whites of three eggs to half a gallon of jelly; stir well; steam for ½ hour) and filter through cotton-wool. Add to jelly a few drops of a weak aqueous solution of crystal violet to remove yellow color (*Bruère and Kaufmann*). To prevent growth of bacteria a small percentage of formol or crystal of phenol may be added. Kaiserling specimens are placed in glass dishes in the melted jelly, and covered with it. When set the dishes containing the mounted specimens may be covered with glass-plates and fastened to these by balsam or cement. I use a deep Petri dish, filling it about two-thirds full with the jelly; over this I pour melted paraffin of a very low melting point so as not to melt the jelly. When the layer of soft paraffin is hard, a thick layer of paraffin of a 52° melting-point is poured over it, and the dish filled even. When the hard paraffin is set, it is varnished with shellac. Liquefaction of the gelatin by bacteria or enzymes constitutes the great drawback to this method.

CHAPTER XX.
THE FIXATION AND HARDENING OF TISSUES.

GENERAL CONSIDERATIONS. For the examination of material that may be injured by freezing, or when very thin sections are required for complicated staining procedures, it becomes necessary to prepare the tissue by *fixation* and *hardening,* so that it can be *imbedded* in some medium permitting the *cutting* on the microtome of as thin sections as may be desired. Fixation is that process by which the appearances of the tissue are preserved as they were when it was taken for examination; hence in order to obtain pictures resembling as closely as possible those of the living tissue the material should be *fixed* immediately upon its removal from the living body by operation, or as soon as possible after death when obtained by autopsy. *Fixing agents* act by coagulating the cell albumins, in this way "setting" or "fixing" the constituents of the cell so that further change is stopped. Fixation, therefore, *hardens* the cell, and all fixatives are also hardening agents. A practical distinction between fixing and hardening is made, however, resting upon the fact that not all fixatives harden the tissue so completely that the proper consistence for the cutting of thin sections is attained. To achieve this the tissue must be dehydrated. Alcohol and acetone are the only reagents fixing and hardening perfectly at the same time, as they remove the water from the tissue; for all other fixing agents an *after-hardening* in alcohol is necessary. In the case of such reagents the division of the process into a *primary fixation* and a *second hardening* stage has been the cause of the divergence in meaning of the two terms.

The best fixing agents are those that kill the cells at once, but cause a slow coagulation with little or no shrinking. They must penetrate and diffuse through the tissues rapidly so that the deepest cells are quickly reached. Acid media, especially those containing small percentages of acetic acid, are therefore better than alkaline solutions. The tissue-elements, particularly the nuclei, must be preserved as perfectly as possible so that they will not be affected by further procedures of microscopic technique. The chemic properties of physiologic and pathologic substances must likewise be preserved. The preservation of karyokinetic figures is a criterion of good fixation. In pathologic work it is also desirable that the fixing agent should preserve the red blood cells, and permit of the staining of bacteria in sections. Since fixing media are more or less selective in their action, it follows that there is no one fixative that gives equally good results in all cases. Especial fixing reagents must be used for the demonstration of certain substances (fat, etc.), or for the use of certain staining methods. Some stains cannot be used at all after certain fixing agents have been employed. For general use that fixing agent having the widest range of usefulness should be employed; and for this reason fixing media composed of several fixing agents are often employed in preference to the use of a single one.

GENERAL RULES FOR FIXING AND HARDENING

The tissue should be put into the fixing fluid as soon as possible after its removal from the body. It must not be allowed to dry. There should be an abundance of the fixing solution, 25-50 times the volume of the object to be fixed. The tissue should never be put into a dry vessel and the fixing fluid poured upon it; the vessel should first be filled with the fixing solution and the tissue then dropped into the latter. A slight agitation of the fluid will prevent the sticking of the tissue to the bottom or sides of the vessel. The size of the pieces must be adapted to the penetrating power of the fixing reagent, but as a rule the pieces should not be more than 2-3 cms. in thickness, and for some reagents 0.5 cm. is as thick as they can safely be. The reagents used should be changed when they become cloudy or discolored. The used solution may be filtered and used again, but some reagents can be used but once. Alcohol may be saved for redistillation. In the case of some reagents (mercuric chloride, chromic acid, osmic acid, etc.), the time limits of the fixation should not be exceeded, as over-fixation will ruin the staining-power of the tissues. Alcohol is practically the only solution in which tissues may be left indefinitely, but even with it there are certain limitations. As a general rule the time required for fixation may be shortened by keeping the reagents at incubator-temperature. As the different fixing reagents vary so greatly as to their especial advantages and disadvantages these will be considered separately. Only the best and most commonly used methods are here included.

1. **ACETONE.** A water-free acetone is employed by placing pure dried white copper sulphate in the bottom of the bottle or vessel in which the fixation-process is carried on. Several layers of filter-paper are put over the copper

sulphate to keep the tissues from touching it, and the acetone is then poured into the vessel. As soon as the copper-sulphate becomes blue it must be again fused. It is only by this method of constant dehydration that acetone can be employed to any advantage as a fixing agent; if fused copper sulphate is not employed the amount of acetone necessary to fix well is so great that the method becomes too troublesome and expensive to be recommended. But with the simple copper-sulphate method of constant dehydration acetone becomes the cheapest, most rapid and one of the best fixing reagents. The use of alcohol is avoided, and the period of infiltration in xylol and in paraffin shortened. For very quick work the entire process of fixation, hardening and dehydration may be achieved by the use of acetone alone, small pieces of tissue being fixed ½-2 hours in acetone and then transferred directly to soft paraffin. For ordinary work pieces of tissue 0.5 cm. thick are put into acetone over fused copper sulphate for 20-60 minutes. A judgment of the degree of fixation can be obtained by pressing the tissue lightly between the fingers; if it is of uniform consistence, and does not give as if the inner portions were softer than the surface, the fixation is complete. From the acetone the tissues may be brought directly into xylol for 5-10 minutes, until they obtain a cloudy transparency, thence into paraffin for 15-30 minutes and then blocked. The whole process of fixation, imbedding, cutting and staining can be carried out in 30 minutes. Acetone may be combined with formol, alcohol or any of the other fixing agents but when it is desired to use any one of these for some especial purpose it is better to fix first with the desired reagent and then to use acetone for the dehydration-process alone, instead of alcohol. We have found that formol-fixation followed by acetone dehydration gives excellent results for general pathologic work. **Formol-acetone** (acetone 100 cc., formol 10 cc.) may be found to have advantages. The quick fixation in water-free acetone causes less contraction than fixation with absolute alcohol; fixation with graded acetone-solutions causes practically none.

Advantages. It is the cheapest and quickest method. It penetrates well and causes little contraction of the tissues, shortens the time in xylol and paraffin and makes more easy the cutting of dense fibrous structures. Cell-division figures are as well preserved as by alcohol fixation, and the staining of bacteria in the tissues can be carried out as well after acetone-fixation as after alcohol. It preserves lecithin, hence can be used for the fixation of nerve-tissues. When combined with formol (formol-acetone) the red blood-cells are well-preserved and take a brilliant eosin stain.

Disadvantages. The disadvantages are practically the same as with alcohol fixation but not so marked. Fat is dissolved, cell-division figures are not so well-preserved as with mercuric chloride and Flemming's solution, and the blood-cells not so well preserved as with formol and mercuric chloride.

2. **ALCOHOL.** Absolute, 95-96 per cent alcohol, or graded alcohols (70, 95 per cent, and absolute) may be used for fixation. For this purpose the stronger alcohols are preferable, as the weaker solutions do not fix quickly enough. On the whole the use of 95-96 per cent is to be advised. The pieces of tissue must not be thick. Plenty of alcohol should be used and it should be changed several times during the process of fixation, which for larger pieces requires several days. For the last change absolute should be used. Very small bits such as uterine curettings can be fixed in one hour, by using three changes of absolute alcohol. Since alcohol both fixes and hardens it has been generally

used, but it is a relatively poor fixative. For after-hardening it is indispensable. Absolute alcohol may be made from 96 per cent by the use of fused copper sulphate. To test the strength of alcohol mix a few drops with pure water-free xylol; if no sediment appears when viewed against a dark background the alcohol is absolute or practically so. Many of the disadvantages of alcohol fixation can be obviated by the use of **formol-alcohol** (95 per cent alcohol 100 cc., formalin 10 cc.).

Advantages. Cheapness, quickness, and ease of method. Can be used for quick diagnostic work. Penetrates well, and can be used for large pieces of tissue. Preserves glycogen, is especially good for the staining of bacteria in sections, and the majority of stains work well with alcohol-fixation.

Disadvantages. Causes much shrinking and loss of finer details; preserves cell-division figures not at all or poorly; destroys the red blood cells; dissolves fat and other chemic products; does not permit of the use of certain specific staining methods (nerve-tissues); causes excessive hardness of fibrous and elastic tissues and makes cutting difficult.

3. **CHROMIC ACID AND SALTS.** Chromic acid is rarely used alone in pathologic work, but is a constituent of Flemming's solution (see below). Its salts are employed in the form of:—

A. **Müller's Fluid** (Potassium bichromate 25.0 grms., sodium sulphate 10.0 grms., water 1,000.0 cc.) This was formerly the favorite fixing solution, but is now used chiefly for the eye and nervous tissues, either alone, or after formol fixation, or mixed with formol. Large pieces may be used, even an entire brain, but the process requires months or even a year for the best results. Even small pieces take several weeks. The process may be hastened in the incubator. The solution should be changed whenever it becomes cloudy. When fixation is complete the fixed and hardened tissue may be cut directly on the freezing-microtome or after-hardened and dehydrated in alcohol or acetone when it is to be imbedded. The dehydration in alcohol should be carried out in the dark and without previous washing of the tissue in the case of nervous tissue. Greenish or brownish chrome precipitates appear if the dehydration takes place in the light; but for ordinary material this precipitate can be avoided by washing the fixed material in running water for 24 hours before transferring to alcohol. Moulds grow luxuriantly in Müller's fluid, but may be inhibited by the use of pieces of camphor, thymol, etc.

Advantages. Cheap, penetrates well, causes little shrinking, permits special nerve-stains, preserves red blood-cells, gives beautiful results with ordinary stains, preserves fat.

Disadvantages. Slowness; does not preserve division-figures; does not permit of staining for bacteria; does not give good results with many special staining methods (fibrin, elastic tissue, reticulum, etc.).

B. **Erlitzky's Fluid** (Potassium bichromate 25.0 grms., copper sulphate 5.0 grms., water 1,000.0 cc.). Used for fixation of nervous tissue. The formation of pigment precipitates may lead to misinterpretation; the artefacts may be removed by hot water or dilute acetic acid.

C. **Orth's Fluid** (Müller's fluid 100 cc., formol 10 cc. Make fresh before using, as the mixture precipitates on standing.). Fix for 3-12 hours in the incubator, or for 24-48 hours at room temperature. Wash in running water for

12-24 hours; cut on the freezing microtome, or after-harden in acetone or alcohol and imbed.

Advantages. Combines the good features of Müller's and formol fixations, and obviates some of the disadvantages. It is a good general fixing solution.

3. **FORMOL OR FORMALIN** (40 per cent solution of formaldehyde gas). Used in a *ten per cent solution* (water or physiologic salt solution nine parts, formalin one part), often incorrectly called 4 per cent formol or formalin, the mistake arising from the confusion with 4 per cent formaldehyde gas. For nerve-tissues it is better to dilute the formol with physiologic salt-solution than with water. Fix for 3-4-12 hours according to size of tissue. As it penetrates well large pieces can be used. Wash in water before after-hardening in alcohol, if tissue is to be employed for general work, otherwise it can be transferred directly to the alcohol without washing. Tissues can be kept in formol for some weeks, but after that time the staining-power is slowly affected, and the finer structures suffer.

Advantages. Probably the best fixing reagent for general pathologic work. It is cheap; easily made and kept in solutions of proper strength for fixing; hardens while it fixes; does not require after-washing; penetrates well; causes little shrinking; permits freezing directly from the fixing solution; preserves fat; permits the use of after-hardening with bichromate solutions for especial nerve-stains; preserves the red blood-cells; gives good results with nearly all stains, and differentiates bile-pigment from hæmatoidin. It is the best fixing reagent when tissues are to be sent some distance, as over-fixation occurs only after several weeks or even months.

Disadvantages. Affects many people unpleasantly, causing coryza, eczema of the hands and arms, and affections of the finger-nails, so that workers having acquired this idiosyncrasy cannot expose themselves to formol vapor; it dissolves glycogen and uric acid; does not fix cell-division figures as well as mercuric chloride or Flemming's solution; causes the precipitation of diffuse hæmoglobin in the form of brown or black pigment-granules that may be taken for melanin, malaria pigment or hæmosiderin; causes a pseudo-ochronosis of cartilages; and, unless thoroughly washed from the tissues before after-hardening in alcohol, it makes carmine-staining difficult or unsatisfactory and affects also the specific staining-reactions for amyloid and mucin; it is not as good as alcohol or mercuric-chloride when the sections are to be stained for bacteria. In spite of these disadvantages it can be recommended as the best general fixing reagent.

For **Orth's fluid, formol-acetone** and **formol-alcohol** see above.

4. **FREEZING AND DRYING.** The fresh tissue is frozen and dehydrated in a vacuum over sulphuric acid, at a temperature of 20-30°C.; when completely dried it is imbedded directly in paraffin. This method has been especially recommended by Altmann on the ground that the tissues are simply deprived of water without any change in volume.

5. **HEAT.** Physiologic salt-solution is heated to 80°C. Thin pieces of tissue are placed in the hot water for two minutes, and then after-hardened in alcohol. For larger pieces of œdematous tissues, cysts, etc., that cannot be cut into thin pieces, the salt-solution should be brought to 100°C and the tissues boiled for several minutes. This method is advised particularly for the coagulation of albumin in cysts, œdematous tissues, for the study of renal casts, etc.

6. **MERCURIC CHLORIDE.** This is used most commonly in the form of a **concentrated water solution** (mercuric chloride 7.5 grms., sodium chloride 0.5 grm., glacial acetic acid 5 cc., water 100.0 cc.), or as **Zenker's solution** (mercuric chloride 5.0 grms., sodium sulphate 1.0 grm., potassium bichromate 2.5 grms., water 100 cc.; dissolve by heating, add 5 cc. glacial acetic acid just before using. The use of a 5 per cent formol solution instead of acetic acid is recommended). The pieces of tissue should not be thicker than 5 mm. Fix 6-24 hours, then wash 24 hours in running water, and after-harden in alcohol. Should the sections show mercuric precipitates they should be treated with Lugol's solution for 30-60 minutes, then washed in a dilute solution of lithium carbonate and thoroughly washed out in water and alcohol. Much better stains can be obtained by this treatment of the sections with Lugol's. The use of iodine in the alcohol during the process of after-hardening is not advisable because of the action of the iodine upon the albuminates of mercury. A 5 per cent solution of **sublamine** in distilled water has recently been recommended by *Klingmüller* and *Veiel*. Fix 1-3 hours, wash and after-harden in alcohol. Precipitates are not formed, and good staining-results are obtained.

Advantages. The mercuric chloride solutions preserve well the red blood-cells, mitotic figures and finer details of cell-structure, and permit the staining of bacteria and animal parasites in the sections. Certain especial staining methods (Mallory's reticulum-stain, etc.) can be used only after mercuric chloride fixation, while many others (Heidenhain's iron-hæmatoxylin, Biondi-Heidenhain triple stain, etc.) give best results after this fixation. For ordinary work the saturated mercuric chloride solution is preferable to Zenker's, as the latter does not give good results with the commonly-used hæmatoxylin stains.

Disadvantages. More troublesome and expensive; require thorough washing and subsequent removal of precipitates, and affect (Zenker's particularly) certain stains.

7. **OSMIC ACID.** Osmic acid is used alone in a 1 per cent solution, or in such combinations as **Flemming's solution** (chromic acid 1 per cent. sol. 15 cc., 1 per cent osmic acid 4 cc., glacial acetic acid 1 cc.), **Hermann's solution** (same as Flemming's, with 15 cc. of a 1 per cent platinic chloride substituted for the chromic acid), **Altmann's solution** (5 per cent potassium bichromate solution 50 cc., 2 per cent osmic acid solution 50 cc), **Marchi's solution** (Müller's fluid 2 parts, 1 per cent osmic acid solution 1 part), and that of **Pianese** (1 per cent sodium-chloroplatinate 15 cc., 2 per cent osmic acid 5 cc., ¼ per cent chromic acid 5 cc., formic acid 1 drop). The pieces of tissue must be very thin, as osmic acid penetrates very slightly. Fix 6-24 hours in the dark, and wash thoroughly in running water, and after-harden in graded alcohols. These solutions have but limited use in pathology, and are used chiefly for the study of fat (oleates) and mitotic figures. Flemming's and Hermann's solutions are the best for the study of mitotic figures, the latter bringing out plasma details more clearly. Marchi's fluid is used especially for the study of nerve-degeneration, and Altmann's for the demonstration of Altmann's granules. The method of Pianese is used for the demonstration of cell-inclusions. The osmic-acid mixtures are all expensive, penetrate poorly, cause precipitates, and affect greatly the staining-power of the tissues, so

that it becomes necessary to use certain stains (safranin, carbol fuchsin, aniline gentian violet, etc.) as counter-stains.

8. **PICRIC ACID.** A saturated water solution of picric acid is usually employed. Fix 12-24 hours, and wash in alcohol, not water, and after-harden in graded alcohols. Preserves mitotic figures, fine details of cell-structure, and is very good for bone and calcified tissues, as it decalcifies and fixes at the same time.

Numerous modifications and combinations of the above methods have been proposed such as *Flemming's chrom-acetic solution, Rawitz's chromic-picric-nitric fluid, Rabl's chrom-formic mixture, Burckhardt's chrom-osmic-nitric solution, Merkel's fluid (chromic acid-platinic chloride), Carnoy's mixture (glacial acetic acid 1, absolute alcohol 6, chloroform 3)*, and many others. They have a limited use in pathologic work.

In the judgment of a section as to its fixation the following points may be of service: in alcohol fixation the red blood cells are haemolyzed, and there is much shrinking; with formol fixation the red cells stain copper-red with eosin; in mercuric chloride fixations the red cells stain rose-red with eosin, and pigment precipitates are present; in bichromate fixation the red cells preserve their natural color, and fat cells show a brownish color; osmic-acid fixation is shown by the black color of the oleates, and the failure of the tissue to stain by ordinary stains.

CHAPTER XXI.
DECALCIFICATION.

Bone and tissue containing deposits of lime must be decalcified before they can be sectioned on the microtome. The decalcification should be carried out after fixation and before the after-hardening in alcohol. Some reagents may combine decalcification with fixation, but this is satisfactory only when the amount of lime-salts is relatively small. Fresh tissues should not be put into any of the stronger acid decalcifying fluids, as they alter unfixed cells so that the staining-power is lost and the fine histologic details destroyed. The fixed tissue cut into small pieces is put into the decalcifying reagent, which is used in large amount and must be frequently changed. It is left in the decalcifying fluid until the calcium salts are removed, as shown by tests with needle or scalpel. The tissue must not be left in the fluid after decalcification is attained, as the staining-power is affected by all decalcifying reagents; it is therefore necessary to make frequent tests in order to judge of the progress of the decalcifying process. After decalcification the tissue should be washed in running water for 24 hours, and then after-hardened in alcohol. Alkaline solutions may be used to remove the acid before washing. Sections of decalcified tissue always stain slowly, and it is advisable to remove any acid remaining in the tissues by soaking the sections in a saturated water solution of lithium carbonate before staining. Numerous formulæ for decalcifying fluids have been recommended; a few of the best methods only are given here.

1. **Combined Fixation and Decalcification.** Picric acid or Müller's fluid may be used for this purpose when the amount of lime-salts contained in the tissues is very small. The process is slow.

2. **Trichloracetic Acid.** Fix tissues in 10% formalin and decalcify in trichloracetic acid 90 cc., formol (40 per cent formaldehyde) 10 cc. Change frequently. Decalcification is rapid, the tissue is but little changed and the staining-power not affected.

3. **Concentrated Sulphurous Acid.** Fix in 10 per cent formol; decalcify in concentrated sulphurous acid for 24 hours or longer if necessary. Wash thoroughly in alkaline water. This is a very good and rapid method; the staining-power is but little affected.

METHODS OF DECALCIFICATION. 233

4. **Haug's Solution.** (Pure nitric acid 3-9 cc., absolute alcohol 70 cc., sodium chloride 0.25 grm., water 30 cc.). For tissues fixed in mercuric chloride.

5. **Phloroglucin.** (Phloroglucin 1 grm., pure nitric acid 10 cc., distilled water 50 cc.). The solution must be carefully dissolved over the flame in a hood. Decalcification is rapid, and the tissue is protected from the acid by the phloroglucin.

6. **Ebner's Fluid.** (Hydrochloric acid 5 cc., sodium sulphate 5 grms., alcohol 500 cc., water 1,000 cc.).

7. **Schaffer's Method.** Imbed the fixed and hardened tissue in celloidin, harden the celloidin preparation in 85 per cent alcohol, then place celloidin block in a 3-5 per cent water solution of pure nitric acid and agitate in Thoma's water wheel, for 12 hours, or longer according to the size of the piece. Transfer block to a 5 per cent solution of lithium carbonate or sodium sulphate for 12-24 hours, changing solution several times, wash in running water for 48 hours, dehydrate in graded alcohols up to 85 per cent, and cut.

CHAPTER XXII.
IMBEDDING.

The most perfect methods of fixation and hardening do not permit the cutting of fine sections on a microtome without the freezing of the tissue, or its **infiltration** and **imbedding** in some substance which surrounds it with a protective coating, and preserves and holds together its structural elements in their relative positions. For the cutting of very thin sections, or for the preparation of serial sections, it is absolutely necessary to employ the process of imbedding. At the present time **paraffin** and **celloidin** are the two substances in general use for this purpose. While each one of these possesses certain advantages over the other, and we find consequently one laboratory worker preferring celloidin and another paraffin for general work, a long and varied experience makes me believe that for a teaching laboratory and for diagnostic work when much material is examined, the paraffin method answers all purposes much better than the celloidin, and that the latter need be employed only in very exceptional cases. Since paraffin sections can be transferred into celloidin by the molasses- or dextrin-fixative method, thus enabling the use of staining-methods that require celloidin sections, very few advantages are left in the favor of celloidin as an imbedding agent. The paraffin method requires a more expensive outfit to start with in the form of a paraffin oven and thermo-regulator, but otherwise the two methods cost about the same. The paraffin method requires more careful attention than the celloidin. As a rule thinner sections can be obtained in paraffin than in celloidin, and for the preparation of serial sections the paraffin method is the only method. Paraffin blocks can be labeled and filed away, and kept indefinitely without any loss of staining-power. With careful attention paid to the different steps of the imbedding process practically everything that can be cut in celloidin can be cut in paraffin. For very large pieces a slow imbedding in celloidin is, however, preferred by most workers. Hard and brittle tissues are as a rule more easily cut in celloidin. For the staining of bacteria in sections paraffin imbedding is necessary. Both methods should be learned and practiced with equal facility; a working knowledge of both is essential in pathologic investigation and diagnosis.

1. **CELLOIDIN IMBEDDING.** The granular form of Schering's celloidin is the best preparation to use, although good results can be obtained by using a cheaper well-washed gun-cotton. In purchasing the latter care should be taken to secure a sample that dissolves easily in alcohol and ether, and does not give off yellow fumes when exposed to the light. Schering's granular celloidin keeps well, and forms on solution a firm, tough, transparent imbedding mass, so that thin sections are obtainable without difficulty. When kept long in stock celloidin becomes hard and dissolves more slowly. For use three solutions are made, thick (10 per cent), thin (2 per cent), and medium (5 per cent). The celloidin granules or shavings are put into a wide-mouthed bottle having a tight stopper, and are covered with absolute alcohol and well shaken, and left for 24 hours. An equal quantity of pure ether is then added, the mixture is well stirred and allowed to stand for another 24 hours, when it is again stirred and evenly mixed, and is then ready for use. When gun-cotton is used it is torn into fine shreds and added to a mixture of equal parts of absolute alcohol and pure ether and shaken until sufficient has been added to give the solution the desired strength.

Slow Celloidin Method.

1. Absolute alcohol 24 hours.
2. Equal parts absolute alcohol and ether 24 hours.
3. Thin celloidin for 1-3 days.
4. Medium celloidin for 1-3 days.
5. Thick celloidin for 1-3 days.
6. Block.

The tissue is blocked by removing it from the thick celloidin on a section-lifter and placing it on a block of vulcanized fiber or wood with enough of the thick celloidin about it to form a good matrix. The preparation is then allowed to evaporate in the air until the surface of the celloidin becomes firm (does not stick to the finger). The block is then placed in 80 per cent alcohol or pure chloroform until hard enough for cutting (1-24 hours). Cork should not be used for blocking, nor should wood unless the tannin has been removed by long treatment with alcohol-ether. The celloidin will adhere more firmly to the fiber block if the latter is dry, and if there is a sufficient layer of celloidin between the tissue and the block. The imbedded tissues may be preserved in 80 per cent alcohol for a long time, but gradually lose their staining power. They may also be kept dry by coating them with melted paraffin. The blocks when preserved in alcohol may be marked with an indelible pencil.

For imbedding large pieces of tissue in celloidin a glass dish may be filled with thick celloidin and the infiltrated tissue placed in it with cutting surface down. The celloidin is then allowed to evaporate slowly under a glass cover, and fresh celloidin may be added as shrinkage occurs. When well-hardened the celloidin is cut out of the dish and the block trimmed to the proper proportions, and attached directly to the object-holder of the microtome or to a block of wood by a few drops of thick celloidin, allowing it to dry for a minute or so and then immersing in 80 per cent alcohol. The block may be cut on the freezing microtome by soaking the hardened celloidin in water to remove the alcohol (when block sinks), then coating it with saturated gum arabic solution, and freezing.

Rapid Celloidin Method.

I have used the following method in my laboratory for a number of years as a regular procedure in practical diagnostic work, and the results have been uniformly good.

1. Fresh tissue cut thin, or uterine curettings, in absolute alcohol 1½ hours, three changes of fresh absolute during this time.
2. Alcohol-ether 1 hour.
3. Thin celloidin at incubator temperature 12 hours (over night).
4. Medium celloidin 1 hour.
5. Block from medium celloidin, evaporating celloidin by blowing, and building up matrix by adding successive layers of celloidin.
6. 80 per cent alcohol 1-3 hours.
7. Cut.

The quick celloidin methods recommended in the literature (Kaufmann, Stepanow, Scholz and others) require more time, and do not give better results. Material received from operative clinics late in the afternoon can be sectioned and stained usually by ten o'clock the next morning.

2. **PARAFFIN IMBEDDING.** A paraffin of a melting-point sufficiently high enough to withstand summer heat is advisable; a 52°C. paraffin answers for this latitude. The use of softer paraffins is not necessary. The paraffin-oven should be regulated at a constant temperature of 54-55°C. Overheating of the tissue while in the oven must be carefully safeguarded, so that in the management of a paraffin-oven the care of the thermo-regulator is the most important thing.

Slow Paraffin Method.

1. Thorough dehydration in absolute alcohol 12-24 hours.
2. Aniline oil to remove alcohol, until tissue becomes transparent or sinks.
3. 1st. Xylol ½ hour, to remove aniline oil.
4. 2nd. Xylol, 1-2 hours, until translucent.
5. 1st. Paraffin, 52°C. in oven, 1 hour, to remove xylol.
6. 2nd. Paraffin, 52°C. in oven, 1-12 hours.
7. Block.

The use of xylol-paraffin is not necessary. For blocking staining dishes, watch-glasses, glass salt-cellars, paper-boxes, metal frames., etc., may be used. A thin smear of tincture of green soap or glycerin is rubbed over the inside of the imbedding box, and it is nearly filled with fresh melted paraffin. With warm forceps the tissue is taken out of the bottle of second paraffin in the oven, and arranged in the melted paraffin in the imbedding dish in the proper position for cutting. Care must be taken that the melted paraffin is not hot enough to "burn" the tissue, else its staining-power may be affected. The surface of the paraffin is then cooled by blowing upon it, and as soon as a film appears upon the surface, the dish is carefully immersed in cold water, so that the paraffin may set quickly. When cool the paraffin-block should slip out of the dish and float to the surface. It is then trimmed to the desired shape, leaving a good matrix of paraffin around the tissue. The paraffin-block is then fastened to a wooden block or to the object-holder of the microtome by means of melted paraffin (a hot knife is drawn along the under-surface of the block and the latter immediately pressed upon the wooden block or object-holder). Chloroform, cedar oil, benzene, carbon bisulphide, etc., may be used instead of xylol, and each one possesses certain advantages for certain purposes. Benzene is advisable for osmic-acid preparations.

Rapid Paraffin Method.

The above method can be greatly shortened for uterine curettings, thin bits of tissue, etc., if the various steps are closely watched, and if the entire process is carried on in the oven. The whole process may be carried out in 1-3 hours, a very great advantage over the quick celloidin method. A simpler and cheaper method is that recommended by *Heller, Henke* and *Brunk*, as follows:—

Acetone Method.

1. Small bits of fresh tissue, or tissue fixed in formol, in water-free acetone over copper sulphate for $\frac{1}{2}$-$1\frac{1}{2}$ hours.
2. Transfer tissue directly to fluid paraffin in the oven for $\frac{1}{2}$-$1\frac{1}{2}$ hours; the acetone evaporates, and the tissue is infiltrated with paraffin; or put into xylol 5-10 minutes, then in paraffin 15-20 minutes.
3. Block.

By this method the entire process of fixing, hardening, imbedding, cutting and staining can be carried out in half an hour, and by it the freezing-microtome can be dispensed with in a large part of quick diagnostic work.

Pyridin Method.

1. Fix in formol.
2. Dehydrate and clear in pyridin.
3. Paraffin.

This method requires a longer time than the acetone method, and is not so good.

Combinations of celloidin and paraffin may be employed by imbedding first in celloidin, transferring block to origanum oil, then xylol and finally paraffin. Formol-agar has been recommended by *Bolton* and *Harris* for simultaneous fixation and imbedding. It offers no especial advantages. *Wright* uses formol-gelatin for imbedding tissues for sectioning on the freezing microtome. The bits of tissue are placed in warm 20 per cent pure gelatin; this is allowed to set, and the block placed in 10 per cent formol for 24 hours; it is then frozen and cut. Soap-gelatin, glycerin-gelatin, gum-glycerin, etc., are now rarely used for imbedding.

NOTE:—When a number of pieces of tissue are blocked at the same time, either in celloidin or paraffin, they may be tagged with paper labels fastened to the tissue with a drop of gum tragacanth or gum arabic. As the gum is not soluble in any of the infiltrating and imbedding media the labels remain attached until the block is ready for cutting.

CHAPTER XXIII.
SECTION-CUTTING.

Fixed and hardened tissues may be sectioned on a microtome without freezing or imbedding, or they may be cut on a freezing-microtome; or, having been imbedded in either celloidin or paraffin, they may be sectioned on any form of microtome suited to the purpose desired. The choice of the microtome depends, therefore, upon the character of the work. For ordinary purposes the small sliding microtomes furnished with a crank are preferable, as they are more easily kept in order and can be used for rapid cutting. For serial paraffin sections the Minot automatic rotary microtome is advised. Especial types of microtomes can be obtained for the cutting of large sections, particularly for brain-sections. The Bardeen freezing-microtome I have already recommended as the most practical instrument for freezing work. In all cases it is absolutely necessary that the instruments be in good order and that they work with precision. The microtome knife must be carefully honed and stropped. A heavy, rigid, biconcave knife-blade should be used, and a good hone and strop are absolute necessities. In honing, the knife is drawn from heel to toe with cutting edge forward; while, in stropping, the motion is reversed, the back of the knife being forward, and the motion from toe to heel. The knife during the honing should be fitted in a knife-holder, and the back of the blade protected from the hone by a knife-back. The knife-blade must be kept free from grease and dirt, and nothing must be permitted to touch its edge. When many sections are cut at one sitting frequent stropping is necessary. When the cutting is finished the knife should be removed from the microtome, carefully cleaned and dried, and placed in its box. The slide and other bearings of the microtome should be well-oiled with the best microtome oil, and kept free from dust.

1. **Cutting of Fixed Tissues Without Imbedding or Freezing.** It occasionally becomes necessary in pathologic work to cut tissues directly upon the microtome without freezing or imbedding. This can be done satisfactorily in the case of very firm substances, such as amyloid liver and spleen, etc. The sectioning is done in the wet, using 80 per cent alcohol, as in celloidin cutting. A large celloidin

knife should be used, and the blade should be flooded in alcohol. A large piece of the tissue, or, better, several pieces, are clamped in the object holder with only a small layer of tissue above the holder. The knife-blade is placed at the least possible angle to the pieces of tissue. To obtain sections of 15-20 microns in thickness the object-holder is raised each time about 25-30 microns. The sections will vary in thickness, some thin, others very thick.

2. **Sectioning of Frozen Fixed Tissues.** Tissues fixed in formol, Müller's fluid or Orth's fluid may be frozen directly on the freezing-microtome without previous washing. For other fixations previous washing is necessary. Tissues in alcohol must have the alcohol thoroughly washed out before freezing. Celloidin blocks may also be cut by freezing after the removal of alcohol. The fixed tissues cut to the proper size are placed on the object-holder of the freezing-microtome in a drop of saturated gum-arabic and the freezing carried out as directed above. (See Page 214.) As the freezing causes little or no damage to fixed tissue, the frozen sections may be transferred directly to alcohol, or floated out on the dilute molasses or sugar-dextrin solution, and stained separately or in sheets, according to the directions given in the next chapter.

3. **Sectioning of Celloidin Blocks.** The celloidin blocks are fastened in the object-holder of the microtome, and the knife-blade (a longer and broader one than for paraffin-sectioning is advisable) set nearly parallel with the longitudinal axis of the microtome, so that the cutting-edge, striking the block at a very slight angle, will be utilized for the greater part of its length in cutting entirely across the surface of the block. Both object and knife-blade must be kept constantly wet with 80 per cent alcohol; a broad camel's-hair brush or a drip-bottle can be used for this purpose. The sections, as they are cut, are transferred from the knife to 80 per cent alcohol by sweeping the finger or brush from above toward the edge of the blade. Care must be taken not to strike the brush against the edge of the blade, and this can be avoided by using the brush always with a downward stroke. As the sections are cut they are guided onto the knife-blade by means of a fine-pointed camel's-hair brush, if the sections show any tendency to curl. They should be smoothed out at once on the knife, and then transferred to the dish of 80 per cent alcohol. Sections 7-10μ thick are easily cut in celloidin, if the process of imbedding has been carefully carried out.

To prepare *serial-sections* from celloidin blocks the sections as they are cut must be arranged in their order on the knife-blade and thence transferred in this order to a slide or glass-plate, to which they are either fastened so that they cannot become loose during the staining process, or they are fastened together by a film of celloidin and stained in one piece. To fasten the celloidin sections to the slide *Mallory* and *Wright* suggest the cutting of the block in 95 per cent alcohol, and the arrangement of the sections in their order on the knife, whence they are drawn on to a dry, clean and numbered slide. Ether vapor from a half-full bottle of ether is then poured over the slide, slowly, to flatten out the sections and fasten down the frilled edges. The slides are then transferred to 80 per cent alcohol to harden the celloidin, and they are kept in this solution until ready for staining. Celloidin sections may also be fastened to the slide by albumin glycerin (equal parts white of egg and glycerin with a crystal of phenol or thymol). The celloidin sections, as they are cut, may be transferred to a dry gelatinized slide or plate (16 grms. gelatin in 300 cc. warm water), and are then covered with a thin celloidin; the slide is then placed in water at 50°C., the gelatin dissolves and the celloidin film floats off; the latter is then stained as one section. Serial sections of celloidin-blocks may also be arranged upon slides or plates covered with a coating of the *Schmorl-Obregia* sugar-dextrin solution or diluted New Orleans black molasses; the slide or plate is flooded with absolute alcohol; drained; a thin celloidin is then poured over it; it is immersed in warm water and the celloidin-sheet containing the sections is liberated, and is then stained as a whole or cut into strips as desired. The molasses method is the cheapest and simplest method, and much to be preferred to the Weigert closet-paper method, by which the sections are arranged upon a strip of moist closet-paper which is either held upon the slide or kept upon a piece of blotting-paper wet with 80 per cent alcohol. A slide or glass-plate is covered with a thin layer of celloidin and the strip of paper containing the sections is laid upon the celloidin surface, the sections down, so that these stick to the slide as the paper is carefully peeled off. The preparation is dried with filter-paper and a thin layer of celloidin poured over the slide and sections. The celloidin is then hardened in 80 per cent alcohol and the sections stained on the slide; or the celloidin film is removed by immersion in warm water, and then treated as one section. Celloidin films may be marked with a brush dipped in a water solution of methylene-blue. This should be done as soon as they are made. *Langhan's method* is advised for the remounting of serial sections from tissues stained in bulk and imbedded in celloidin. The sections are cut in origanum-alcohol (1 part absolute alcohol to 3 parts origanum oil) and placed on a slide in a layer of origanum oil, blotted and mounted in balsam. Should sections become milky in the oil, renew the latter until they are cleared.

4. **Sectioning of Paraffin Blocks.** The paraffin block trimmed to the proper proportions, leaving a rim of paraffin about 2-3 mm. wide all about the tissue, is fastened to the wooden block by melting the under side of the paraffin by drawing a hot knife across it, and then immediately pressing the block upon the wood. The wooden block is then clamped into the object-holder. If desired the paraffin block can be fixed directly to the metal plate of the object-holder in the same manner. The block is raised until the level of the edge of the knife is reached. The knife is placed transversely or at a slight angle, and the cutting done with a relatively small portion of the edge. The paraffin block may be breathed upon to warm slightly the upper layer when a hard paraffin is used, and the knife is then drawn carefully through the block, guiding the section onto the knife-blade by means of a fine-pointed camel's-hair brush held in the left hand. It is preferable, I think, to have a wider rim of paraffin at one corner of the block and to place the block with that corner at a slight angle to the knife, so that the edge of the blade will first engage the block at that point. The tip of the camel's-hair brush moistened in water catches the corner of the section as the knife begins to cut, and pushes it over onto the blade, thus holding the section flat and preventing curling. When entirely cut through, the section is removed from the knife by the brush, still holding it at the corner first touched, or if necessary it is again moistened and applied to the upper side of the section, lifting the latter off the knife. The block is trimmed down to the proper level by cutting thick sections first, then sections of the desired thickness when the level of the entire block is reached. The sections are then transferred, with their shiny side down, just as they come off the knife, to a slide, sheet of paper, warm water, warm molasses or sugar-dextrin solution, or 70 per cent alcohol, and treated further according to the directions given in the next chapter. The presence of ridges on the cut surface of the block is an indication that the knife needs stropping. The knife must cut the paraffin, not scrape it. Crumbling of the paraffin is the result of imperfect infiltration during the imbedding process; water, alcohol, aniline oil or xylol may be left in the tissue, the paraffin may contain oil, or the cooling

process may have been delayed. Curling of the sections can be prevented by using a sharp knife and slightly warming the surface of the block by breathing upon the block, use of a warm knife or spatula, heat-focus, etc. For ordinary work paraffin sections 5-7μ thick are easily obtained; for especial work 1-2μ sections may be obtained by especial care in imbedding, using graded paraffins and finally imbedding in a 56°C. paraffin. The pieces of tissue should be small, and the sections may be cut with a knife wet with water or alcohol. *Serial paraffin sections* are easily obtained; in fact, paraffin imbedding is by far the best method for serial cutting. To cut ribbons of sections upon the ordinary slide microtome the block must be clamped into the object-holder so that the edge of the block facing the knife, as well as the opposite side of the block, is parallel with the knife-edge. The knife should be placed at right angles to the microtome. If the paraffin has the right consistency the edges of the sections as they are cut will adhere, and a ribbon of serial sections will be pushed up over the knife. This ribbon can be cut into pieces of the desired length and mounted according to the directions given in the next chapter. The Minot automatic rotary microtome is especially well adapted for the cutting of ribbon sections. Failure of sections to adhere to each other is usually the result of too hard consistence of the paraffin, and this can be remedied by warming slightly, according to the method given above. If the paraffin is too soft the sections fold together. The block may be cooled in ice-water, or the sections may be cut with a cooled knife. Paraffin knives so constructed that they may be cooled by a stream of ice-water are supplied by dealers in microtomes. The conditions essential for successful paraffin cutting are perfect infiltration and imbedding, sharp clean knives and a certain degree of skill in manipulation that can only be secured by practice.

CHAPTER XXIV.
THE PREPARATION OF MOUNTED SECTIONS.

Sections of fresh material, unimbedded or imbedded tissues must be treated by a series of processes before they are finally permanently mounted and ready for use. These processes in general are: **preparation for staining, staining, differentiation, washing, dehydration, clearing and mounting.** The general procedure will be modified to some extent by the character of the tissue, manner of preparation (fixed or unfixed, imbedded or unimbedded, unstained or stained), character of stain (affected by alcohol, xylol, etc.), and the mounting agent (glycerin, balsam, damar, colophonium). Two or more of these steps may be combined in one; the same agent may differentiate, dehydrate and clear. Several stains may be combined in one solution, or it may be necessary to use them in succession. The very greatest variation is possible in pathologic technique; in fact, practically every laboratory worker modifies methods according to the light of his individual experience. The really important thing is to be master of the method, and not allow the method to control the situation. One of the greatest attractions about laboratory work is the infinite possibility of variation and improvement of methods and the invention of new ones.

I. PREPARATION FOR STAINING.

a. **Frozen Sections of Fresh Tissue.** Frozen sections of fresh tissues, as well as those obtained by the single or double razor, may be stained by floating the section on a slide, staining it directly (carbol-kresyl-echt-violett or carbol-thionin), examining in the stain or washing, dehydrating, clearing and mounting; or the section may be fixed to the slide with molasses or sugar-dextrin solution, covered with a celloidin-film, and treated according to the methods followed for paraffin or celloidin sections. Sections of fresh tissue may be fixed in formol or alcohol, and then treated by the same methods as celloidin sections. (See also Page 220.)

b. **Sections of Unimbedded Tissues.** These may be handled for staining in the same way as paraffin, celloidin or fresh-tissue sections, either when sectioned directly or after freezing. The sections may be stained directly, on the slide, cover-slip, or in the staining solution, or they may be transferred into celloidin sheets by the same methods employed in the preparation of paraffin sections.

c. **Celloidin Sections.** These may be transferred from water or alcohol directly to the stain. It is not necessary to remove the celloidin. If not stained soon after cutting they should be preserved in 95 per cent alcohol. Celloidin sections may be stained on the slide by simply blotting the section firmly on the slide, without permitting it to become dry, and manipulating it carefully through the various solutions; or the section may be fixed to the slide by the use of 95 per cent alcohol, ether-vapor and fixation in 80 per cent alcohol; or the section may be fixed to the slide by the methods given above under the cutting of serial sections of celloidin blocks. The most common method of preparation of celloidin sections for staining is to transfer the sections from alcohol into water to straighten them out, and then to transfer on the spatula into the stain. For the treatment of serial celloidin sections see above.

d. **Paraffin Sections.** Paraffin sections may be stained directly *without removing the paraffin.* This is especially advisable in the staining of tuberclebacilli and in other cases where the use of alcohol is to be avoided. For many stains this method cannot be used. The sections as they are cut are floated directly into the warm stain, on which they flatten out, and are then transferred to the other solutions on the section-lifter, finally dried on the slide, in the incubator or over the flame, cleared in xylol and mounted in balsam. Paraffin sections may also be stained without removing the paraffin by being transferred directly from the knife on to 80 per cent alcohol, stained, washed, dehydrated in absolute alcohol or by drying, cleared and mounted. The section is transferred from one solution to another on the slide or spatula. The paraffin is removed during the clearing in xylol in both of these methods. The treatment with xylol must be on the slide, else the section may go to pieces. The staining of the section in the paraffin usually takes more time than staining after the paraffin has been removed, but the process can be hastened by heating the stain.

Slide and Cover-slip Preparations. Paraffin sections may be affixed to a slide smeared with a thin film of albumin-glycerin (equal parts of filtered beaten white of egg and glycerin, with crystal of phenol or thymol, or 1 grm. of sodium salicylate to 100 grms. of the mixture as a preservative). A drop of fixative is placed upon a clean slide, and is rubbed over the slide in a fine film with the back of the finger. The dry paraffin section with glossy side down is placed upon the smeared slide, flattened with a brush and then pressed firmly against the slide with the ball of the thumb. The albuminfixative is then coagulated in the incubator or over the flame; the paraffin is melted over the flame without overheating the section and the slide covered at once with xylol to remove the paraffin. It is then put into 95 per cent alcohol, thence into the stain; and after staining, the section is washed, dehydrated, cleared and mounted. *Cover-glass* preparations of paraffin sections are made by floating the sections with glossy side downward on warm water (just below the melting-point of the paraffin) until they straighten out and are perfectly flat. They are then floated on to cover-slips covered with a thin film of albumin-glycerin, the albumin having previously been coagulated by passing the smeared cover-slips through the flame quickly so that they do not scorch or burn. The cover-slips with the adherent sections are then placed in the incubator for 12 hours. The paraffin is then removed by xylol, the xylol is washed out in 95 per cent alcohol, and the cover-slips are then carried through the processes of staining, washing, dehydration, clearing and mounting. The cover-slips must be handled with forceps and the section side should always be uppermost. Slides covered with a film of albumin-glycerin may be used instead of cover-slips. The albumin-glycerin film may be omitted, and the sections with glossy side down floated in warm water on to clean covers or slides; the water is drained off and the slides or covers are put in the incubator for 12 hours. Sections adhere fairly well by this method (*capillary attraction method*). Bubbles are removed by careful heating. Serial ribbons of the size desired can be floated and mounted on slides by the albumin-glycerin or the capillary attraction method.

By far the best method of preparing paraffin sections for staining is the *molasses plate method,* a modification, originating in my laboratory, of the *Schmorl-Obregia* sugar-dextrin method. When many sections are to be stained at once it is the most convenient method and gives uniform results. In the preparation of sections for class-work it has no equal. It can be used also for giving out unstained sections. When many sections must be stained in diagnostic work the method saves much time and labor. Fifty sections can be stained as easily as one. It combines all the advantages of the celloidin and paraffin methods, as does the *Schmorl-Obregia* sugar-dextrin method, but is much cheaper than the latter.

Schmorl advised the use of a sugar-dextrin solution (cane sugar solution [1:1] 300 cc., 80 per cent alcohol 200 cc., yellow dextrin solution [1:1] 100 cc.) to be run over a perfectly clean glass plate or slide until the entire surface is covered with an even layer. The paraffin sections as they are cut are arranged in order on the wet plate, and when the plate is full, it is heated sufficiently to flatten and smooth the sections. The plate is then placed in an incubator for 3-12 hours to harden and dry. When dry it is immersed in xylol to take out the paraffin, then treated with absolute alcohol for 10-15 minutes, the alcohol drained off, and the plate covered with a thin layer of celloidin (celloidin or photoxylin 10, absolute alcohol 100, ether 100). As soon as the celloidin sets (1-2 minutes) the plate is immersed in warm water and the celloidin film containing the sections is detached. It can now be carried through the staining, washing, dehydrating and clearing solutions as one section, and in the clearing solution cut into strips or single sections, as desired, for mounting. *Huber and Snow* improved the method greatly by floating the paraffin sections directly on to warm dilute sugar-dextrin (a 10 per cent solution of Schmorl's stock-solution will suffice), and plating the sections directly from the latter. This method of using the dilute solution is less expensive, much cleaner, and saves time in drying in the incubator. The results are in every way better than with the Schmorl solution in full strength. The formation of bubbles and crystals is almost wholly prevented, and less dust is caught on the plate. In my laboratory we have modified the method still further by using a 10 per cent solution of New Orleans black (or baking) molasses instead of the more expensive sugar-dextrin solution. As the molasses costs but 20 cents a gallon, a gallon of the dilute solution costing 2 cents can be used indefinitely if fermentation be prevented by a crystal of phenol or thymol. The paraffin sections are floated on to this dilute molasses solution warmed sufficiently to smooth out the sections; 4 x 5 glass plates (old negatives) thoroughly cleaned and kept in alcohol are immersed in the warm molasses solution and the sections arranged on them as desired, lifting out of the solution that part of the plate covered with sections as they are drawn upon it. As soon as the plate is covered it is drained, and is then flooded with absolute alcohol. After 1-2 minutes the alcohol is drained off and the plate flooded with thin celloidin, which is allowed to set for a minute or so, and the plate then immersed in warm water in which the celloidin film containing the paraffin sections is detached. This film is then handled by catching it at the two corners of one end with the fingers, or better still by a pair of forceps held in each hand. The film is put first into xylol to remove the paraffin, then into 95 per cent alcohol, then into water and thence into the staining solution. After staining the film is washed, dehydrated and cleared, and in the clearing solution is cut into strips or single sections by means of the wheel-shaped paper-cutter used by paper-hangers. The pieces are then mounted. A dilute sugar-dextrin solution can be used instead of the molasses-solution, but the latter is much cheaper and does just as well. Aside from this advantage our method of transferring the paraffin-sections into the celloidin film without first removing the paraffin saves a great deal of time, as it is not necessary to wait for the plates to dry in the incubator. The same method can be applied to the staining of single paraffin sections on the slide. The conversion of the paraffin section into a celloidin preparation without any loss of time for drying is so quickly and easily carried out that I advise it above all others. The same method may also be applied to the staining of fresh and fixed tissues cut on the freezing microtome or sectioned without imbedding. The success of the plate-method will depend largely upon the state of the glass-plates when put into the molasses solution. They must be perfectly clean or the celloidin sheet will not separate well. It is best to keep them in alcohol until they are needed. The celloidin must be of the right consistency, the layer must be thin, and cover the entire plate uniformly. It must not be allowed to harden too much before immersion in water or it will be tough and will shrink. Handling of the celloidin-sheets with the bare hands is not advisable because of the large number of epithelial cells adhering to the celloidin. The sheets are easily changed from one solution to another by catching them with forceps; the use of a glass-plate to transfer them is not necessary. When it is desired to preserve sections for future staining the celloidin sheet containing the paraffin-sections can be kept in 80 per cent alcohol indefinitely.

NOTE:—If the glass-plate is numbered with a blue wax-pencil after the paraffin sections are floated on, the marking will be transferred to the celloidin sheet, and the latter will retain the marking through all solutions.

II. STAINING AND DIFFERENTIATION.

Staining is necessary to bring out clearly the constituent elements of the tissues and their relations with each other, and for the demonstration of histologic structures or chemical substances that would otherwise be nearly or wholly invisible. The technique of staining depends upon the fact that stains or dyes possess certain affinities for the tissue–elements or for certain simple or complex substances present in the tissues (*microchemic reactions*). These affinities vary greatly with the dye. Some dyes have an affinity only for single constituents of the tissue (*elective* or *specific stains*); others have an especial affinity for the nucleus (*nuclear stains*), others stain all the tissue-constituents diffusely (*diffuse* or *protoplasmic stains*). There are but few pure elective stains for single tissue-elements; the majority of stains will stain more than one of the tissue elements, but may show an especial affinity for certain ones. As a result of these variations in the affinities of dyes for the constituents of the tissues it becomes possible to manipulate the dyes or to combine them in such a way that a specific differentiation of many tissue-elements is possible through the use of different *methods of staining.* These methods are based in part upon the use of different mordants, the employment of several stains in combination or in succession, the mixture of stains to form a new staining compound, the phenomenon of *metachromasia,* the differentiation of certain tissue-elements by the removal of the stain from the structures for which it possesses a weaker affinity, and by the employment of different microchemic reactions. The two most commonly employed methods are the *progressive,* in which the stain is allowed to act until the affinities of certain tissue-elements have been satisfied when the staining process is interrupted; and the *regressive,* in which the tissue is overstained, and the dye withdrawn from the tissue-elements for which it possesses the weakest affinities leaving the other elements stained. This latter process is usually called *"differentiation,"* and the chief substances used for such differentiating are dilute acid, acid alcohol, acid stains, aniline oil, aniline-xylol and alcohol. Some workers use the regressive method for such simple stains as hæmatoxylin, overstaining, and then differentiating with acid alcohol before counter-staining with eosin. The results obtained in this way are much less satisfactory than is possible with the progressive method.

Tissues may be stained in the body during life (*intravital staining*), or immediately after removal from the body (*supravital or survival staining*), either before or after sectioning. (See Page 217.) Fixed tissues may be stained in bulk or in sections.

Staining Tissues in Bulk.

This method is not often used in pathologic work. The fixed and hardened tissue is cut into small pieces, placed in the staining solution for several days, washed thoroughly, dehydrated in alcohol, imbedded, cut, and mounted without further staining. Alcoholic solutions penetrate best; hæmatoxylin, hæmalum, carmine and alcoholic solutions of the aniline stains may be used. *Metallic impregnation* (gold or silver salts) of fresh or fixed tissues is but little used in pathology. (See Staining of Nervous System, and Spirochætes.)

Staining of Sections.

Celloidin sections are lifted from water or alcohol into the stain by the needle or section-lifter. The use of the latter is advised, as by it the section can be floated flat on to the staining solution. When many celloidin sections are to be stained at once they can be stained in small tea-strainers and transferred in these from one solution to another. **Paraffin sections** may be floated directly on to the stain without removing the paraffin; or they may be stained on the slide or cover-glass after removing the paraffin, the stain being dropped on to the section, or the slide or cover-slip is immersed in the stain. Special staining-dishes for the staining of paraffin sections on slides and covers can be obtained. Paraffin sections transferred to celloidin sheets by the plate method can be put into the staining-solution while on the glass-plate, or the films can be detached and transferred from one solution to another by means of forceps. This is the easier way, and it is not necessary to touch the films with the fingers.

General Rules for Staining.

1. The stain should be filtered just before being used, in order to remove precipitates, moulds, etc. Unless they have been diluted most of them can be used over and over again, hence after using they should be filtered back into the stock bottle.

2. A liberal amount of stain should be used. Slides and cover-slips are given enough stain to cover completely the section, when the staining is done on the slide, or they may be immersed in staining-dishes. Plates and celloidin sheets should be stained in large trays. Sections and celloidin films should be flat without folds or wrinkles, and they should not touch one another when several are stained at the same time. Transference of the section from water or dilute alcoholic solutions to dilute or stronger alcohol respectively for a moment and then back again will usually straighten out curled or wrinkled celloidin sections.

3. Stain until the section is properly stained. Control this by removing it from the staining-solution and examining it in water on a glass-slide without a cover-slip, using the low-power. Sections will always appear more deeply-stained when cleared than when examined in water, hence due allowance should be made. Celloidin sheets can be examined on glass-plates. The time-limits given in staining methods are only approximate; no absolute rules can be laid down as to the length of time necessary to obtain a good stain. The methods of fixation and hardening, age of the tissue, age of the stain, etc., affect the staining power. Some stains lose their staining-power after a time; others require a period of ripening before they yield the best results. As a rule staining may be intensified or hastened by staining in the incubator or at a higher temperature, by concentrating the stain, or by the use of such substances as aniline oil. When differentiation is necessary the process should also be controlled by frequent examination of the section, as above for staining. Usually the section can be examined in the differentiating fluid.

III. WASHING.

Thorough washing after staining is necessary after nearly all stains. The washing should usually be done by soaking the sections in several changes of distilled water, although tap-water, alcohol, alum-water, and other solutions may be used to intensify the staining effects. When this is done a final washing in distilled water or alcohol is usually necessary. Differentiating fluids should always be thoroughly removed from the section before mounting. Sections should not be allowed to lie in wash-water that is colored by the stain; as soon as the wash-water becomes colored it should be replaced by fresh. When sections are left lying in the wash-water for some time the vessel containing them should be covered to prevent the settling of dust on the sections, as it is practically impossible to remove from the latter dust or other precipitates that may become attached to them. Some stains give better results after long washing; others are easily washed out if the sections are left standing in the wash-water. The time-limits of washing will depend upon the character of the stain employed.

IV. DEHYDRATION.

Dehydration of the sections is usually produced by passing them through two alcohols, 80 per cent and absolute, or 80 per cent and 95 per cent. For certain clearing reagents (xylol) it is necessary to use absolute alcohol. When carbol-xylol is used as a clearing reagent absolute alcohol is not necessary, and 95 per cent can be used instead for the second dehydrating solution. Usually a minute in each alcohol is sufficient for the dehydration of single sections.. If dehydration with alcohol is not desirable because of its action on the stain it is possible to dehydrate and clear in xylol by repeatedly blotting the section with absorbent paper, covering the section several times with xylol and then blotting. The section should never be allowed to become perfectly dry. Dehydration with alcohol may also be avoided by staining paraffin sections without removing the paraffin, drying in the incubator or over the flame, removing the paraffin in xylol, and mounting. Imperfect dehydration is shown by the presence of white spots or a milky cloud in the section when it is put into the clearing fluid.

V. CLEARING.

After dehydration, sections must be cleared in some solvent of balsam before they can be mounted in the latter medium. When 95 per cent alcohol has been used for the final dehydration the sections may be completely dehydrated and cleared at the same time by the use of carbol-xylol (xylol, 3 parts; melted crystals of carbolic acid, 1 part; add melted carbolic acid to the xylol to prevent formation of crystals). The sections (on the slide or cover-slips, in celloidin sections or films) are transferred from the alcohol, draining or blotting off excess of the latter, into the carbol-xylol, and left until perfectly clear. This can be most easily determined by viewing the sections against a dark background. Carbol-xylol cannot be used for sections treated with aniline stains. These are dehydrated in 95 per cent alcohol, and the final dehydration and clearing accomplished by repeatedly placing xylol upon the slide and blotting it out until the sections are transparent. Turpentine, chloroform, benzine, toluol, the oils of bergamot, cloves, thyme, lavender, origanum cretici, and cedarwood, aniline oil, and various mixtures of these oils are also used as clearing agents. The majority of these will clear from 95 per cent alcohol, but not so readily as carbol-xylol; they have individual disadvantages of taking out the eosin, affecting aniline colors, dissolving celloidin, making sections brittle, slow action, clinging odor, etc. Chloroform and benzine may be used for clearing osmic-acid preparations; oil of turpentine is also good for clearing sections stained with kresyl-echt-violett, and Wright's blood-stain. With but few exceptions carbol-xylol and xylol meet all requirements better than any other clearing reagents. There is but one disadvantage in the case of carbol-xylol; some of the phenols in the market cause a fading of eosin and hæmatoxylin stains. *DeWitt* has shown that this fault can be corrected by redistillation, stopping the distillation as soon as the temperature begins to rise above the constant boiling point of the phenol; or the carbol-xylol that fades the stains can also be corrected by supersaturating it with a mixture of sodium bicarbonate one part, and sodium-potassium tartrate two parts. Sections kept in xylol or carbol-xylol should be protected from dust and evaporation; it is not a good plan to keep them in these solutions for more than 24 hours.

VI. MOUNTING.

Permanent mounts are made in glycerin, potassium acetate, lævulose, glycerin gelatin, balsam, damar or colophonium. For celloidin and paraffin sections a solution of **Canada balsam** in xylol is most commonly used for mounting. Celloidin sections (celloidin films are best cut into strips and single sections when in the carbol-xylol; the wheel-shaped paper-cutter used by paper-hangers is the best instrument for this purpose) are lifted onto the slide from the clearing-fluid; folds or wrinkles in the celloidin are straightened or removed by cutting the celloidin at right angles to the section in order to relieve the tension, and the section is then blotted firmly against the slide by means of a pad of absorbent paper. The greatest care should be taken to prevent wrinkling, folding or turning over of the edge of the section. As soon as the pad is removed a drop of balsam is placed upon the section and the cover-glass put over it. There should be just enough balsam used to fill the space between cover-slip and slide, so that air-bubbles are not formed. The balsam must not be so thin that the cover-glass will float about on the liquid, or so thick that it does not spread well. In the latter case warming the slide may cause it to spread more readily, but care must be taken not to injure the stain by over-heating. Paraffin sections on the slide are similarly blotted and covered with balsam and cover-glass; those on cover-slips are blotted between folds of absorbent paper and immediately placed with section-side downward upon a drop of balsam that has been put upon the slide.

Xylol-damar may be used in place of Canada balsam; it is cheaper and colorless, but it tends to become cloudy. **Colophonium** is the cheapest of the three and has but little color; it is highly recommended by many workers. In a xylol-solution it may be used for aniline stains; a chloroform solution is advisable for the mounting of osmic-acid preparations; while a solution in turpentine and shellac is recommended for Weigert's neuroglia method, Wright's blood-stain, and other special staining methods.

Glycerin, potassium acetate, laevulose and **glycerin-gelatin** are used for the preservation of amyloid-, mucin- and fat-stains, as well as for other preparations that do not permit the use of alcohol and xylol. **Glycerin-gelatin** is probably the best medium for this purpose. It is made according to *Kaiser* by soaking 7 grms. of gelatin for 2 hours in 42 cc. distilled water, then adding 50 grms. glycerin and 1 grm. carbolic acid; the mixture is warmed 10-15 minutes, stirring constantly, and filtered while hot. It is also made by taking water, 200 cc.; gelatin, 20 grms.; powdered white shellac, 2 grms.; Farrant's solution (gum arabic, glycerin, solutio acidi arsenicosi conc., aa. 30.0 grms.), dissolve by warming, and filter while warm. To mount in this medium the section is placed on the slide, and blotted with absorbent paper. A drop of warm glycerin-gelatin is then placed on it and the cover-slip affixed. The drop spreads evenly beneath the cover-glass and becomes solid as it cools. Mounts in glycerin, glycerin-gelatin, potassium acetate and laevulose must be cemented around the borders of the cover-slip with asphalt, wax, paraffin, gold size, etc., using a brush or glass rod for this purpose.

VII. SUMMARY OF METHODS OF PREPARATION OF CELLOIDIN SECTIONS.

1. Fixation of the tissues in alcohol, formol, etc.
2. Wash 24 hours, when necessary.
3. After-harden in 80 and 95 per cent alcohols for 1 to several days.
4. Complete dehydration in absolute alcohol for 24 hours.
5. Equal parts of pure ether and absolute alcohol, 24 hours.
6. Thin celloidin, 1-3 days.
7. Thick celloidin, 1-3 days.
8. Block. Harden block in 80 per cent alcohol.
9. Cut; keep sections in 80 per cent alcohol.
10. Stain; differentiate.
11. Wash thoroughly.
12. Dehydrate in 80 and 95 per cent alcohols.
13. Final dehydration and clearing in carbol-xylol.
14. Place on slide and blot with absorbent paper.
15. Mount in xylol-balsam or xylol-colophonium.

VIII. SUMMARY OF METHODS OF PREPARATION OF PARAFFIN SECTIONS.

1. Fixation of the tissue in alcohol, formol, etc.
2. Wash 24 hours, when necessary.
3. After-harden in 80 and 95 per cent alcohol for 1 to several days.
4. Complete the dehydration in absolute alcohol for 24 hours.
5. Aniline-oil until tissue becomes transparent.
6. 1st. Xylol, ½ hour, to remove aniline oil.
7. 2nd. Xylol, 1-2 hours, until translucent.
8. 1st. Paraffin (52°C.), ½ hour in oven, to remove xylol.
9. 2nd. Paraffin (52°C.), 1-12 hours in oven, until infiltrated.
10. Imbed and block; cool quickly.
11. Cut sections; mount on slides or covers.
12. Remove paraffin in xylol.
13. Remove xylol in absolute alcohol.
14. 80 per cent alcohol, for a few minutes.
15. Stain; differentiate; wash.
16. Dehydrate in 80 and 95 per cent alcohols.
17. Clear in carbol-xylol.
18. Mount in Canada-balsam or colophonium.

IX. ARTEFACTS IN MOUNTED SECTIONS.

A mounted section, after passing through the various stages indicated above, must of necessity present some appearances that are the result of the technical methods employed. The number and degree of such artefacts will depend upon the character of the methods employed and the care exercised in their performance. The trained observer ignores the presence of artefacts as having nothing at all to do with the significance of the section itself; but to the beginner in microscopic work they often appear to be the most important thing in the preparation, and are given a pathologic interpretation. How frequently do we see students, undergraduates and postgraduates, take up a section and pick out a fold, wrinkle, tear, staining-defect, precipitate, dirt, etc., as pathologic features! It is necessary, therefore, for the student to acquaint himself with the nature of artefacts so that he may ignore them and not give them an incorrect interpretation. The most important artefacts are as follows:—

1. **Artefacts due to fixation** (mercuric, chromic, osmic, etc., precipitates; alterations in blood-pigment due to formol; loosening of cells from basement membrane due to contraction [kidney tubules, etc.; loosened endothelium in blood-vessels, particularly confusing to students]; destruction of red blood cells, as in alcohol fixation; poor staining due to overfixation).

2. **Artefacts due to hardening** (contraction, desquamation of cells, etc.).

3. **Artefacts due to imbedding and cutting** (tears, holes, ragged edges, irregular thickness, knife-streaks, compression of soft structures, dislocation and tearing-out of firm tissues or material, wrinkles, folds, etc.).

4. **Artefacts due to poor staining** (uneven, spotted or streaked staining, overstaining, understaining, poor differentiation, precipitates, insufficient washing, fading, poor contrasts, defective staining due to presence of paraffin, dextrin, etc., in section).

5. **Artefacts due to poor mounting** (imperfect dehydration and clearing, cloudiness, milkiness or opacity of section; folds; wrinkles; turned-over edges; tears in section caused by striking it with balsam-dropper or needle; air-bubbles; lack of balsam).

6. **Dirt and foreign-material** (opaque and translucent dirt, above or below section; coloring-matter in balsam; ink; pigment from pencil; cotton-, silk, wool-, linen-, vegetable and paper-fibres, hairs, desquamated squamous epithelium, portions of insects, etc.)

CHAPTER XXV.
STAINS AND STAINING METHODS.—NUCLEAR AND PROTOPLASMIC STAINS.

THEORIES OF STAINING. The exact nature of the process of staining has not yet been determined. Various theories have been advanced, explaining the affinity of the tissues for certain dyes, on the ground of a chemical, mechanical or chemicophysical action. The chemical theory assumes the formation of an insoluble compound through the chemical combination of tissue and stain; the physical theory is based upon the assumption that the process is purely physical or mechanical, while the chemicophysical theory holds that it is neither purely physical nor purely chemical. The process is not controlled by the molecular weights alone of the substances concerned, but does depend upon the conditions controlling the formation of solutions in general. Therefore, the theory most widely accepted at the present time is the solution-theory, which assumes that the staining-process is a solution of the dye in the tissue, and that the stained tissue-element is a fixed solution of the stain in its substance. This solution of the dye in the tissues may be a direct action between the two (direct or substantive stains); or it may be brought about only by the interaction of a third substance (indirect or adjective stains). The third substance is called a *mordant,* and the combination of the dye with the mordant is known as a *lake.* The mordant may be added to the stain or to the tissue, either before or at the time of staining. Many of the fixing-fluids are mordants, particularly those containing chromic acid or its salts. Alum, iron, and many of the metals are the most commonly used mordants. In a general way acid mordants are used for basic colors, and basic mordants with acid colors.

The **stains** most commonly used in pathologic work are:—
1. **Natural Dyes:**—Hæmatoxylin and Carmine.
2. **Aniline Dyes:**—*a, Acid.*—Eosin, erythrosin, acid fuchsin, orange G, picric acid, sudan III, and scarlet R (Fett-ponceau).

b, Basic.—Methylene blue, methylene violet, thionin, toluidin blue, kresyl-echt-violett, methyl violet, gentian violet, crystal violet, basic fuchsin, dahlia, aniline blue, methyl green, iodine green, safranin, Bismarck brown, and vesuvin.

In a general way it may be said that basic stains are nuclear stains, and acid stains are protoplasmic. Neutral stains are usually diffuse stains; when formed by the combination of acid and basic dyes they usually act as selective stains for some especial tissue-element or cell-constituent. **Metachromasia**, in its narrowest sense, is the term applied to that staining-phenomenon, in which a single-chemical entity gives different colors to different tissue-elements. In this sense iodine, in its action upon glycogen and amyloid, is a true metachromatic substance. The majority of the so-called metachromatic stains, however, do not possess true metachromasia, since their metachromatic powers are dependent upon a mixture of two or more dye-stuffs in the one compound. The most important stains of this class are gentian violet, methyl violet, crystal violet, dahlia, thionin, toluidin-blue, polychrome methylene blue, methylene azure, and kresyl-echt-violett. The chief *chromotropic* substances are amyloid, mucin, mast-cell granules and cartilage. Metachromatic reactions are at their best usually when examined in water; they are affected by alcohol and usually destroyed by carbol-xylol. Sections stained by metachromatic stains should be quickly dehydrated by absolute alcohol and blotting, and cleared in xylol, when mounted in balsam.

I. NUCLEAR STAINS.

1. **Haematoxylin** ($C_{16}H_{14}O_6$) is an ether extract of the wood of *Hæmatoxylon campechianum*, a tree found in the West Indies and Central America. In itself not a dye, it becomes one of the most valuable when odidized to hæmatein ($C_{16}H_{12}O_6$), and combined with alum, iron or other mordants to form a lake. It then stains nuclei a deep violet-blue or black color that is practically permanent. Mucin, lime-salts, bacteria, and colonies of actinomyces are also stained varying shades of blue. If the staining process is prolonged the entire tissue, as well as celloidin, becomes more or less heavily stained blue. A pure nuclear stain is obtained by interrupting the stain at the right time (examine in water); or if the sections are overstained they may be differentiated in acid alcohol (1 per cent hydrochloric acid in 70 per cent alcohol). Hæmatoxylin stains well after all fixing-solutions except òsmic acid; some of its staining-formulæ stain slowly after fixation in Zenker's fluid. On the whole, it is by far the best general nuclear stain for laboratory and diagnostic work. It is employed in numerous staining formulæ, the most useful of which are given here. These formulæ differ chiefly in the time of staining, "ripening" of the stain (oxidation of hæmatein), intensity of stain, necessity of differentiation, etc.

a. Böhmer's Alum-haematoxylin.

Dissolve 5 grms. of hæmatoxylin crystals in 50 cc. of absolute alcohol; add this drop by drop, while stirring, to 1,000 cc. of a 1 per cent solution of potassium alum. Expose in open vessel to air and light for 1-2 weeks. Filter before using.

THE HÆMATOXYLIN STAINS. 255

b. Hansen's Haematoxylin.

To 200 cc. of alum-hæmatoxylin solution brought to the boiling-point add 2 cc. of a concentrated solution of potassium permanganate. Cool quickly; filter when cold. Can be used at once without further ripening. It tends to stain diffusely.

c. Delafield's Haematoxylin.

To 400 cc. of a saturated solution of ammonia alum add a solution of 4 grms. of hæmatoxylin in 25 cc. of absolute alcohol. Expose mixture to air and light for 3-4 days; filter; then add 100 cc. of glycerin and 100 cc. of 95 per cent alcohol, and filter. Expose to light until solution is dark enough, then keep in tightly-stoppered bottle. It is a strong stain, and may be diluted with distilled water when desired. The solution keeps well.

d. Ehrlich's Acid-haematoxylin.

Dissolve 2 grms. of hæmatoxylin in 100 cc. of absolute alcohol. Add this to a saturated solution of potassium alum in water 100 cc., glycerin 100 cc., and glacial acetic acid 10 cc. Allow mixture to stand for a week exposed to air and light; then filter. Keep in well-stoppered brown bottles. The solution stains best when it is six months old, and may be kept for several years. It does not overstain, and on the whole is more useful than Böhmer's, Hansen's or Delafield's.

e. Mayer's Haemalum.

Dissolve 1 grm. of hæmatein in 50 cc. of 90 per cent alcohol and warm. Add this solution to a solution of 50 grms. of potassium alum in 1,000 cc. of distilled water dissolved by heating. Mix warm, cool, and filter. With hæmatein no ripening is required, and the solution can be used at once. Hæmalum is a more precise nuclear stain, but stains more slowly than the formulæ given above.

It may be prepared directly from hæmatoxylin crystals by dissolving 1 grm. of hæmatoxylin in boiling water; add water up to 1 litre, and cool. Add 0.2 grm. sodium iodate and 50 grms. potassium alum, dissolving at room temperature; 50 grms. chloral hydrate and 1 grm. citric acid may be added to make solution keep better.

f. Mayer's Acid-haemalum.

Add 2 cc. glacial acetic acid to 100 cc. of hæmalum solution. It stains the nuclei more precisely than hæmalum.

g. Weigert's Iron-haematoxylin.

Dissolve 1 grm. of hæmatoxylin in 100 cc. of 96 per cent alcohol. Allow to ripen several days, but this solution should not be kept longer than six months. Make a second solution of 4 cc. of liq. ferri. sesquichlor. (German Pharmak. IV, sp. gr. 1,124), 1 cc. of concentrated hydrochloric acid and 100 cc. of water. Mix equal parts of each solution just before staining. The mixture stains well for 5-8 days, so that a quantity of stain sufficient for this time only should be made up. The two stock solutions are easily made and keep well. The nuclei stain quickly and deeply, and differentiation and long washing are unnecessary when hydrochloric acid is included in the second solution, as given above. After-staining with eosin, picric acid or the Van Gieson's mixture gives better results with Wiegert's iron-hæmatoxylin than with any other hæmatoxylin.

Method of Staining with Haematoxylin.

1. Stain 1-15 minutes, controlling progress of stain by examination of section in water, on slide, using low-power.

2. If sections are overstained, differentiate in ½-1 per cent potassium-alum or in acid alcohol.

3. Wash thoroughly in tap water, until a good blue is obtained. Exposure to ammonia vapor or washing for a few seconds in lithium-carbonate solution will hasten the development of the blue color. If these reagents are used the section should afterwards be thoroughly washed in water.

(Stain with a plasma stain, if contrast is desired.)

4. Dehydrate in 80 and 95 per cent alcohols.

5. Clear in carbol-xylol.

6. Mount in balsam.

Over-ripened hæmatoxylins may stain reddish or even brownish, and too diffusely. In such cases the celloidin will be deeply stained. The addition of alum-water to the stain may counteract the fault. Alum-hæmatoxylins must always be filtered before using, as precipitates are constantly formed as the result of oxidation.

2. Carmine. Carmine is the coloring matter of cochineal, the dried bodies of the female *coccus cacti*, and is obtained chiefly from Honduras. The coloring principle is carminic acid ($C_2H_{22}O_{12}$). When combined with alum, borax, lithium, etc., carmine gives a good, permanent nuclear stain, varying from reddish violet to deep scarlet. It is used chiefly in pathology to give a contrasting nuclear stain to the various pigments, and when specific blue stains have been used for fibrin, mucin, bacteria, elastic tissue, etc., or when a blue injection-mass has been used. Alum-carmine is the most precise nuclear stain. Differentiation with acid-alcohol is necessary after staining with borax- or lithium-carmine. Lithium-carmine is on the whole the best of the three for use as a contrast-color to the various pigments.

a. Alum Carmine.

Carmine ½-1 grm., 1-5 per cent alum solution 100 cc.; boil 20 minutes; cool; filter. Add crystal of thymol as preservative.

1. Stain 15 minutes to several hours.
2. Wash thoroughly in distilled water.
3. Dehydrate in 80 and 95 per cent alcohols; clear in carbol-xylol; mount in balsam. Nuclei are a light reddish violet; the plasma is slightly stained (muscle) or not at all.

b. Lithium Carmine.

2-5 grms. of carmine to 100 cc. of a cold saturated water solution of lithium carbonate; filter.

1. Stain 1-3 minutes; transfer directly to acid alcohol (1 cc. of hydrochloric acid to 100 cc. of 70 per cent alcohol) without putting section into water; differentiate ¼-6 hours, until nuclei alone retain the color. Control differentiation by examination on the slide in acid alcohol.

2. Wash thoroughly in water.

(Use plasma stain, as picric acid, if desired.)

3. Deyhdrate in 80 and 95 per cent alcohols; clear in carbol-xylol; mount in balsam.

c. Borax Carmine.

Dissolve by boiling 0.5-0.75 grm. carmine and 1-2 grms. of borax in 100 cc. of water. To the hot solution add 5 cc. of a 0.5 per cent acetic acid until solution is deep red. After 24 hours filter and add crystal of thymol.

Stain and differentiate as with lithium-carmine, but leave the sections somewhat longer in the stain (15 minutes).

3. **Basic Aniline Stains.** The basic aniline stains are used as general stains for bacteria in sections, and at the same time stain the nuclei. Methylene blue and fuchsin are employed especially for this purpose. The metachromatic dyes (thionin, kresyl-echt-violett, etc.) are also used as nuclear stains in combination with their metachromatic reactions with mucin, amyloid, mast-cells, etc. Methylene blue is used in the study of the blood-forming organs, cell-inclusions, parasites in the tissues, etc. Safranin and fuchsin are used for staining mitotic figures. (See Staining of Mitoses.) Bismarck brown is employed sometimes in preparing sections for microphotography. Methyl green is an intense chromatin stain and is used in various combinations. Since these dyes are not very permanent, and are easily washed out in dehydrating and clearing fluids, as well as "running" in balsam mounts, they are rarely employed as pure nuclear stains in pathologic work.

When the basic-aniline stains are used a saturated water or concentrated alcoholic solution (1½-2 per cent in 40 per cent alcohol) may be employed as stock-solution and diluted 1:5 or 1:10, as desired. The sections are stained 3-5 minutes, then differentiated in absolute alcohol, cleared in xylol, and mounted in balsam. Methylene-blue is used by some workers as a nuclear stain contrasted with eosin for tissues fixed in Zenker's solution, giving better effects with this fixation than the hæmatoxylins. **Unna's alkaline methylene-blue formula** is employed (methylene-blue 1 grm., carbonate of potassium 1 grm., water 100 cc.). Dilute 1:10 or 1:5 for staining. Stain 10-15 minutes, wash quickly in water, differentiate in 95 per cent alcohol; dehydrate in absolute, clear in xylol, mount in balsam. When celloidin sections are used, 95 per cent alcohol may be used for dehydrating, blotting on the slide with several changes of xylol.

The **nucleolus** has an affinity for the acid stains. With the modifications of the Romanowsky methylene-blue-eosin methods the nucleolus stains red, the nucleus blue.

II. DIFFUSE OR PLASMA STAINS.

The most commonly used diffuse stains are eosin, erythrosin, acid fuchsin, orange G, and picric acid. They are practically never used alone, but are employed as contrast-stains to the nuclear stains. Eosin, orange G, acid fuchsin and picric acid may be used as counterstains for hæmatoxylin; picric acid is used as the best contrast to the carmines, while eosin and orange G are employed as counterstains for methylene blue. The combination of hæmatoxylin and eosin is by far the best general staining method for laboratory and diagnostic work, except for tissues fixed in Zenker's solution; for these the combination of methylene blue and eosin is preferable. Ammonia carmine is sometimes used as a diffuse stain for bone and the central nervous system. The majority of the diffuse stains wash out easily in water, alcohol and xylol, hence sections thus stained should not be allowed to remain too long in these fluids.

a. **Eosin.** Two forms of eosin are obtainable, one soluble in water, the other in alcohol. Saturated solutions of both kinds should be kept as stock solutions and diluted as occasion demands. For use after hæmatoxylin a ½ per cent solution is advisable; with Zenker's fixation a more dilute solution may be used, as tissues so fixed stain intensely in eosin. If used as a contrast-stain to methylene-blue, eosin is used first in a 5 or 10 per cent solution, as the basic nuclear stain takes out some of it. Some workers express a preference for the aqueous solution of eosin, others for the alcoholic; the alcoholic solution stains more uniformly and with less differentiation than the other. Eosin is particularly good as a contrast-stain for tissues containing red blood cells when fixed in formol, mercuric chloride or Zenker's.

b. **Orange G.** Used in a 1 per cent water solution. Requires longer time for staining than eosin.

c. **Acid Fuchsin.** A saturated water solution is kept in stock and diluted as needed. Must be used in weaker solutions than eosin, as it more quickly overstains, and cannot be washed out so well.

d. **Picric Acid.** Keep in stock either a saturated water or saturated alcoholic solution, and dilute as needed. As it washes out more readily than eosin, the staining solution should be stronger than for the latter, and the sections somewhat overstained to allow for some loss of stain. Picric acid gives a brownish tint to nuclei stained with hæmatoxylin or carmine, and will take out the stains completely, if allowed to act too long.

e. **Ammonia Carmine.** One grm. of carmine is dissolved, without heating, in 50 cc. of distilled water and 5 cc. of strong ammonia water. The fluid is then exposed in an open dish until the odor of ammonia is lost; it is then filtered. When ready for use dilute by filtering 1-2 drops into 20 cc. of distilled water.

III. COMBINED NUCLEAR AND DIFFUSE STAINS.

The diffuse or plasma stains may be combined with the nuclear in one staining solution, or used in succession. The latter method gives better results. The nuclei are stained first, the diffuse stain being used after the washing-out following the use of the nuclear stain, except in the methylene-blue and eosin method in which to obtain the best results it is necessary to stain with the eosin first. Nuclear hæmatoxylin may also be followed by a combination of plasma stains, as in the Van Gieson's mixture of picric acid and acid fuchsin, Delépine's mixture of rubin and orange, White's erythrosin and picric acid mixture, etc. In these mixtures the different affinities of the plasma-stains give rise to differential or selective staining effects.

a. Haematoxylin and Eosin.

1. Stain in any one of the hæmatoxylins.
2. Wash thoroughly.
3. Stain in dilute water or alcoholic eosin until section is bright rose-red.
4. Differentiate eosin-staining, as desired, by rapid or slow washing in water.
5. Dehydrate quickly in 80 and 95 per cent alcohols.
6. Clear quickly in carbol-xylol. (If carbol-xylol takes out eosin too rapidly add some of the dry eosin stain to it. Hæmatoxylin-stained sections can be placed in such eosin-carbol-xylol and will take up the eosin beautifully.)
7. Mount in balsam.

Hæmatoxylin and eosin can also be combined in one stain, but the results are not as good as those obtained by successive staining.

b. Haematoxylin and Picric Acid.

1. Stain with Weigert's iron-hæmatoxylin, or overstain with any other hæmatoxylin.
2. Wash thoroughly.
3. Stain in saturated water solution of picric acid, diluted one-half, until sections are a bright yellow. If left too long in the stain, the hæmatoxylin will become brown or may be wholly lost.)
4. Wash, dehydrate and clear quickly, as for eosin. (Dry picric acid may be added to the carbol-xylol.)
5. Mount in balsam.

c. Haematoxylin and Acid Fuchsin.

Stain with hæmatoxylin, and after washing use a 1 per cent water solution of acid fuchsin, until section is sufficiently red; wash; dehydrate; clear; mount.

d. Haematoxylin and Orange G.

Stain with hæmaotxylin, and after washing use a 1 per cent water solution of orange G, staining ¼-3 hours. Treat otherwise as for eosin-staining.

e. Carmine and Picric Acid.

Stain with borax- or lithium-carmine; differentiate in acid alcohol and wash thoroughly. Then counterstain with picric acid, as for hæmatoxylin and picric acid. Carmine and picric acid may also be combined in one stain, as picro-carmine, but this is rarely used at the present.

f. Eosin and Methylene-blue.

(For tissues fixed in mercuric chloride or Zenker's.)

1. Stain in a 5-10 per cent aqueous eosin for 20 minutes or longer, until a deep eosin-stain is obtained.
2. Wash out excess of eosin in water.
3. Stain in Unna's alkaline methylene-blue, diluted 1-4 or 5 with water, 10-15 minutes.
4. Wash in water.
5. Differentiate in 95 per cent alcohol, keeping the section in constant motion to obtain a uniform decolorization. Control process under microscope. *Wolbach* advises the use of a 0.75-1-5 per cent solution of colophonium in methyl alcohol as a differentiating medium instead of 95 per cent alcohol. For tissues fixed in formol or alcohol a 10 per cent solution should be used.
6. When the background is pink, dehydrate quickly with absolute alcohol, or in 95 per cent by blotting on slide with xylol, until clear.
7. Clear in xylol.
8. Mount in balsam.

g. Van Gieson's Method.

1. Stain in Weigert's iron-hæmatoxylin, or overstain if any other hæmatoxylin is used. (Weigert's gives the best results, as it does not decolorize so readily.)
2. Wash thoroughly.
3. Stain in Van Gieson's mixture (acid fuchsin 1.5 grms., saturated water solution of picric acid [0.6 per cent] 150 cc. This mixture keeps well. Add 1 cc. of this stock solution to 10 cc. of saturated water solution of picric acid. Stain in this for 10 seconds).
4. Wash quickly; dehydrate in alcohol; clear in xylol or carbol-xylol; mount in balsam.

I have obtained the best results by making the Van Gieson's mixture by taking an ordinary small staining-dish nearly full of saturated water solution of picric acid, and adding to this, drop by drop, sufficient saturated water solution of acid fuchsin to make the solution just dark enough so that the finger cannot be seen through the staining-dish. The hæmatoxylin-stained section is put into this mixture for a few seconds, until it appears to become lighter. The section is then washed in 95 per cent alcohol, dehydrated, cleared and mounted.

The Van Gieson method is extremely valuable in pathologic work, because of its varied differential reactions. The nuclei are brown or black, protoplasm is ochre-yellow, connective-tissue light red, voluntary and involuntary muscle yellow, axis-cylinders red, connective-tissue hyalin deep rose-red, epithelial hyalin yellow, orange or brownish, amyloid yellow or brownish pink, mucin yellow or brownish, fibrin yellow or brown, necrotic areas yellow or brownish, lime-salts brown to brownish blue or violet.

Combinations of rubin and orange (Delépine) and erythrosin and picric acid (Powell White) are also advised as differential combination stains, but are not so useful as Van Gieson's. Other combination methods are to be found in the various modifications of the Ehrlich triple stain.

CHAPTER XXVI.

SPECIAL STAINING METHODS FOR DEMONSTRATION OF PATHOLOGIC CONDITIONS IN CELLS OR TISSUES.

I. AMYLOID. The best selective staining of amyloid is obtained with relatively fresh tissues; long preservation in alcohol or formol tends to weaken the reactions. Probably the best effects are obtained by formol-fixation for 24 hours, and sectioning on the freezing-microtome. Good results may be produced, however, after any of the ordinary fixing and hardening methods by cutting the sections on the freezing-microtome, without imbedding, or imbedding in paraffin. The metachromatic reactions are not satisfactory with celloidin sections. With hæmatoxylin and eosin the amyloid substance stains a light red or bluish-pink; Van Gieson's stains it a yellow or brownish-pink color, giving it practically the same color that it does epithelial hyalin. The different tissue-relations of the two substances serve to distinguish them. The most important specific amyloid stains are:—

1. Iodine.

1. Stain in Lugol's solution 5-10 minutes.
2. Dehydrate in absolute alcohol 4 parts, tincture of iodine 1 part.
3. Clear and mount in origanum oil. Seal preparation with paraffin, gold size or shellac.

The iodine reaction is also applied to fresh tissues by pouring Lugol's solution over a freshly cut surface, and is a good gross test for amyloid. In both microscopic and macroscopic preparations iodine gives a mahogany brown color to amyloid; other tissue is yellow. The iodine reaction may be intensified by placing the sections in a 1 per cent sulphuric acid; the brown color may be changed to blue, violet or green.

2. Methyl Violet.

1. Stain in 0.5 per cent methyl-violet solution ½ to several minutes. Examine in water.
2. Wash in water.
3. Differentiate in 2 per cent acetic or dilute hydrochloric acid 1-2 minutes.
4. Wash thoroughly in water.
5. Mount in lævulose or glycerin-gelatin. Amyloid ruby red; tissue blue-violet.

3. Gentian Violet.

Use same method as for methyl violet. The same color-effects are produced.

4. Methyl Green.

Use methyl green in the same way as methyl violet. Amyloid sky-blue or violet; tissue is green.

5. Iodine Green.

1. Stain for 24 hours in a ⅓ per cent water solution of iodine green.
2. Wash in water.
3. Mount in lævulose, glycerin or glycerin-gelatin. Amyloid red violet; tissue green.

6. Birch-Hirschfeld's Method.

1. Stain in a 2 per cent alcoholic solution of Bismarck brown for 5 minutes.
2. Wash in absolute alcohol.
3. Wash in water.
4. Stain in a 2 per cent water solution of methyl-violet (or a 20 per cent gentian violet) for 5 minutes.
5. Differentiate in 1 per cent acetic acid until the non-amyloid parts are brown.
6. Wash thoroughly in water.
7. Mount in lævulose, glycerin or glycerin-gelatin. Nuclei are brown; amyloid ruby red.

7. Green's Method.

To a few cc. of hæmalum in a watch-glass add a saturated solution of methyl-violet, drop by drop, until the mixture shows a faint purple-red tinge at the edge of the glass.

1. Stain sections 15-30 minutes.
2. Differentiate in acid alcohol until the purple begins to fade.
3. Wash thoroughly in water.
4. Mount in glycerin. (Sections may be blotted and dehydrated in pure liquid paraffin; the latter is then removed by blotting with xylol, and then mount in pure white vaseline.)

Nuclei are blue, amyloid ruby-red.

8. Kresyl-echt-violett (Morse's Method).

Kresyl-echt-violett (R. extra) 1 grm., 5 per cent carbolic acid 80 cc., alcohol 20 cc. Mix, stirring well; filter. Solution keeps well, and can be diluted as desired without precipitating.

1. Stain 1-5 minutes.
2. Wash thoroughly in distilled water, differentiating, if necessary.
3. Blot with filter paper.
4. Dehydrate in absolute alcohol as quickly as possible.
5. Clear in turpentine. Blot nearly dry before mounting.
6. Mount in balsam.

Formol, mercuric chloride and Zenker's all give good results. Paraffin imbedding, with staining of sections on the cover-glass (albumin-fixative method), is the best method of staining for permanent mounts, although good preparations can be obtained by the use of the freezing-microtome. Carbol-xylol cannot be used for clearing. Nuclei are blue, protoplasm pale blue, amyloid ruby-red.

As a specific reaction for amyloid and mucin this method has been used in my laboratory for the last ten years in preference to any other. The stains are permanent if not exposed to the action of light.

Thionin, toluidin-blue, polychrome-methylene-blue, and other metachromatic dyes are also used to give similar reactions with amyloid, but are not as satisfactory as the kresyl-echt-violett method. Amyloid may also be stained with **scarlet R** or **sudan III**, according to the method of Herxheimer, but the results are rarely satisfactory.

II. ATROPHY. Good pictures of atrophic tissues are obtained with formol-Müller's, mercuric chloride or Zenker's fixation, and staining with Van Gieson's, to bring out the stroma which is usually relatively or absolutely increased. In the case of pigment-atrophy the sections should be very thin and stained with alum- or lithium-carmine.

III. CALCIFICATION. Deposits of lime-salts appear in fresh tissue as gritty, refractive areas that are bright and shining by reflected light, and dark by transmitted. They are soluble in acids, solution of the carbonate being accompanied by the formation of bubbles of carbonic acid gas. Hæmalum and the alum-hæmatoxylins show a specific reaction with the phosphates and carbonates of lime, giving them a deep blue or reddish-violet stain. Fresh calcification usually stains diffusely blue; older deposits are deep-blue about the borders of the deposits, lighter or unstained in the center of the mass. Tissues containing much calcium must be decalcified before imbedding. If the process of decalcification is not carried too far the specific staining reaction is not lost.

Von Kossa's Silver Method for Calcium Phosphate.

1. Fix in alcohol or formol; imbed; cut.
2. Place section in 1-5 per cent silver nitrate solution, and expose to daylight 5 minutes to 1 hour.
3. Wash in distilled water.
4. Transfer section to a 5 per cent solution of sodium hyposulphite, to remove excess of silver nitrate.
5. Wash thoroughly in water.
6. Dehydrate in absolute alcohol.
7. Clear in xylol; mount in balsam.

Calcareous deposit black, as the result of the formation of phosphate of silver and its reduction by the action of light. Alum carmine may be used as a nuclear stain before the sections are treated with silver nitrate, or safranin may be used after the sodium sulphite has been washed out.

IV. CELL GRANULES AND CELL INCLUSIONS.

The granules and cell-inclusions here included fall within the class of special protoplasmic structures found particularly in neoplasms and inflamed tissues, and which have been supposed to be parasites. For the staining of other cell-granules see Blood and Blood-forming organs.

1. Altmann's Granules.

1. Fix small, thin pieces of fresh tissue in equal parts of 5 per cent potassium bichromate and 2 per cent perosmic acid for 24 hours. Wash in running water for several hours. After-harden in alcohol, and imbed in paraffin. Cut very thin and mount on cover-glass; remove paraffin.
2. Stain in aniline-water-acid-fuchsin (acid fuchsin 20 grms., aniline water 100 cc.), warming until vapor is given off.
3. When cool remove the fuchsin with a mixture of 1 part saturated alcoholic picric acid and 2 parts of water.
4. Renew the picric acid solution and warm on the paraffin oven for 30-60 seconds.
5. Dehydrate in alcohol; clear in xylol; mount in balsam.

Protoplasm yellow; Altmann's granules red; fat black.

2. Russell's Bodies.

1. Fix and harden in Müller's; wash; after-harden in alcohol; imbed in paraffin; mount on cover-glass.
2. Stain sections in a saturated solution of fuchsin in 2 per cent carbolic acid 10 minutes or longer.
3. Wash in water.
4. Wash in absolute alcohol for 30 seconds.
5. Counterstain in iodine green (1 grm. in 100 cc. of a 2 per cent carbolic acid) for 5 minutes.
6. Dehydrate quickly in absolute alcohol.
7. Clear in xylol; mount in balsam.

Nuclei are green; Russell's fuchsin-bodies light-red; Altmann's granules light-red.

3. Pianese's Method.

1. Fix in Pianese's solution (see methods of fixation) 6 hours; wash in running water for 12 hours; after-harden in graded alcohols; imbed in paraffin; mount on cover-glass.
2. Stain 30 minutes in a staining mixture consisting of malachite green 0.5 grm., acid fuchsin 0.1 grm., Martius yellow 0.01 grm., distilled water 150 cc., 96 per cent alcohol 50 cc.
3. Dehydrate in absolute alcohol; clear in xylol; balsam.

Nuclei are green; protoplasm reddish; cell-inclusions light-red.

4. Method for Staining "Plimmer's Bodies."

1. Fix in Hermann's fluid for 12-24 hours. Imbed in paraffin. Mount sections on cover or slide.
2. Transfer sections to hydrogen peroxide for 15-30 seconds.
3. Wash in water.
4. Transfer to a 4 per cent ferric alum solution for 2 hours.
5. Wash in water.
6. Stain in 0.5 per cent watery hæmatoxylin solution for 30 minutes. Differentiate in the ferric alum solution until the nuclei are dark and protoplasm colorless; control under the microscope.
7. Wash in water 3-6 hours.
8. Counterstain in 1 per cent solution of Ehrlich's neutral red until section is yellow-red.

Nuclei blue-black; cell-inclusions yellow- to copper-red.

V. CHOLESTERIN. Cholesterin is soluble in absolute alcohol, xylol, ether and glacial acetic. It occurs in the tissues in characteristic rhombic plates often showing a square notch in one corner. In sections from which the cholesterin has been dissolved its presence may be told by the appearance of "cholesterin-clefts" in the tissue, or often in the protoplasm of large foreign-body giant-cells ("cholesterin-giant-cells"). With concentrated sulphuric acid, sections or material containing cholesterin become yellow and then rose-pink. Lugol's gives it a brown color which turns blue-violet after the addition of sulphuric acid, and exhibits a play of colors, blue, green, to red.

VI. CLOUDY SWELLING. This is best seen in the fresh state in cells obtained by scraping or teasing, or by the examination of frozen sections. Osmic acid, sudan III, scarlet R, ether, alcohol and acetic acid may be used to differentiate from fatty degeneration. The ordinary fixing and staining methods give good pictures, except for slight degrees of the change. These are sometimes wholly lost as the result of the contraction due to the fixation.

VII. COLLOID. (See Epithelial Hyalin.)

VIII. CORNIFICATION. Horn takes the plasma stains (eosin, picric acid, etc.). Van Gieson's makes a good differential stain. With Gram's method horn stains deep blue, and with the Ehrlich-Biondi-Heidenhain method it stains red. After fixation in Flemming's it may be stained with safranin or gentian-violet. **Keratohyalin** occurs as fine granules in the cells of the stratum granulosum. They stain by hæmatoxylin, carmine and Gram's method, or may be demonstrated by means of special stains. **Eleidin** stains with carmine and the fat-stains, but not with hæmatoxylin.

1. Buzzi's Method of Staining Eleidin and Keratohyalin.
1. Harden, imbed, cut.
2. Stain in Congo red (2-3 drops of a 1 per cent water solution added to small basin of water) for 2-3 minutes.
3. Wash thoroughly in water.
4. Stain in hæmatoxylin, and wash.
5. Dehydrate in absolute alcohol; xylol; balsam.

Keratohyalin blue, eleidin red.

2. Fick's Method of Staining Keratohyalin and Keratin.
1. Harden in alcohol, imbed, cut.
2. Stain in saturated water solution of kresyl-echt-violett for 3-4 minutes.
3. Wash thoroughly in water.
4. Differentiate in 95 per cent alcohol until connective-tissue is colorless.
5. Dehydrate in absolute alcohol; xylol; balsam.

Keratohyalin red, keratin dark violet; nuclei blue-violet, plasma light blue-violet.

IX. FAT. When alcohol has been used in the preparation of the tissue, the fat-contents of the latter are dissolved out, and their presence can alone be told by the presence of vacuoles. When osmic acid is used as a fixing agent the oleates and oleic acid are blackened. The tissue should then be washed in running water and cut upon the freezing-microtome, or it may be imbedded in celloidin or paraffin if this is done as quickly as possible to prevent the loss of the fat. Chloroform or benzene should be used in place of xylol, as the last-named dissolves out the fat. Safranin should be used as a stain after fixation with any fluid containing osmic acid. Frozen sections are to be mounted in glycerin-gelatin; when balsam is used it should be warm melted Canada balsam without xylol. Formol fixation preserves fat, and tissues so fixed may be cut on the freezing-microtome and the sections stained with osmic acid, sudan III or scharlach R, with nuclear counterstaining when desired. For the demonstration of fat-embolism, fatty degeneration or fatty infiltration the following methods are advised:—

1. Staining of Fat with Osmic Acid.
1. Fix in formol for 24 hours.
2. Wash; freeze; cut.
3. Place sections in 1 per cent osmic acid, Flemming's or Marchi's fluid for 1-24 hours.
4. Wash in water, changing frequently.
5. 80 per cent alcohol ½-2 hours.
6. Wash in water.

7. Place section flat on slide; blot; add a drop of warmed glycerin-gelatin; cover quickly. Ringing or sealing is not necessary.

Or, to mount section in balsam:—

After 6, counterstain with hæmatoxylin or safranin; wash again; dehydrate quickly with absolute alcohol; clear in pure benzene; mount in pure melted Canada balsam (containing no xylol).

2. Staining of Fat with Sudan III or Scharlach R.

Staining-solutions of these dyes may be made, as follows:—

a. Dissolve stain in 70-80 per cent boiling alcohol, keep in the incubator over night, and use warm.

b. Make a solution of absolute alcohol 70 cc., 10 per cent caustic soda solution 20 cc., water 100 cc. Saturate this with the stain, slightly heating.

c. Make a mixture of 70 per cent alcohol 50 cc. and pure acetone 50 cc.; saturate this with the stain.

All solutions of these dyes should be filtered before using, and should be kept covered to avoid evaporation and subsequent precipitation.

1. Formalin fixation 24 hours; cut on freezing-microtome.
2. Place sections in 70 per cent alcohol.
3. Stain in the simple solution 20-30 minutes; in the acetone or alkaline alcoholic solutions 2-3 minutes.
4. Wash in 50-70 per cent alcohol, differentiating as needed.
5. Transfer to water; thence to slide; blot, and mount in glycerin gelatin.

When a nuclear counter-stain is desired, put the sections in water after 4; then stain in hæmatoxylin; differentiate quickly in acid alcohol; wash in water; place in weak ammonia or lithium-carbonate solution; wash in water; transfer to slide; blot; mount in glycerin gelatin.

Sudan III and scarlet R stain the smallest particles of fat yellowish-red to deep scarlet; scarlet R on the whole gives the best results. The contrast with the blue nuclei when stained with hæmatoxylin gives beautiful preparations.

3. Staining of Fat with Indophenol.

Stain sections with lithium-carmine; wash; then stain 20 minutes in a saturated solution of indophenol in 70 per cent alcohol. Fat blue; nuclei red.

4. Staining of Fatty Acids and Soaps.

a. Benda's Method. Fix in 10 per cent formol. Transfer tissue to Weigert's copper-fluorchrom mordant (neutral copper acetate 5 grms., fluorchrom 2.5 grms., water 100 cc.; boil and add 5 cc. of 36 per cent acetic acid) in the incubator for 2-4 days. Cut on the freezing-microtome. Stain sections in sudan III or scharlach R, and then in hæmatoxylin. Nuclei are blue, normal fat red, necrosed fat green due to formation of fatty acid copper salt. Soaps give the same reaction when converted into insoluble salts by fixing in formol saturated with calcium salicylate. Through comparison of tissue hardened in this way with another portion fixed in formol alone soaps and fatty acids may be differentiated.

b. Smith's Method. Stain in concentrated water solution of Nile blue sulphate for 10 minutes. Fat stains red, nuclei dark blue, protoplasm light blue, fatty acids dark-blue. Differentiate in 1 per cent acetic acid; wash in water; mount in glycerin-gelatin.

  X. FIBRIN. Fibrin stains with the acid aniline dyes, except in areas of necrosis containing diffused chromatin, under which conditions it stains deep blue with hæmatoxylin. In Van Gieson's mixture it stains yellow or brownish; in Mallory's reticulum stain it stains red, and with Mallory's chloride of iron hæmatoxylin it is grayish to dark blue. The best selective method by far is Weigert's, and it is the only really practical method giving a good differentiation.

  ### 1. Weigert's Fibrin Stain.

  I have obtained the best results by making this stain as follows: 10 cc. of aniline oil and 100 cc. of water are shaken together violently for several minutes, and then filtered through a moist filter. The filtrate must contain no drops of aniline. Add to the filtrate sufficient dry gentian-violet or methyl-violet to produce a metallic shimmer on the surface of the solution after the dye is dissolved by shaking. The solution will keep for several months.

  Weigert advised the use of two stock solutions, I (absolute alcohol 33 cc., aniline oil 9 cc., methyl violet in excess) and II (saturated water solution of methyl violet). These solutions will keep for years. When ready to use stain take 3 cc. of Sol. I and 27 cc. of Sol. II. This staining mixture will keep for about 2 weeks.

  1. Fix in alcohol, formol, acetone, mercuric chloride or Müller's. Imbed in celloidin or paraffin: the latter preferably. Mount sections on cover-glass with albumin fixative. Celloidin sections must be fastened to slide by thin film of celloidin to prevent shrinkage. Sections fixed in chromic mixtures (and sometimes after formol fixation) must be oxidized in potassium permanganate and then reduced in oxalic acid to give good results. (Transfer sections to a 1 per cent solution of potassium permanganate to which 2 volumes of water have been added; oxidize for 10 minutes; then wash in water, and reduce for several hours in a 5 per cent water oxalic acid solution.)
  2. Wash in water.
  3. Stain in lithium carmine; differentiate in acid alcohol; wash thoroughly in water.
  4. Stain on the slide or cover-glass in the aniline-methyl-violet (or gentian-violet) solution for 10 minutes. Wash off stain with physiologic salt solution.
  5. Blot section with absorbent paper.
  6. Cover section with Lugol's (300-2-1) or a 5 per cent watery potassium iodide saturated with iodine. Leave on section for 1-5 minutes.
  7. Blot off iodine.

8. Differentiate in aniline xylol (equal parts of xylol and aniline oil) until the nuclei become red.
9. Wash in xylol, blotting with absorbent paper. Repeat until section is transparent; then mount in balsam. All aniline oil must be removed before using the balsam.

Nuclei are red; fibrin deep blue; bacteria, mucin, keratin and Altmann's granules also blue. The differentiation must be carefully controlled under the microscope, and should be stopped before the finest threads of fibrin begin to be decolorized.

XI. GLYCOGEN. Glycogen is soluble in water; and fixation and hardening must be carried out with absolute alcohol to prevent the solution of the glycogen. Tissue must be fixed immediately after death, as glycogen is quickly broken up. Its reaction with iodine is similar to that of amyloid, but it does not give the iodine-sulphuric-acid reaction that the latter substance does.

1. Best's Iodine Method.
1. Fix and harden in absolute alcohol; imbed in paraffin; cut.
2. Stain somewhat deeply with hæmatoxylin.
3. Wash in water.
4. Stain in iodine 1, potassium iodide 2, water 100.
5. Dehydrate in iodine 2, absolute alcohol 100.
6. Differentiate in origanum oil, 1-2 hours.
7. Wash thoroughly with xylol.
8. Arrange on slide and dry in air.
9. Mount in pure melted balsam (no xylol).

Nuclei are blue, glycogen brown.

2. Best's Carmine Method for Glycogen.
1. Fix in absolute alcohol; imbed in celloidin; cut.
2. Stain in hæmatoxylin; differentiate in acid alcohol.
3. Wash in water.
4. Stain in filtered carmine mixture (carmine 1 grm., ammonium chlorate 2 grms., lithium carbonate 0.5 grm., water 50 cc.; bring to boiling point, and when cool, add 20 cc. of strong liquid ammonia. Keep in dark; can be used after 2-3 days and gives good results up to 14 days) 2 parts, strong ammonia 3 parts, methyl alcohol 6 parts. Make fresh each time it is used, as it soon precipitates; do not filter; stain few sections at a time ¾-1 hour.
5. Differentiate 1-2 minutes in a mixture of absolute alcohol 4 parts, methyl alcohol 2 parts, water 5 parts.
6. Wash in 80 per cent alcohol.
7. Dehydrate in absolute alcohol.
8. Clear in xylol; mount in balsam.

Glycogen is stained red; nuclei blue; dense connective-tissue, mast-cell granules, protoplasm of gastric glands, etc., red; but these can all be distinguished morphologically from glycogen. This is by far the best method for the staining of glycogen.

XII. HYALIN. Epithelial hyalin (colloid) stains red or violet with hæmatoxylin and eosin; it takes the other acid dyes and stains to some degree with basic aniline stains. Van Gieson's stains it a yellow, orange or brownish-pink. Kresyl-echt-violett gives it a deep indigo-blue color or a more green robin-egg blue. *Connective-tissue hyalin* stains deep brilliant red with Van Gieson's; this is the best method for differentiating connective-tissue hyalin from amyloid or epithelial hyalin. Russell's method also stains hyalin red.

XIII. HYDROPIC DEGENERATION. Fix by heat or formol-alcohol. Imbed in celloidin; stain with hæmatoxylin and eosin.

XIV. HYPERTROPHY. Fix in Müller's or mercuric chloride for simple staining; for study of nuclei fix in Flemming's and stain with safranin.

XV. INFLAMMATION. The process of inflammation may be studied to advantage in the mesentery, web or tongue of the curarized living frog, by stretching these parts over a cork-ring attached to a glass plate on which the animal rests. The exposed tissues must be kept moist with physiologic salt solution. Heat, chemicals or other irritants may be employed to produce the inflammatory reaction. For the study of the inflammatory process in sections the ordinary fixations may be employed, but for the study of the nuclei, mitotic figures and cell-granulations fixation in Flemming's, Zenker's, etc., is advised. Safranin, methylene blue and eosin, the various stains used in the study of blood-cells, etc., may be used.

1. Staining of Mast-cells.

a. Kresyl-echt-violett used as for amyloid or mucin is the best stain for mast-cells. The cell-granules stain bright rose-red.

b. Ehrlich's Dahlia Method.
1. Harden in absolute alcohol; imbed; cut.
2. Stain with saturated water solution of dahlia.
3. Wash in water.
4. Dehydrate in absolute alcohol.
5. Clear in xylol; mount in balsam.

c. Unna's Method for Mast and Plasma Cells.
1. Harden in absolute alcohol; imbed; cut.
2. Stain in Unna's polychrome methylene blue ¼-12 hours.
3. Wash in water.
4. Differentiate in Unna's glycerin-ether mixture (Grübler) 15 seconds to several minutes.

5. Wash carefully in water.
6. Dehydrate in absolute alcohol; clear in xylol; mount in balsam.

Mast cell granules are red; plasma cell granules blue.

d. Various modifications of the *Romanowsky method* stain mast- and plasma-cells very well.

XVI. IODINE. For the demonstration of iodine in tissues the following method has been advised by **Justus.** The experience of other workers with it has not been satisfactory.

1. Harden in absolute alcohol; imbed in celloidin; cut.
2. Soak in water to remove alcohol.
3. Put section in wide-mouthed, stoppered bottle in freshly prepared green chlorine-water for 1-2 minutes.
4. Transfer section on a glass needle to a vessel containing 500 cc. water and 1 cc. of a 1 per cent solution of silver nitrate for 2-3 hours. The section is colored yellow-green, and a precipitate of silver chloride appears.
5. Transfer section to a warm saturated solution of sodium chloride until it becomes light.
6. Wash in distilled water.
7. Transfer to a concentrated solution of mercuric chloride.
8. Examine in pure glycerin.

Iodine should be red.

XVII. MITOTIC FIGURES. Various histologic methods devised for the study of mitoses can be applied to the demonstration of these in neoplasms, inflammation and regeneration. Flemming's solution or mercuric chloride fixation gives best results, although formol, or even absolute alcohol, when used quickly and carefully gives fair results if tissue is very fresh.

1. Flemming's Solution and Safranin.

1. Fix small pieces of fresh tissue in Flemming's, in the dark, for 24 hours; wash 24 hours; after-harden in graded alcohols; imbed and cut.
2. Stain in 1 per cent water solution or saturated aniline water solution of safranin, or 1 per cent water methyl violet for 12-24 hours, or carbol-fuchsin for one hour.
3. Differentiate quickly in a 0.5-0.0001 HCl in 70 per cent alcohol and then in absolute alcohol until stain no longer comes away in clouds and nuclei have right shade.
4. Clear in xylol; mount in balsam.

Fat is black; mitoses stand out sharply; tubercle-bacilli may be stained black or red.

STAINING OF MITOTIC FIGURES.

2. Fixation in mercuric-chloride may be followed by **Ehrlich-Biondi-Heidenhain's stain** (saturated aqueous orange 100 cc., saturated aqueous acid fuchsin 20 cc., saturated aqueous methyl green 50 cc.) 12 grms. of Grübler's prepared stain dissolved in 100 cc. of distilled water, for stock solution. For staining take 1 cc. of stock solution, water 30 cc., ½ per cent watery acid fuchsin 3 cc., and 2 per cent acetic 5-6 drops. Stain 2-24 hours; wash in 90 per cent alcohol; dehydrate in absolute; clear in xylol; balsam.

Resting nuclei are bluish; mitoses and fragments of leukocyte nuclei dark green; red blood cells orange red; protoplasm and connective-tissue fuchsin red.

3. Benda's Iron-Haematoxylin Method.

1. Fix in osmic acid, mercuric chloride or other fixative.
2. Stain sections by placing them in liq. ferri. sulfur. oxyd. (Germ. Pharm.) diluted with double its volume of water, for 24 hours; wash carefully in distilled water and then in tap water; stain in 1 per cent watery hæmatoxylin until section is black. Wash in water. Differentiate in 10-30 per cent acetic acid, or in liq. ferri. sulfur. oxyd. diluted with distilled water 1-20. A 10 per cent solution of ferric sulphate may be used instead of the persulphate.

4. Heidenhain's Iron-Haematoxylin.

1. Imbed in paraffin after fixation in mercuric chloride.
2. Immerse section in a 1.5 per cent solution of iron-alum sulphate (violet-colored salt) or iron-ammonium sulphate for ½-3 hours.
3. Wash in water.
4. Stain in 0.5 per cent watery hæmatoxylin or hæmatein for 12-18 hours.
5. Wash in water.
6. Differentiate in the iron-alum or iron-ammonium solution until the section becomes deep blue (control under microscope) and nuclear structures stand out distinctly.
7. Wash in running water for 15 minutes.
8. Absolute alcohol; xylol; balsam.

Instead of the watery hæmatoxylin solution a mixture of hæmatoxylin 1 grm., alcohol 10 cc., and water 90 cc. may be used. Keep four weeks before using. Stain 24-36 hours. For contrast staining a weak solution of Bordeaux red may be used before the iron-alum and hæmatoxylin, staining 24 hours.

XVIII. MUCIN.

Mucin stains a deep blue or reddish-violet with an over-ripe hæmatoxylin. When counterstained with picric acid very beautiful preparations can be obtained. Mucin also gives a metachromatic reaction with kresyl-echt-violett, thionin, toluidin-blue and polychrome methylene-blue, staining red with these stains. Water or carbolic-acid solutions of these stains may be used; dehydrate in absolute alcohol, clear in xylol, and mount in balsam. In my opinion **Morse's Carbol-kresyl-echt-violett** method as given above for amyloid is the best of these metachromatic reactions. Muchæmatein and mucicarmin give the most delicate reactions.

1. Mayer's Muchaematein.

1. Absolute alcohol fixation is preferable.
2. Stain sections in Mayer's solution (hæmatein 0.2 grm. mixed with a few drops of glycerin, 0.1 grm. of aluminum chloride, 40 cc. of glycerin, 60 cc. of water) for 5-10 minutes.
3. Wash in water.
4. Dehydrate in absolute alcohol; xylol; balsam.

Carmine may be used for counterstaining; mucin is blue. Should the mucin swell in the stain replace water and glycerin with 100 cc. of 70 per cent alcohol and 1-2 drops of nitric acid.

2. Mayer's Mucicarmin.

Make staining solution by mixing 1 grm. carmine, 0.5 grm. aluminum chloride, 2 cc. water and 100 cc. of 50 per cent alcohol, heating over the flame for 2-3 minutes until mixture darkens. Let stand 24 hours and filter. The stock solution may be diluted 1-10. Stain 10 minutes. If it does not stain well add 0.5-1 grm. of aluminum chloride. Mucin alone should be stained red. Counterstain with hæmatoxylin.

XIX. MYELIN. This appears in the form of doubly refractive granules, that stain with less intensity with the fat dyes, but may be differentiated from fat in that it loses the power of reducing osmic acid after being mordanted for eight days or more in bichromate solutions, while fat does not.

XX. NECROSIS. Hæmatoxylin and eosin, and Van Gieson's give good pictures. Use Weigert's fibrin stain for coagulation-necrosis, and Benda's method for the demonstration of fatty acids for the staining of fat-necrosis. Recent necrotic areas stain diffusely blue with hæmatoxylin; older areas may take the plasma stains alone. Use various methods for the demonstration of micro-organisms in the necrotic areas.

XXI. NEOPLASMS. Use hæmatoxylin and eosin, and Van Gieson's for ordinary diagnosis. To differentiate sarcoma and carcinoma use Van Gieson's, Mallory's or other reticulum stains. For the study of cell-inclusions use Altmann's, Russell's, Plimmer's and Pianese's methods. Special fixation or Zenker's is necessary. Methylene-blue and eosin after Zenker's give excellent pictures. For the demonstration of mitoses the methods given above should be employed.

XXII. PIGMENT. Use the carmines for contrasting melanin, hæmofuscin, lipochromes, hæmatoidin, hæmosiderin, bilirubin and all yellow, brown, blue, black, etc., extrinsic pigments. In tissue fixed in mercuric chloride or formol bilirubin is green, and can thus be differentiated from hæmatoidin. The lipochromes give weak fat-reactions, and this is used to distinguish them from other yellow or brown pigments. Alcohol fixation is the best for pigment study, although the other fixing solutions may be used. Formol sometimes produces pseudo-pigments by its action upon hæmoglobin. The iron-reactions are obtained best in sections cut on the freezing-microtome, although both paraffin and celloidin imbedding may be used. In testing for iron glass needles should be used and all traces of iron should be removed from staining-dishes, slides, etc., by treating with hydrochloric acid, distilled water and alcohol.

1. Potassium Ferrocyanid Test for Iron.

1. Stain sections in lithium carmine for several hours.
2. Differentiate in acid alcohol, stopping short of the desired complete differentiation of the nuclei.
3. Wash in water.
4. Saturated solution of potassium ferrocyanid 1-3 hours.
5. Acid alcohol until iron-pigment becomes blue ($\frac{1}{2}$-12 hours). Complete differentiation of nuclei.
6. Wash in water.
7. Dehydrate in absolute alcohol.
8. Clear in xylol; mount in balsam.

Hæmosiderin is blue (Berlin blue); nuclei are red. Lithium carmine may be used after the iron-test, if desired.

2. Ammonium Sulphide Test for Iron.

1. Fix in alcohol; imbed; cut.
2. Treat sections with yellow ammonium sulphide for 5-60 minutes.
3. Wash quickly in water.
4. Dehydrate in absolute alcohol.
5. Clear in xylol; mount in balsam.

Stain with lithium carmine either before or after the reaction with ammonium sulphide. Iron is grayish-black to black.

3. Combined or Masked Iron.

1. Treat tissues with Bunge's fluid (95 per cent alcohol 95 cc., 25 per cent hydrochloric acid 10 cc.) for 1-2 hours at 50-60°C., until inorganic iron is all removed.
2. Place tissues in acid alcohol (sulphuric acid 4 cc. in 100 cc. alcohol 95 per cent.
5. Wash sections in acid alcohol, then pure alcohol, and finally in distilled water.
6. Transfer to ammonium sulphide (5-60 minutes) or to potassium ferrocyanid and 0.5 HCl for 5 minutes.
7. Wash in water.
8. Counterstain in eosin or safranin; wash; dehydrate in absolute alcohol; clear in cedar-oil; mount in benzene balsam. Keep preparations in the dark.

4. Staining of Chromophilic Cells.

1. Fix in a chromic solution. In this the chromophilic cells become yellow or brown.
2. Stain in polychrome methylene blue; the cells become grass-green in color.

5. Tests for Silver, Lead and Mercury.

Use ammonium sulphide as for iron. Black sulphides are formed.

6. Test for Copper.

Treat with potassium ferrocyanid and hydrochloric acid; copper gives a dark yellow-brown coloration.

XXIII. PSEUDOMUCIN. It is not precipitated by acetic acid. It has a greater affinity for the diffuse stains than mucin, and gives weaker metachromatic reactions.

XXIV. REGENERATION AND REPAIR. For the staining of mitoses, cell granules and cell-inclusions see methods given above. See also methods for staining of epithelium, reticulum, neuroglia, etc.

XXV. URIC ACID AND PURIN BASES:—

1. Courmont and Andre's Method.

1. Fix in absolute alcohol; imbed; cut.
2. Treat sections with 1/100 ammonia solution or very weak sodium hyposulphite solution.
3. Transfer to 1/100 silver nitrate solution.
4. Wash.
5. Develop with a photographic developer.
6. Wash in water; stain with hæmalum and eosin; dehydrate; clear in xylol; balsam.

Uric acid and xanthin or purin bases appear as black granules.

CHAPTER XXVII.
THE STAINING OF PATHOGENIC MICRO-ORGANISMS IN TISSUES

Rapid fixation and hardening are requisites for the successful staining of micro-organisms in sections. Alcohol, Zenker's, mercuric chloride and formol give best results; Müller's because of its slow action is not good, although formol-Müller's may be used because of the more rapid fixation with this fluid. In the case of formalin-fixation staining with Weigert-Gram's method may not give good results unless the sections are oxidized in potassium permanganate solution and then reduced in oxalic acid. (See Staining of Fibrin.) Preservation of the tissue for a long time in alcohol impairs the staining power of micro-organisms contained within it. The tissue should be imbedded preferably in paraffin, as very thin sections must be obtained. The freezing-microtome may be employed and the thinnest sections selected for staining. Celloidin stains very heavily with the aniline dyes and retains the color, so that bacteria in celloidin sections do not stand out very distinctly. On the whole paraffin sections, floated on slide or cover, and fastened by albumin-fixative, give the best results, though for the micro-organisms stained in carbol-fuchsin and decolorized in nitric acid it is best to float the sections directly onto the warm stain without removing the paraffin, and mount without the use of alcohol. This method may be employed for all stains that are taken out by alcohol. The stains used for film preparations are as a rule applicable to sections. The basic aniline dyes, particularly methylene-blue, fuchsin, methyl or gentian violet, kresyl-echt-violett, thionin, and Bismarck brown, either in saturated alcoholic solutions or dilutions of such, or in combination with alkalies, aniline oil or phenol, are usually employed. The various modifications of the Romanowsky method are very useful. The time required for staining in sections is usually much longer than for films; but the staining can often be accelerated or strengthened by warming over the flame or in the incubator. Contrast staining of the nuclei with lithium-carmine or Bismarck brown is advisable after the use of staining methods in which the nuclei are decolorized. Xylol or origanum oil should be used for clearing.

I. THE STAINING OF BACTERIA IN TISSUES.

According to their staining-reactions bacteria may be very conveniently grouped in three classes: 1, *Staining with Gram-Weigert's method;* 2, *Not staining with Gram-Weigert's;* 3, *Staining with the tubercle-bacillus method (acid-resisting).*

1. BACTERIA STAINING BY THE GRAM-WEIGERT METHOD.

Weigert's modification of Gram's method, as given above for the staining of fibrin, is the best for the staining of bacteria that stain by this method. (See Fibrin, Chapter XXVI.) The differentiation with aniline-xylol is slower and safer than with alcohol. Acetone-xylol (1:5) has been recommended in place of aniline-xylol. Wolbach recommends the use of a 5-10 per cent colophonium-alcohol for differentiation. Contrast staining with watery Bismarck brown, dilute carbol-fuchsin or eosin may be carried out if desired. The aniline-xylol may be saturated with eosin and the section stained during the differentiation. *Carbol-gentian-violet* may be used instead of aniline-gentian-violet; it keeps much better than the latter.

Staining by Gram's Method (Gram-positive).

Staphylococcus pyogenes aureus.
Staphylococcus pyogenes albus.
Staphylococcus pyogenes citreus.
Streptococcus pyogenes.
Micrococcus tetragenus.
Diplococcus pneumoniæ.
Bacillus aërogenes capsulatus.
Bacillus of diphtheria.
Bacillus of anthrax.
Bacillus of leprosy.
Bacillus of tetanus.
Bacillus of tuberculosis.
Bacillus of rhinoscleroma.
Bacillus of mouse septicæmia.
Bacillus of swine erysipelas.
Oïdium albicans.
Mycelium of actinomyces.

2. BACTERIA NOT STAINING BY GRAM'S METHOD.

For the bacteria belonging to this class Löffler's methylene-blue, carbol methylene-blue, a watery solution of methylene-blue or gentian-violet, Leishman's or Wright's modification of Romanowsky's methylene-blue eosin method (see page 290), Unna's alkaline methylene-blue solution preceded by eosin after Zenker's fixation (see page 260), aniline gentian-violet, Zieler's method and carbol fuchsin are most commonly used as stains. Wolbach advises the use of a 5-10 per cent acetone-colophonium solution for the differentiation of Gram-negative bacteria in tissue fixed in formol.

1. Löffler's Methylene-blue.

1. Saturated alcoholic solution of methylene-blue 30 cc.; potassium hydrate solution (1 in 10,000) 100 cc.
2. Stain 5 minutes to 24 hours.
3. Wash in water.

STAINING OF GRAM-NEGATIVE BACTERIA.

4. Differentiate in 1 per cent acetic acid, 10-30 seconds.
5. Wash in 90 per cent alcohol, 2-5 minutes; dehydrate in absolute alcohol; clear in xylol; mount in balsam.

2. Gentian-violet.

1. Stain sections in a 2 per cent watery gentian-violet for 5-20 minutes.
2. Wash in water.
3. Decolorize in 70 per cent alcohol until stain ceases to come away.
4. Dehydrate in absolute alcohol; clear in xylol; balsam.

3. Zieler's Method.

1. Fix in Orth's solution, or any fixing solution except those containing osmic acid; imbed in paraffin or celloidin.
2. Stain in Pranter's solution (orcein D 0.1 grm., hydrochloric acid 2.0 cc., 70 per cent alcohol 100 cc.) for 8-24 hours.
3. Wash rapidly in 70 per cent alcohol.
4. Wash in water.
5. Stain in polychrome methylene-blue 10 minutes to several hours.
6. Wash in distilled water.
7. Differentiate in glycerin ether until no more clouds of color come away and section is light blue.
8. Wash in distilled water.
9. 70 per cent alcohol for a few seconds; absolute 5-10 minutes; xylol; balsam.

Protoplasm is gray-brown; bacteria dark-blue; background colorless. Zieler's method is especially good for the staining of the glanders, typhoid and chancroid bacilli and the gonococcus.

For Unna's methylene-blue eosin and the modifications of the Romanowsky method see Pages 260 and 290 respectively. Pappenheim's methyl-green-pyronin method is also recommended for the staining in sections of Gram-negative bacteria.

Not Staining by Gram's (Gram-negative).

Gonococcus.
Micrococcus melitensis.
Meningococcus (in sections).
Bacillus of bubonic plague.
Bacillus of chancroid.
Bacillus coli communis.
Bacillus dysenteriæ.
Bacillus of epidemic conjunctivitis (Koch-Weeks).
Bacillus of influenza.
Bacillus mallei.
Bacillus pneumoniæ.
Bacillus proteus.
Bacillus of malignant œdema.
Bacillus pyocyaneus.
Bacillus of typhoid fever.
Bacillus of fowl cholera.
Bacillus of rabbit septicæmia.
Bacillus of swine plague.
Spirillum of Asiatic cholera.
Spirochæte pallida.

3. BACTERIA STAINING BY THE TUBERCLE-BACILLUS METHOD. (ZIEHL-NEELSEN.)

1. Tubercle-bacillus.
2. Lepra-bacillus.
3. Smegma-bacillus.
4. Lustgarten's bacillus.

1. Stain sections by floating thin paraffin sections directly on to warm carbol-fuchsin (fuchsin 1 grm., absolute alcohol 10 cc., cryst. carbolic acid, 5 grms., water 100 cc.) for 1-3 minutes.
2. Transfer on spatula to water, agitating so as to wash off excess of stain.
3. Transfer section to 30 per cent nitric acid and water alternately, until section has a pale lilac tint.
4. Wash in water.
5. Float on warm watery methylene-blue for 1 minute.
6. Wash in water.
7. Float section on slide; dry over flame or in oven; melt over flame, and put section at once into xylol to remove paraffin.
8. Balsam.

Various staining-methods have been recommended for the staining of the most important pathogenic bacteria in tissues. The most useful of these methods are here given:—

a. Cocci.

1. **Pyogenic Cocci.** Stain by Gram-Weigert's, contrast with Bismarck brown or lithium-carmine.

2. **Pneumococcus.** Stains with ordinary water solutions, carbol-fuchsin and Gram-Weigert's. The staining of the capsule in sections is not very satisfactory.

3. **Gonococcus.** Gram-negative. Stains in sections with Zieler's method, Löffler's methylene-blue, or dilute carbol-fuchsin with differentiation in alcohol.

4. **Micrococcus Catarrhalis.** Stains like the gonococcus.

5. **Diplococcus Intracellularis Meningitidis.** Smear preparations often Gram-positive, in sections usually Gram-negative. Use same stains as for gonococcus.

6. **Micrococcus Tetragenus.** Stain with Gram's or watery solutions of basic aniline dyes.

b. Bacilli.

1. **Anthrax-bacillus.** Stain with Gram-Weigert's and contrast with Bismarck brown or lithium-carmine. Stains also with strong watery gentian-violet solution, with differentiation in strong alcohol.

2. **Bacillus of Malignant Oedema.** Gram-negative. Stain with watery solution or gentian-violet.

3. **Bacillus of Tetanus.** Gram-positive. Stains with watery solutions of basic aniline dyes.

4. **Bacillus Aërogenes Capsulatus.** Gram-positive. Stains with other aniline stains.

5. **Bacillus Pyocyaneus.** Stains with Gram's and other aniline dyes.

6. **Bacillus of Influenza.** Gram-negative. Fix tissue in alcohol. Stain with dilute carbol-fuchsin and differentiate in dilute acetic acid.

7. **Koch-Week's Bacillus.** Gram-negative.

8. **Bacillus of Bubonic Plague.** Gram-negative. Stain by *Gaffky's method* (Fix in alcohol or a mixture of glacial acetic acid 10.0, chloroform 30.0, and 96 per cent alcohol 60.0, imbed in paraffin, stain 2-3 hours in weak watery methylene-blue, dehydrate quickly in absolute alcohol, xylol, balsam). It may also be stained by 24 hours in concentrated solution of fuchsin in glycerin, rapid differentiation in weak acetic; alcohol; xylol; balsam. Alcohol or mercuric chloride fixation should be used, as formol fixation does not give good staining.

9. **Typhoid Bacillus.** Löffler's methylene-blue or carbol-fuchsin, staining 24 hours, decolorizing in dilute acetic and washing rapidly in alcohol. Zieler's method may also be used. It is Gram-negative.

10. **Paratyphoid Bacillus.** Stains like the typhoid bacillus.

11. **Colon Bacillus.** Gram-negative. May be stained with Löffler's methylene-blue or carbol-fuchsin.

12. **Diphtheria Bacillus.** May be stained in sections of diphtheritic membranes with Löffler's methylene-blue, watery aniline stains, or with Gram's if the decolorization is not carried too far.

13. **Bacillus of Chancroid.** Gram-negative. Stain according to *Unna's method:*—
   1. Fix in alcohol.
   2. Stain 5-10 minutes in a mixture of a solution of methylene-blue 1 grm., potassium carbonate 1 grm., alcohol 20 cc., water 100 cc., and a solution of methylene-blue 1 grm., borax 1 grm., water 100 cc.
   3. Place sections on slide; blot.
   4. Decolorize in Unna's glycerin-ether mixture.
   5. Dry; dehydrate in alcohol.
   6. Xylol; balsam.

14. **Bacillus of Glanders.** Gram-negative. Stain with Zieler's method or with Löffler's methylene-blue, differentiating in weak acetic.

Noniewicz's Method.
1. Stain with Löffler's methylene-blue 2-5 minutes.
2. Wash in water.

3. Differentiate for about 5 seconds in a mixture of ½ per cent acetic acid 75 cc., ½ per cent watery solution tropaeolin 25 cc.
4. Wash in water; dry by blotting; xylol; balsam.

Bacilli deep-blue; tissues light-blue.

15. **Bacillus of Rhinoscleroma.** Gram-positive. Fix in alcohol for *Wolkowitsch's method:*—
    1. Stain in aniline gentian-violet 24-48 hours.
    2. Wash in water.
    3. Treat with Lugol's 1-4 minutes.
    4. Decolorize in absolute alcohol.
    5. Remove more color by oil of cloves.
    6. Xylol; balsam.

In tissues fixed in osmic acid and then stained in hæmatoxylin the bacilli are dark blue with light blue capsules. The hyaline substance of rhinoscleroma stains with basic stains.

16. **Friedländer's Bacillus.** Gram-negative. Stains with ordinary aniline dyes. For staining the capsules the following method is advised:—
    1. Stain for 24 hours in the incubator in a mixture of a concentrated alcoholic solution of gentian-violet 50 cc., glacial acetic acid 10 cc., and distilled water 100 cc.
    2. Wash in a 1 per cent acetic acid solution.
    3. Alcohol; xylol; balsam.

Bacilli deep-blue; capsules light-blue.

17. **Tubercle-bacillus.** Gram-positive. Stain in sections on warm carbol-fuchsin without removing paraffin, as given above. Alcohol and mercuric chloride fixation give best results. Aniline-gentian-violet may also be used, staining with a warm solution for 15-30 minutes, and decolorizing in 20 per cent nitric acid followed by 70 per cent alcohol, counterstaining in Bismarck brown, dehydrating in alcohol, clearing in xylol and mounting in balsam. The Weigert-Gram method may be used for the demonstration of the branched or streptothrix forms of the tubercle bacillus. For celloidin sections *Mallory and Wright* advise the following:—
    1. Stain rather lightly in alum-hæmatoxylin.
    2. Wash in water.
    3. Dehydrate in 95 per cent alcohol.
    4. Attach sections to slide by ether-vapor method.
    5. Stain in steaming carbol-fuchsin 2-5 minutes.
    6. Wash in water.
    7. Acid alcohol ½-1 minute.
    8. Wash thoroughly in several changes of water to remove acid completely and to bring back blue color to nuclei.
    9. 95 per cent alcohol to remove fuchsin.
    10. Aniline-oil, followed by xylol, blotting.
    11. Xylol; balsam.

Celloidin is colorless, nuclei blue, tissue colorless, tubercle-bacilli red. Orange G may be used as a diffuse stain.

18. **Lepra Bacillus.** Gram-positive. Stain paraffin sections on warm carbol-fuchsin, as for the tubercle-bacillus. To differentiate from the tubercle-bacillus, stain 6-7 minutes in a dilute alcoholic solution of fuchsin, and decolorize in acid alcohol (nitric acid 1, alcohol 10). Lepra-bacilli stain; tubercle-bacilli do not.

c. Trichomycetes.

1. **Actinomyces.** Alcohol and formol fixation are best. Good preparations can be obtained with hæmatoxylin and eosin, Van Gieson's or Weigert-Gram's. The special staining methods advised give no better results than these simpler stains. Differential staining of clubs and mycelium may be obtained by *Mallory's method:—*

 1. Stain lightly in alum-cochineal. (Powdered cochineal 6 grms., ammonia alum 6 grms., water 100 cc. Boil half an hour, add water lost by evaporation, filter, add crystals of thymol.)
 2. Saturated watery eosin 10 minutes.
 3. Wash in water.
 4. Stain in aniline gentian-violet 2-5 minutes.
 5. Wash in physiologic saline solution.
 6. Transfer sections to Lugol's for 1 minute.
 7. Pass rapidly through water.
 8. Dry thoroughly between folds of filter-paper.
 9. Cover section with aniline-oil until clear.
 10. Xylol; balsam.

Clubs pink; mycelium blue.

2. **Nocardia, Cladothrix, Streptothrix and Leptothrix.** Löffler's methylene-blue and carbol-fuchsin give good results. The Nocardiæ are acid-fast with dilute acids. They give good preparations with Weigert's fibrin stain and lithium-carmine.

d. Vibrios.

1. **Cholera Vibrios.** Gram-negative. Sections may be stained with fuchsin or methylene-blue.

e. Spirilla and Spirochætes.

1. **Spirillum of Recurrent Fever.** Stain in sections with Levaditi's silver-method, or with Nikiforoff's method:—

 1. Fix for 24 hours in equal parts of a 5 per cent water solution of potassium bichromate and a saturated solution of mercuric chloride in 0.6 per cent sodium chloride.
 2. After-harden in graded alcohols in the incubator.
 3. Imbed in paraffin.
 4. Stain 24 hours in a mixture of alcoholic 1 per cent solution of tropæolin 5 cc., concentrated watery methylene-blue solution 10 cc., caustic potash solution (1:1000) 2 drops.
 5. Wash in water.
 6. Dip several times in a mixture of equal parts of absolute alcohol and ether.
 7. Oil of bergamot; xylol; balsam.

The spirillum of *African relapsing fever* stains with the same stains as the spirillum Obermeieri. The *spirochætes of Vincent's angina* and *fowl-spirillosis*, and the *spirochæte refringens* stain with watery aniline dyes and with Giemsa's stain; in section they are stained by the Levaditi method.

2. **Spirochaeta Pallida (Treponema Pallidum).** This organism is best examined in the living condition by means of the dark-field illumination (dark-field condenser). A very simple method of dark-field illumination consists of the use of India ink. The suspected discharge or serum is placed on a slide and an equal quantity of ink (Günther's or Higgin's) added. The serum and ink are rapidly mixed and spread over the slide to dry in a pale brown smear. The oil for the immersion is placed directly on the smear. The spirochætes appear as white spirals against a brownish-black field. The best results are obtained with serum: the presence of mucus or fibrin interferes with the clearness of the picture obtained.

Smears of serum from syphilitic lesions may be dried in the air and fixed in absolute alcohol or equal parts of absolute alcohol and ether for 15-20 minutes. They may then be stained by Giemsa's (old formula) stain (azur II-eosin 3 grms., azur II 0.8 grm., glycerin [Merck's chemically pure] 250 grms., methyl-alcohol [Kahlbaum I] 250 grms.). This solution can be obtained from Grübler. Ten drops of the stain are mixed with 10 cc. of distilled water immediately before the staining. The fixed preparation is covered with the diluted staining fluid and warmed over the flame until a slight steam arises. It is then allowed to cool for about 15 seconds, when the stain is poured off and replaced by fresh, and the process repeated four or five times, when the preparation is washed, dried and mounted in balsam. Spirochætes are dark red. Slide or cover-glass and forceps must be absolutely clean. Smears may also be fixed and stained by *Wright's blood-stain*.

For the demonstration of the treponema in sections the method of *Levaditi* gives the most satisfactory results:—

1. Fix thin pieces of tissue 24 hours or longer in 10 per cent formol. (Formol-Müller's and alcohol-fixation may also be used.)
2. 24 hours in 96 per cent alcohol.
3. Transfer to distilled water until tissue sinks.
4. Impregnation for 3 days in incubator, in a 1.5-3 per cent silver nitrate solution.
5. Wash for a short time in water.
6. Reduce for 48 hours, in the dark, at room-temperature, in pyrogallic acid 4 grms., 40 per cent formol 5 cc., distilled water 100 cc.
7. Wash in water. Cut on freezing-microtome, or imbed in celloidin or paraffin. Toluidin-blue or safranin may be used as a contrast-stain.

The spirochætes are dark brown to black. Silver precipitates occur chiefly in the outer portions of the tissue. The reticulum is brown; other parts of the tissue are yellowish. Levaditi's more recent modification of this method does not give so good results as the original.

Schmorl's Staining of Sections with Giemsa's Stain.

1. Fix in 10 per cent formol. Cut very thin sections on freezing-microtome.

2. Place the sections in a staining dish containing a measured amount of distilled water. To each cc. of water add one drop of Giemsa's stain. Use clean glass-needles to manipulate the sections. After 1 hour transfer sections to a fresh solution, in which they are left 5-12-24 hours.
3. Wash quickly in a concentrated solution of potassium alum, then quickly in water.
4. Mount in glycerin-gelatin; or dry on the slide until nearly perfectly dry, then xylol, and balsam, or cedar oil. Alcohol must not be used.

II. THE STAINING OF PATHOGENIC YEASTS AND MOULDS IN SECTIONS.

1. **Blastomycetes.** The parasites of blastomycetic dermatitis can be demonstrated unstained in pus treated with a weak sodium hydroxide. In sections they are easily found after treatment with ordinary staining methods. The various modifications of the Romanowsky method, or other methylene-blue-eosin staining, give better staining of the parasite than can be obtained by hæmatoxylin and eosin.

2. **Oïdium Albicans.** Staining with Weigert-Gram's and lithium-carmine gives beautiful preparations.

3. **Moulds.** These are best examined in the unstained condition, by treating the material with equal parts of alcohol and ether, followed by a 3 per cent potassium hydroxide solution. The organisms and spores are brought out distinctly. Löffler's methylene-blue may be used for staining. In the case of sections stain 1-2 hours and contrast with eosin. For the examination of hairs or horny scales for fungi, *Unna's method* may be used:—

1. Add glacial acetic acid to hair or epidermis; make cover-glass preparations, drying by heat.
2. Ether and alcohol equal parts.
3. Stain in borax 1 grm., methylene-blue 1 grm., water 100 cc., ½-5 minutes.
4. Wash in water; dry; balsam.

If the horny elements are too deeply stained, decolorize in 1 per cent acetic for 10 seconds, or in 1 per cent oxalic, citric, or arsenious acid for 1 minute.

III. THE STAINING OF ANIMAL PARASITES.

1. **Amoeba Coli.** Examine fresh material from fæces, abscesses or cultures, in physiologic saline solution, on a warm stage. Stain under the cover with methylene-blue and carmine. Make permanent mounts by removing excess of stain and running in 50 per cent glycerin. In fixed preparations the nuclei of the amoebæ do not stain with ordinary nuclear stains. *Mallory's method* may be used:—

1. Fix in alcohol.
2. Stain sections in a saturated aqueous solution of thionin 3-5 minutes.
3. Differentiate in a 2 per cent aqueous solution of oxalic acid for ½-1 minute.

4. Wash in water; dehydrate in absolute alcohol; clear in xylol; mount in xylol-balsam.

Nuclei of the amœbæ and granules of the mast-cells are brownish-red; nuclei of cells blue.

2. **Trichomonas vaginalis and intestinalis; Cercomonas coli; Megastoma entericum; Balantidium coli; Pyrosoma bigeminum; Trypanosoma; Leishman-Donovan bodies,** and allied forms are best stained with the modifications of Romanowsky's stain; the chromatin is red-violet (macro-nucleus red, micro-nucleus black, flagellum red, protoplasm blue, basophilic granules black). For staining in sections mercuric chloride or Zenker's fixation followed by staining with polychrome methylene-blue, Giemsa's or the modifications of the Romanowsky method may be employed.

3. **Plasmodium Malariae.** For films make medium smears (not too thin); fix with equal parts of absolute alcohol and ether for $\frac{1}{2}$-1 hour; or fix and stain in the same solution (Leishman-Romanowsky, Wright's stain, etc.). For single staining methylene-blue, carbol-thionin, etc., may be employed; for double staining eosin and methylene-blue, Ehrlich's tri-acid, or any of the eosin-methylene-blue combinations may be used (particularly the Leishman-Romanowsky or Wright's). With the Romanowsky methods the body of malarial organism is stained blue, the chromatin varying shades of lilac, red, purplish-red or almost black. When the blood contains but few parasites 1 cc. may be drawn, mixed with 20 cc. of distilled water and centrifugated. Smears are then made of the sediment. For the staining of the plasmodium in imbedded tissues the following method is recommended by *Bignami*. The tissue should be fixed in formol or mercuric chloride, preferably a mixture of mercuric chloride 1 grm., sodium chloride 0.75 grm., acetic acid 0.75 grm., water 200 cc. Fix for 2 hours; after-harden in alcohol and iodine-alcohol, changing the alcohol each day for seven days. Dehydrate in absolute alcohol, and imbed in celloidin or paraffin. Stain in a saturated watery solution of magenta or in a mixture of equal parts of saturated alcoholic mixtures of magenta and orange G. Good results may, however, be obtained with Löffler's methylene-blue. Clear in xylol; mount in balsam.

4. **Coccidia and Sarcosporidia.** The ordinary fixations give good results. Imbed in paraffin or celloidin. Weigert's iron-hæmatoxylin and Van Gieson's give as good pictures as any of the special methods advised.

5. **Negri Bodies of Rabies.** Examine in smears or make sections. Take portions of gray brain-substance from the cortex in the region of the fissure of Rolando (in the dog from around the crucial sulcus), from the hippocampus, and from the cerebellum. Smear cover or slide by taking a thin slice of the gray matter and compressing it between two slides, or cover and slide, or by drawing the cover across the cut surface in order to get some of the cells. Dry in the air; stain with watery methylene-blue; wash; stain with watery acid fuchsin; wash in water; blot dry; mount in balsam. Negri bodies fuchsin-red (about size of red blood cells); everything else blue. When dried in the air and then fixed in methyl alcohol for 5 minutes the smears may be stained by Giemsa's method. For the demonstration of

the bodies in sections fix in Zenker's, imbed in paraffin, and stain by the eosin-methylene-blue method. The bodies take the eosin stain. Formol fixation, freezing-microtome and Romanowsky stain give quick results. *Mann's method* for the staining of Negri bodies in sections is strongly recommended by many workers. Fix material in mercuric chloride or Mann's fluid (1 grm. picric acid and 2 grms. tannin dissolved in 100 cc. concentrated water solution of mercuric chloride) for 24 hours; wash thoroughly in running water; imbed in paraffin. Stain in Mann's mixture (1 per cent aqueous methyl-blue [not methylene-blue] 35 parts, 1 per cent aqueous eosin 35 parts) for 24 hours; wash in water; rinse in absolute alcohol; place in alkaline alcohol (absolute alcohol 50 cc., 4 drops of a 1 per cent solution of sodium hydroxide) for 15-20 seconds until sections become reddish; wash quickly in alcohol; wash about 2 minutes in water until superfluous color is removed; place in weak acidulated water (acetic acid) 1-2 minutes until sections are blue; quick dehydration in alcohol; xylol; balsam. Cells are blue, nucleoli and blood-vessels red; Negri bodies bright red. For quick diagnosis use acetone fixation and imbedding, stain in Mann's fluid 2-4 minutes, and proceed as in the Mann's method. While these bodies possess a great diagnostic importance for rabies, their exact nature must still be regarded as unsettled; they are most probably not parasites.

6. **Vaccine Bodies.** Fix in Flemming's, mercuric chloride or Zenker's; imbed in celloidin or paraffin. Stain with Heidenhain's iron-hæmatoxylin (bodies black) or Biondi-Heidenhain mixture (bodies blue, nuclei of leukocytes and mitoses green, nuclei of epithelium and connective-tissue blue, protoplasm and connective-tissue red). These bodies are probably not parasites, but may be products of cell-degeneration.

7. **Vermes.** The *heads, proglottides* and *ova* are best examined in the fresh state, in physiologic saline or glycerin. Acetic acid may be used to bring out details. Berlin-blue or methylene-blue may be injected through the genital pore for the demonstration of the excretory and genital organs. *Scolices* and *hooklets* of *echinococcus* may be obtained by scraping the cyst-wall; examine in glycerin. Permanent preparations of *cestodes, nematodes* and *trematodes* may be made by fixing in mercuric chloride, formol or Flemming's, after-hardening in alcohol, staining in orange G, borax carmine, alum hæmatoxylin, hæmatoxylin and eosin, etc., mounting in glycerin gelatin; or dehydrating, clearing in xylol and mounting in balsam. For sections imbed in paraffin or celloidin. *Trichinæ* may be studied by teasing the fresh muscle; by digesting with pepsin and hydrochloric acid and examining the freed trichinæ on a warm stage; or by imbedding in paraffin or celloidin and staining with hæmatoxylin and eosin. Permanent mounts of the embryos of *filaria* may be made by fixing cover-glass preparations of blood or chylous fluid by heat or mercuric chloride, and staining for a few seconds with Löffler's or a 2 per cent aqueous thionin.

CHAPTER XXVIII.
THE STAINING OF SPECIAL ORGANS AND TISSUES.
I. BLOOD AND BLOOD-FORMING ORGANS.

The **blood** may be examined by means of *films, stained* or *unstained,* or by *sections, celloidin* or *paraffin.*

A. FILMS. The blood may be obtained from the pulp of the ring finger, from the skin over the knuckles, or from the posterior aspect of the lobe of the ear. The place selected should be carefully cleansed with water, soap and 1/1000 mercuric chloride solution, and finally with alcohol and ether. A puncture is made with a sterilized triangular needle or knife, or a stub-pen with one point broken off. The last-named makes a most useful and inexpensive instrument for this purpose. The puncture should be made by a quick and deep stab, so that sufficient blood can be obtained from one stab-wound. Pressure should not be employed to force blood from the wound. Bleeding may be encouraged by letting the arm hang down, or by applying pressure in the furrow of the terminal joint of the finger. The first drop of blood should be wiped away with a clean towel. When the second drop reaches the size of a pin-head touch it with the under side of a perfectly clean cover-glass, held by forceps, not by the fingers; place this cover-glass immediately upon another clean cover, so that the blood will spread out between the two covers in a thin film. The covers are then separated by sliding them apart without pressing or squeezing; place covers with film side upward, and dry in the air. The films should not be touched with the hands; forceps alone should be used to handle them. If the blood does not dry as quickly as it is spread the film will be too thick. Films may be made upon slides in the same way, or the drop of blood may be caught upon the edge of a clean cover, slide or "spreader" and then drawn rapidly across a slide. The dried film may be marked by scratching with a needle-point the number and date on the film itself. Blood-films may be fixed *without drying* by exposure to the vapor of formol or osmic acid for several seconds and then dropping into absolute alcohol. Formol alcohol, saturated mercuric chloride solution or Flemming's solution may also be used for the fixation of wet films, fixing for

5-10 minutes, and washing thoroughly after each of the last two solutions. The *dried film* may be fixed by exposure to heat (110-115°C.) for 5-10 minutes for Ehrlich's triple stain, and for 2 hours for the methylene-blue-eosin methods; 30-60 seconds at a temperature of 120°C. may suffice; the film should be brought at once into the required temperature. Heat-fixed films are improved by dipping them for a few minutes in mercuric chloride solution and then washing well before staining. *Acetone-free methyl alcohol* (1-2 minutes), *absolute alcohol and ether in equal parts* (½-12 hours), *formol-alcohol* (1-2 minutes), *alcoholic mercuric chloride* (absolute alcohol 25 cc., ether 25 cc., 5 drops of a 2 grms. mercuric chloride solution in 10 cc. of absolute alcohol) for 2-5 minutes, and *formol-vapor* are the chief solutions used for fixing the air-dried film. For ordinary work methyl alcohol, formol alcohol, and the absolute-alcohol and ether mixture give good results; heat fixation brings out the granules well, and mercuric chloride is a good fixative for the leukocytes. The combination of fixation and staining, as in Leishman's or Wright's modification of the Romanowsky method, is also recommended for general work.

For the *staining of blood-films* an almost endless variety of staining-methods can be found in the literature. Many of these represent slight deviations in the method of making the stain or in its application, such deviations marking stages of improvement in the development of the method. It is not necessary, therefore, to give all of these methods, but to consider only the latest modifications of value. In a general way *blood-stains* may be divided into five classes:—

1. HAEMATOXYLIN AND EOSIN.

Fix in equal parts of absolute alcohol and ether for at least 30 minutes; stain with hæmalum and eosin, or Ehrlich's acid hæmatoxylin and eosin. By adding 0.5 grm. of eosin to the formula for Ehrlich's acid hæmatoxylin, a combination stain can be made that is very good for blood-films fixed by heat or absolute alcohol and ether. Stain 2-24 hours, wash, dry and mount in xylol balsam.

2. EOSIN AND METHYLENE-BLUE.

Fix by formol (dried film over 40 per cent formol for 1 minute); absolute alcohol for 1 minute; stain 5 minutes in a 1 per cent watery eosin; then without removing eosin place in watery methylene-blue for 2 minutes; wash quickly; dry in air; balsam.

3. MIXTURES OF EOSIN AND METHYLENE-BLUE.

The numerous mixtures of methylene-blue and eosin are not very stable, can be kept for a few days only, and give varying results. *Jenner* improved this method of staining greatly by collecting the precipitate formed by the addition of eosin to methylene-blue, and dissolving it in pure methyl alcohol, thus giving a solution that fixes and stains at the same time. The *May-Grünwald* method is practically the same.

Jenner's Method.

a. Water-soluble eosin, 1.25 grms.
Distilled water, 100 cc.
b. Medicinal methylene-blue, 1 grm.
Distilled water, 100 cc.

Mix equal parts of *a* and *b* in an open basin, stirring with a glass rod. Let stand for 24 hours; filter; dry the residue at 50°C. Wash residue thoroughly with distilled water and again dry thoroughly. Take 0.5 grm. of the dried powder and dissolve in 100 cc. of pure methyl alcohol. Filter. Solution keeps well.

1. Make blood-film. Dry in air. Do not fix.
2. Cover film with stain, keeping under watch-glass to prevent evaporation. Stain 2 minutes.
3. Wash in distilled water until the film has a pink color. Dry in air. Mount in xylol-balsam.

Neutrophile granules are red, eosinophile rose red, basophile granules violet, red blood cells and central portion of blood-platelets are terra-cotta, leukocyte nuclei and granules in red blood cells are blue, protoplasm of nuclei and outer portion of platelets light blue.

4. MODIFICATIONS OF THE ROMANOWSKY METHOD.

A large group of stains has resulted from various applications of the Romanowsky idea of uniting equimolecular proportions of methylene-blue and eosin, and the solution of the dyes so obtained in some suitable solvent. These dyes consist of mixtures of methylene violet, methylene azure, eosinate of methylene blue, etc., and can be obtained from Grübler and Co. under various names, such as *Azur-blau, Bleu Borrel, Giemsa's stain, Leishman's stain,* etc. Hastings, Leishman, *Wright* and others have combined the Romanowsky method with that of Jenner by dissolving the new dyes obtained by their various modifications in pure methyl alcohol, so as to form a solution that will fix and stain at the same time. *Hastings' stain* is a modification of *Nocht's stain;* *Wright's stain* is a modification of the *Leishman-Romanowsky* method. The revised directions given by *Wright* for making and using his stain are here given. Wright's method and the Giemsa stain possess all of the staining advantages afforded by the variations of the Romanowsky method, and are alone given here. The former is recommended for blood-work, the latter for the staining of protozoa.

Wright's Blood-stain.

To a 0.5 per cent aqueous solution of sodium bicarbonate add methylene-blue (B.X or medicinal) in the proportion of 1 grm. of the dye to each 100 cc. of the solution. Heat the mixture in a steam sterilizer at 100°C. for one full hour, counting the time after the sterilizer has become thoroughly heated. The mixture should be placed in a flask of such size and shape that the fluid will not be more than 6 cm. deep. After heating, allow the mixture to cool, placing the flask in cold water if desired, and then filter it to remove the precipitate. When cold the fluid should have a deep purple-red color when viewed in a thin layer by transmitted yellowish artificial light. It does not show this color while warm.

To each 100 cc. of the filtered mixture add 500 cc. of a 0.1 per cent aqueous solution of yellow water-soluble eosin, and mix thoroughly. Collect on a filter the abundant precipitate which immediately appears. When the precipitate is dry, dissolve it in pure methyl alcohol (Merck's) in the proportion of 0.1 grm. to 60 cc. of the alcohol. To facilitate solution the precipitate is to be rubbed up in a porcelain dish or mortar with a spatula or pestle. This alcoholic solution is the staining solution. It should be kept in a tightly-stoppered bottle. Should it become concentrated through evaporation methyl alcohol in proper quantity should be added.

1. Cover film with a given quantity of staining fluid by means of a medicine dropper.
2. After 1 minute add to the staining fluid on the film the same quantity of distilled water by means of the medicine dropper, and allow the mixture to remain for 2-3 minutes according to the intensity of the stain desired. A longer period of staining may produce a precipitate. Eosinophile granules show best after short staining. The quantity of diluted stain on the preparation should not be so great that some of it runs off.
3. Wash the preparation in water for 30 seconds or until the thinner portions of the film become yellow or pink in color.
4. Dry, and mount in balsam.

Films more than a few hours old do not stain as well as fresh ones.

The *red cells* are orange or pink in color. Polychromatophilia and punctate basophilia or granular degeneration are well shown. Nucleated reds have deep-blue nuclei, and their cytoplasm is usually bluish. The *lymphocytes* have dark purplish-blue nuclei and cytoplasm of a robin's-egg blue, in which a few dark-blue or purplish granules are sometimes present. The nuclei of the *polynuclear neutrophilic leukocytes* are dark-blue or dark lilac-colored, the granules reddish-lilac. The *eosinophiles* have blue or dark lilac nuclei, a blue cytoplasm and eosin-red granules. The *large mononuclear leukocytes* have a dark lilac or blue nucleus, cytoplasm pale blue or blue with dark-lilac or deep purple granules. Mast-cells have purplish or dark-blue nuclei, bluish protoplasm and coarse dark purple or black granules. *Myelocytes* have dark blue or lilac nuclei, blue cytoplasm, and dark-lilac or reddish-lilac granules. *Blood platelets* are blue with small violet or purplish granules in their central portions. *Malarial parasites* have a blue body and lilac or red chromatin. *Spirochæte pallida* is pale blue.

Giemsa's Method.

a, One per cent water solution of azur-blau; *b*, one per cent watery solution of eosin. For staining take 1 cc. of *b*, add 10 cc. of water, and then 1 cc. of the azur-blau solution. Stain 10 minutes to 1 hour.

Giemsa's Old Method.

Azur II—Eosin .... 3.0 grm.
Azur II .... 0.8 grm.
Glycerin (Merck's pure) ....250.0 cc.
Methyl-alcohol (Kahlbaum I) ....250.0 cc.

To 1 cc. of distilled water in a small, perfectly clean graduate add 1 drop of the stain, shaking very gently. Make very thin film; dry in air; fix 15-20 minutes in absolute alcohol. Cover preparation with a thin layer of the freshly diluted stain for 10-15 minutes, renewing stain at end of 10 minutes. Wash in a stream of water. Differentiate over-stained preparations in distilled water. Dry with absorbent paper; mount in balsam. Stains the *spirochæte pallida* and *malarial organisms*. The Giemsa solution may be obtained from Grübler. A more intense staining can be obtained by adding to the water used for diluting the stain 1-2 drops of a 0.1 per cent solution of potassium carbonate.

5. SPECIAL ELECTIVE STAINS FOR THE BLOOD.

1. Ehrlich's Triple Stain.

Saturated watery solution of Orange G.................120 cc.
Saturated watery solution of acid fuchsin .... 80 cc.
Saturated watery solution of methyl green ....100 cc.
Glycerin .... 50 cc.
Distilled water ....300 cc.
Absolute alcohol ....180 cc.

Mix gradually; allow to stand for several months; do not shake or filter. Remove stain with pipette. Fix by heat, or pure methyl alcohol for 5 minutes. Stain 5-10 minutes; wash thoroughly, dry and mount in balsam. Neutrophile granules violet; eosinophile, a bright red; nuclei of the neutrophilic and eosinophilic cells greenish-blue; nuclei of the lymphocytes deep-blue; nuclei of the large mononuclears pale blue; those of red cells intense blue; red cells copper red. The Aronson-Philipp modification is more variable and less satisfactory.

Pappenheim's Stain for Lymphocytes.

3-4 parts of polychrome methylene-blue or methyl green to 1-2 parts of pyronin. Fix in absolute alcohol. Nuclei blue-green; protoplasm bright red.

Staining of Blood-platelets.

The blood-platelets may be examined in the fresh state by coating a cover-slip with Deetjen's agar-solution (boil 5 grms. agar-agar in 500 cc. distilled water, filter hot, and to each 100 cc. of the filtrate add 0.6 grm. sodium chloride, 6-8 cc. of a 10 per cent solution of sodium phosphate and 5 cc. of a 10 per cent solution of sodium diphosphate). Place drop of blood on this coating and examine on warm stage. For permanent stained preparations bleed into a fixing and staining fluid (equal parts alcohol and ether and Romanowsky's stain) or use Wright's stain.

Bremer's Diabetic Reaction.

Take a clean cover-glass, smear one-half with normal blood, the other half with diabetic blood. Fix for 2 hours at 120°C., or in equal parts of absolute alcohol and ether at 60°C. for 4 minutes. Stain in a 10 per cent watery methylene-blue for 2 minutes, wash off the stain in water, and stain for 10 seconds in a ⅛ per cent watery eosin. Wash, dry and mount in balsam. In diabetic blood the red cells are green; in normal blood red. While this reaction is constant in diabetic blood it also occurs in leukæmia, Hodgkin's disease, exophthalmic goitre and multiple neuritis. A 1 per cent solution of *Biebrich scarlet* stains diabetic blood intensely, normal blood but slightly. On the other hand, a *1 per cent methylene-blue* and a *1 per cent Congo red* stain normal blood intensely and diabetic blood slightly.

Staining of Glycogen in Leukocytes.

To a solution of Lugol's (100:3:1) add sufficient gum arabic to make a syrupy mixture. Keep tightly corked. Place a drop of this solution upon an air-dried film. After 1 minute dry with blotting paper. Examine with oil immersion. A positive reaction is shown by the presence of a diffuse brown or reddish-brown coloration or granules in the cell-body of the polymorphonuclear leukocytes.

Staining of Fat in Blood.

Stain in solutions of scharlach R or sudan III in 70 per cent alcohol.

Staining of Blood-parasites.

The *malarial parasites, trypanosomes, Leishman-Donovan bodies, sporidia, piroplasma bigeminum, spirilla* and *spirochætes* and the *filaria* may all be stained with Wright's or Giemsa's modification of the Romanowsky method, or by any of the modifications of this method. (See also Staining of Animal Parasites.)

B. SECTIONS. The blood is allowed to drop directly into Flemming's solution and allowed to stand for 24 hours. It is then washed in water by repeated decanting, or the coagulum may be placed in a bottle covered with muslin, and then exposed to running water. It is after-hardened in alcohol and imbedded in paraffin. Safranin should be used to stain the sections. This method is especially good for the demonstration of mitoses in the blood-cells.

Bone-marrow.

Prepare films and fix and stain, as for blood films. For sections, fix the marrow in formol-Müller's, mercuric chloride, Zenker's, etc.; imbed in paraffin; cut very thin sections; stain with Ehrlich's triple stain or Wright's modification of Leishman's stain. To distinguish the young forms of erythrocytes and leukocytes *Trambusi* fixes in Flemming's, stains the sections in a 1 per cent thionin solution in aniline-water (4:100), differentiates in acid-alcohol, and then brings the sections into a watery eosin and finally an alcoholic eosin, and mounts in xylol-balsam.

Spleen and Lymph-nodes.

Fresh material may be obtained by means of a trocar, and may be examined in the fresh state, or films may be prepared, fixed and stained, as for blood-smears. Sections of fixed tissues may be obtained by the use of the same fixing and staining methods employed in the study of the blood or bone-marrow. For the study of the reticulum Mallory's reticulum stain or the digestion-method may be used. In ordinary work formol-fixation followed by eosin-staining is of great value in distinguishing hæmolymphnodes and lymphatic glands.

II. BONE.

For ordinary work decalcification is necessary except for those pathologic conditions in which the lime-salts have been lost (see Chapter XXI). Imbed in celloidin preferably. When decalcification has been carried out place sections in an alkaline solution before staining, and stain for a longer period than usual. Methylene-blue and eosin stain osteoblasts and osteoclasts very well. Van Gieson's is an especially useful stain for ordinary work; osteoid tissue is red, calcified areas yellow. Sections of bone without decalcification can be prepared by fixing, hardening and staining in bulk; the bone is then sawn in the dried condition, and the sections ground down to the required thickness. *Schmorl's* methods for the preparation of bone-sections have practically superseded all other staining methods.

Schmorl's Thionin-picric-acid Method.

1. Fix in formol or formol-Müller's preferably.
2. Decalcify in formol-nitric acid or Ebner's alcoholic HCl acid solution.
3. Wash thoroughly in water. After-harden in increasing strengths of alcohol; freeze or imbed in celloidin (not paraffin); cut.
4. Transfer sections to water for 10 minutes.
5. Stain sections, well spread out, for 5-10 minutes in a solution of 2 cc. of a saturated solution of thionin in 50 per cent alcohol and 10 cc. of water, to which 1-2 drops of ammonia are added.
6. Wash in water.
7. Stain ½-1 minute in hot saturated and cold filtered watery-solution of picric acid.
8. Wash in water.
9. Differentiate in 70 per cent alcohol until the color ceases to come away in blue-green clouds, 5-10 minutes or more.
10. Dehydrate in 96 per cent alcohol.
11. Clear in phenol xylol; xylol; balsam.

Lacunæ and canaliculi dark brown to black; bone cells red; ground substance yellow or brownish yellow. Calcified areas take a darker yellow than non-calcified. This method consists in an impregnation with a fine precipitate rather than a staining. Should the precipitate be too heavy in portions of the section it may be removed by thorough washing between 9 and 10.

Schmorl's Thionin and Phosphotungstic or Phosphomolybdic Acid Method.

1. Fix thin pieces of fresh bone in formol, then in Müller's for 6-8 weeks, or 3-4 weeks in the incubator. Fixation is best at 37°C.
2. Decalcify in Ebner's hydrochloric acid solution. Wash thoroughly. After-harden in alcohol. Imbed in celloidin or paraffin. Cut very thin sections.
3. Water for 10 minutes.
4. Stain in the alkaline-thionin solution, as in previous method, for 3 minutes.
5. Wash in water.
6. With glass needles transfer sections to a saturated watery solution of phosphotungstic or phosphomolybdic acid for a few seconds.

7. Wash 5-10 minutes, until section is sky-blue in color.
8. Fix the stain for 3-5 minutes in ammonia 1 part, water 10 parts.
9. Transfer directly to 90 per cent alcohol; change twice.
10. Dehydrate; clear in carbol-xylol; balsam.

If the ground-substance is too dark differentiate in acid alcohol before dehydrating, and then wash thoroughly before beginning the dehydration.

Outlines of lacunæ and canaliculi are dark blue; ground-substance a light or greenish blue; cellular elements a diffuse blue. Schmorl advises this method for growing bone; in rickets the well-ossified areas alone stain well. Both of the Schmorl methods can be used for the study of **teeth** as well.

Staining of Sharpey's Fibres (Kölliker).

1. Harden, decalcify, imbed, cut.
2. Place section in strong acetic acid until it becomes transparent.
3. Stain in a saturated watery solution of indigo carmine for 15-16 seconds.
4. Wash in water; mount in glycerin.

Fibres red; ground-substance blue.

III. CARTILAGE.

Cartilage stains deeply with hæmatoxlyin; with Weigert's fibrin stain it holds the blue; with thionin and polychrome methylene-blue stains for mucin cartilage stains metachromatically red.

IV. CONNECTIVE TISSUES.

a. **Connective-tissue Fibrils.** The demonstration of connective-tissue fibrillæ or reticulum is of great importance in the differential diagnosis of sarcoma and carcinoma. *Van Gieson's* method is the best stain for the coarser fibrils, but does not bring out the finer reticulum as well as Mallory's aniline-blue method.

1. Mallory's Reticulum Stain.

1. Fix in mercuric chloride or Zenker's. After-harden in alcohol; imbed in celloidin or paraffin; cut.
2. Stain in 1/10 aqueous acid fuchsin 5-10 minutes.
3. Transfer directly to the following solution and stain for 20 minutes or longer:—
   Aniline-blue, water-soluble (Grübler).........0.5 grm.
   Orange G (Grübler).........................2.0 grms.
   1 per cent aqueous solution of phosphomolybdic
        acid ....100 cc.
4. Wash and dehydrate in several changes of 95 per cent alcohol; dry with absorbent paper.
5. Clear in xylol or origanum oil.
6. Mount in balsam.

Fibrils and reticulum of connective tissue, amyloid, mucin and connective-tissue hyalin are blue; nuclei, protoplasm, fibroglia fibres, axis cylinders, neuroglia fibres and fibrin are red; elastic fibres are pink or yellow; red blood-cells and myelin-sheaths are yellow.

2. Mall's Method for Reticulum.

1. Digest frozen sections of fresh tissue for 24 hours in a solution of Parke, Davis and Co.'s pancreatin 5 grms., soda bicarbonate 10 grms., water 100 cc.
2. Wash carefully in water.
3. Place section in test-tube half-full of water and shake thoroughly to remove cells.
4. Spread out on slide and allow to dry.
5. Allow a few drops of the following solution to dry on slide:—picric acid 10 grms., absolute alcohol 33 cc., water 300 cc.
6. Stain for 30 minutes in the following mixture: acid fuchsin 10 grms., absolute alcohol 33 cc., water 66 cc.
7. Wash in the picric acid solution for a second.
8. Dehydrate in absolute alcohol; xylol; balsam.

3. Unna's Method for Collagen.

1. Harden in absolute alcohol; imbed; cut.
2. Stain 5–15 minutes in polychrome methylene-blue.
3. Wash in water.
4. Differentiate in 1 per cent neutral orcein in absolute alcohol, 15 minutes.
5. Dehydrate in absolute alcohol.
6. Clear in xylol; mount in balsam.

Nuclei dark blue; protoplasm light blue; collagen dark red; plasma-cell granules greenish-blue; mast-cell granules red.

4. Mallory's Fibroglia Method.

1. Fix thin, small, fresh pieces of tissue in Zenker's fluid; harden in alcohol; imbed in celloidin or paraffin; cut.
2. Stain sections in 1 per cent aqueous acid fuchsin for 12 hours in the cold, or 20–30 minutes at 50–56°C.
3. Wash in water for 5 seconds.
4. Differentiate in 0.25 per cent aqueous potassium permanganate solution 10–20 seconds.
5. Wash in water for 5 seconds.
6. Dehydrate in alcohol; clear in xylol or origanum; mount in balsam.

Fibroglia fibrils and cell-nuclei intensely red; contractile elements of striped muscle, smooth muscle, neuroglia fibres, cuticular surfaces of epithelial cells and fibrin are also red; connective-tissue fibres brownish-yellow or colorless; elastic fibres, unless degenerated, bright yellow.

b. **Elastic Fibres.** Weigert's method is so superior to the Unna orcein-stain that it alone is given here. It is our best elective stain; gives permanent preparations, and is in every way practical. The stain keeps well.

Weigert's Method for Staining Elastic Fibres.

Preparation. Boil in a porcelain dish resorcin 4 grms., fuchsin (Grübler) 2 grms., and water 200 cc. After the mixture has boiled a few seconds add 25 cc. of liquor-ferri sesquichlor., Pharm. Germ. III. Stir well and boil for 5 minutes. When cool, filter. Carefully loosen the filter from the funnel, transfer it to the same porcelain dish which still contains a small amount of sediment, and add 200 cc. of 94 per cent alcohol. Boil and stir carefully. Remove the filter-paper when all the sediment is dissolved. Cool, filter; make up the filtrate to 200 cc. with 94 per cent alcohol, and to these 200 cc. add 8 cc. of hydrochloric acid. Resorcin-fuchsin may be obtained from Grübler, but the freshly-prepared stain gives better results.

1. Fix in any ordinary solution; imbed; cut.
2. Stain with lithium-carmine and differentiate in acid alcohol; wash thoroughly.
3. Stain in the resorcin-fuchsin mixture for 20-60 minutes.
4. Wash rapidly in acid alcohol.
5. Dehydrate and differentiate in absolute alcohol until section is red.
6. Clear in xylol; balsam.

Nuclei are red; elastic fibres blue-black. Should the stain when old give a diffuse staining differentiate for a longer time in acid alcohol.

c. **Fat Tissue.** Use same methods as advised for the demonstration of fatty degeneration and infiltration (osmic acid, scharlach R, sudan III).

V. EAR.

Remove temporal bone; fix in formol-Müller's; decalcify in trichloracetic acid; wash; after-harden in alcohol; imbed in celloidin. For nerve-endings use Golgi's and methylene-blue methods.

VI. EYE.

Fix in Müller's, formol-Müller's, Zenker's, formol, Flemming's or Marchi's solution. Aid fixation by incisions into sclera. The eye should not be left in formol for more than 3 days. Section as desired; imbed larger pieces in celloidin, small ones in paraffin. Use alum-carmine, iron-hæmatoxylin, Van Gieson's, Weigert's elastic stain, Levaditi's silver-method, Golgi's nerve-stain, methylene-blue method, etc., according to the object of the investigation.

VII. LIVER.

For the demonstration of the bile-capillaries *Weigert's neuroglia method* gives the best results. (See Page 300.) This method may be used with sections cut on the freezing-microtome after fixation in formol. Such sections are placed in a ½ per cent solution of chromic acid for 1 hour, transferred to the neuroglia mordant for 5-6 hours, washed well with water, and then treated as for the neuroglia method. Van Gieson's method may also be used for frozen sections of formol-fixed tissue. The walls of the capillaries show as fuchsin-colored streaks.

VIII. MUSCLE.

Van Gieson's is the best general stain for both striped and unstriped muscle, as it differentiates the muscle perfectly from the connective-tissue. Mallory's reticulum stain may also be used for the same purpose. For the study of myoglia fibrils the tissue must be fixed within a few minutes after its removal from the living body. Autopsy material cannot be used. These fibrils can be demonstrated by Mallory's fibroglia stain, or by Mallory's phosphotungstic-acid hæmatoxylin stain for neuroglia. (See below.)

IX. NERVOUS SYSTEM.

It is impossible in a book on general pathologic technic to consider all of the numerous staining methods that have been devised for the study of the nervous system. I have attempted, therefore, to pick out the best selective methods for the staining of the more important nervous structures, so as to cover adequately the general field of nervous pathology. Formol has now replaced Müller's for the preliminary fixation of nervous tissue, because of its quick action, and because after its use chromic acid may be employed to mordant the tissue, when it is desired to use certain staining methods requiring such mordanting. *Celloidin imbedding* is preferable, although paraffin may be used for general work. *General stains,* such as *hæmatoxylin and eosin,* and *Van Gieson's* are used for general impressions.

1. METHODS FOR STAINING GANGLION CELLS.

A. Lenhossék's Method.

1. Fix in equal parts of saturated watery picric acid and mercuric chloride (Rabl's mixture); after-harden in absolute alcohol; imbed in paraffin; cut.
2. Stain in saturated watery solution of toluidin blue, or thionin blue, for 12 hours.
3. Wash rapidly in water.
4. Differentiate carefully in absolute alcohol, or in aniline-alcohol (1-10).
5. Carbol xylol; xylol (quickly); balsam.

Nissl's granules are blue. This method is easy, and the best for general work.

B. Nissl's Method.

1. Fix in 96 per cent alcohol for 2-5 days; mount tissue in gum arabic on block; harden in 96 per cent alcohol; cut; place sections in 96 per cent alcohol.
2. Stain in methylene-blue soap mixture (methylene-blue B 3.75 grms., Venetian soap shavings 1.75 grms., water 1,000 cc. Shake well. Keep 3 months before using. Shake and filter before using.), warming, until bubbles arise.
3. Differentiate in aniline alcohol (aniline oil 10 parts, 96 per cent alcohol 90 parts) very rapidly.
4. Arrange section on slide; dry with blotting-paper; cover with cajuput oil.
5. Blot; wash off oil with benzene.
6. Remove benzene; mount the wet section in xylol colophonium, slightly warming; press on cover, and remove excess of colophonium.

Nuclei of ganglion cells light blue; granules dark blue. Toluidin blue, thionin, dahlia, Bismarck brown or neutral red may be used instead of methylene-blue, and often give better results.

2. METHODS FOR STAINING MYELIN SHEATHS.
A. Weigert's Method.
1. Fix in formol 2-3 days.
2. Primary mordant (potassium bichromate 5 grms., fluorchrom 2.5 grms., water 100 cc.; boil and filter) 4-6 days.
3. Without washing after-harden in graded alcohols, in the dark.
4. Imbed in celloidin.
5. Secondary mordant (neutral copper acetate 5 grms., fluorchrom 2.5 grms., water 100 cc., boil and add 36 per cent acetic 5 cc.) for 1 day at 37°C.
6. Transfer to 70-80 per cent alcohol.
7. Cut.
8. Stain in Weigert's iron-hæmatoxylin, 24 hours.
9. Wash in water, 30 minutes or longer.
10. Differentiate in borax-potassium ferricyanide (potassium ferricyanide 2.5 grms., borax 2 grms., water 100 cc.) until the gray substance appears yellow to white. Control under microscope.
11. Wash thoroughly in water.
12. Dehydrate in absolute alcohol; clear in xylol; mount in balsam.

Myelinated fibres, blue-black, upon a colorless or light yellow background; red blood cells may be blue-black. Weigert's method is better than any of the numerous modifications.

B. Orr's Osmic-Acid Method.
1. Place fresh tissue from cerebral cortex or cord, not more than ⅛ inch in thickness, in 1 per cent acetic, 2 cc., and 2 per cent osmic acid 8 cc., for 48 hours. If mixture is darkened at end of 24 hours, renew.
2. Transfer to 10 per cent formol for 3 days, in order to complete reduction and hardening.
3. Imbed in celloidin or paraffin; cut.
4. Remove paraffin; alcohol; water; differentiate in ⅛-1/12 per cent potassium permanganate.
5. Transfer to a 1 per cent oxalic acid solution, until sections become yellowish-green.
6. Wash; dehydrate; xylol; balsam.

Nerves and fat black; tissue yellowish-green. A very reliable method.

3. STAINING OF AXIS CYLINDERS.
Stain with Van Gieson's (red), Mallory's aniline blue method (red), lithium carmine (red), or

Williamson's Modification of Bielschowsky's Method.
1. Fix in Müller's; imbed; cut.
2. Place sections in 10 cc. of tap water containing a few drops of formalin, 5 minutes.
3. Wash in water.

4. Place in the following silver bath 5-10 minutes: 3 drops of liq. ammoniæ (B.P.) are dropped into a test tube. Add 10 per cent silver nitrate solution, drop by drop, until a brownish precipitate is formed. Dissolve the latter by adding ammonia, drop by drop, until the fluid is quite clear. Add tap water up to 10 cc.
5. Wash thoroughly in water.
6. Transfer to the dilute formol solution until sections become grayish-black (1-3 minutes).
7. Place in the following solution for a few minutes: To 10 cc. of water add 2 drops of 1 per cent watery solution of chloride of gold, a few drops of saturated borax solution, and a few drops of a 10 per cent solution of potassium carbonate.
8. Transfer to a 10 per cent aqueous solution of sodium hyposulphite for a few minutes.
9. Wash in water; dehydrate in alcohol; clear in oil of cajuput; xylol; balsam.

Axis-cylinders, intracellular fibrils and Golgi's network are stained.

4. STAINING OF NEURO-FIBRILLAR STRUCTURES.

These are stained by Bielschowsky's method, and by acid fuchsin after fixation with osmic acid. The special methods (Apathy's gold method, Bethe's molybdic method, the silver methods of Ramon y Cajal and Robertson) have little practical application in pathologic work, and are used chiefly in the study of normal histology.

5. THE STAINING OF NEUROGLIA.
A. Weigert's Method.

1. Fix small pieces of fresh tissue in 10 per cent formol for 24 hours.
2. Mordant, 8 days at room temperature (4 days at 37°C.) in copper acetate 5 grms., fluorchrom 2.5 grms., acetic acid 5 cc., water 100 cc.

Or, harden and mordant at the same time in 9 parts of the copper mordant, and 1 part of commercial formol for 8 days, changing on the second day, and once again later.

3. Wash in water; after-harden in alcohol; imbed in celloidin; cut.
4. Place sections in ½ per cent aqueous solution of potassium permanganate.
5. Wash in two changes of water.
6. Place in the following reducing mixture, 2-4 hours: Chromogen 5 grms., formic acid (sp. gr. 1.2) 5 cc., water 100 cc.; filter; to 90 cc. add 10 cc. of 10 per cent sodium sulphite solution just before using.
7. Wash twice in water.
8. Place sections in 5 per cent carefully filtered aqueous chromogen solution 10-12 hours. (The glia fibres become darker, and a yellowish contrast is obtained for the ganglion and ependymal cells and thicker axis cylinders. Connective-tissue is stained red.)
9. Wash in water.

10. Place section on a slide freshly cleaned with alcohol; dry with filter paper; stain in the following mixture for about 30 seconds: Saturated solution of methyl violet in 70-80 per cent alcohol 100 cc., oxalic acid 5 per cent solution, 5 cc.
11. Remove excess of stain; dry with filter paper; cover slide with saturated solution of iodine in 5 per cent potassium-iodide solution, 30 seconds.
12. Remove iodine solution; dry with filter paper; differentiate in a mixture of equal parts aniline oil and xylol until no more heavy clouds of stain are given off. Control under microscope.
13. Dry section with filter-paper; add xylol; blot; repeat three times.
14. Mount in balsam or turpentine colophonium.

Neuroglia fibres and nuclei, blue; connective-tissue, blue-violet; thicker myelin sheaths, ganglion and ependymal cells, yellowish. This is the best method, none of the modifications giving as good results. No method, however, will stain every neuroglia-fibre.

B. Mallory's Neuroglia Method.

1. Fix small pieces in 10 per cent formol, 4 days.
2. After-harden in saturated watery picric solution 4-8 days; or combine 1 and 2 by using formol 10 cc. with 90 cc. saturated picric acid solution.
3. Place in a 5 per cent aqueous solution of ammonium bichromate, 4-7 days at 37°C., changing solution on second day; or 3-4 weeks at room-temperature.
4. Without washing, harden in alcohol; imbed in celloidin or paraffin; cut.
5. Place sections in ¼ per cent aqueous solution of potassium permanganate, 15-30 minutes.
6. Wash in water.
7. Immerse in 5 per cent aqueous oxalic acid, 5-30 minutes.
8. Wash in several changes of water.
9. Stain in following solution, 1-several days: Hæmatoxylin 0.1 grm., 10 per cent phosphotungstic acid 20 cc., hydrogen peroxide 0.2 cc., water 80 cc.
10. Wash rapidly in water.
11. Differentiate in freshly prepared 30 per cent alcoholic solution of ferric chloride, 5-20 minutes.
12. Wash in water.
13. Dehydrate in 95 per cent and absolute alcohol or blot with xylol.
14. Clear in xylol; balsam.

When Zenker's fixation is used, omit 2 and 3, and after cutting sections treat with Lugol's to remove mercury and then with 95 per cent alcohol to wash out iodine; then wash in water and proceed with 5.

Neuroglia, nuclei and fibrin, dark-blue; all else is pale yellow or gray. If the differentiation in 11 is omitted, the axis-cylinders and ganglion-cells are rose-pink; the connective-tissues, dark red-pink.

6. COMBINED STAINING OF SEVERAL NERVOUS STRUCTURES.

Various methods of impregnation with silver, gold or lead are used in histologic work, the Golgi methods and their modifications in particular. They have but little application in pathologic work, and for that reason are omitted here, as is also a consideration of Ehrlich's vital methylene-blue method and its modifications. Full details of these methods can be found in laboratory textbooks on histology.

7. METHODS FOR THE DEMONSTRATION OF NERVE-DEGENERATION.

A. Marchi's Method.

1. Harden small fresh pieces of tissue in Müller's fluid for at least 8 days. Handle tissue very carefully to prevent mechanical injury. The tissue may be placed first in formol, and then later transferred to Müller's fluid.
2. Place in freshly prepared Marchi's fluid (Müller's fluid 2 parts, 1 per cent osmic acid solution 1 part) for about 8 days in the incubator at 37°C. The brain requires a longer time. When the mixture loses the osmic acid smell renew it.
3. Wash in running water, 24 hours.
4. Harden in graded alcohols.
5. Imbed in celloidin; cut; dehydrate; clear; mount.

Degenerated nervous tissue (fat) is black; all else brownish gray. Contrast stain in Van Gieson's, lithium carmine, etc. This method is good for the demonstration of early degenerations.

B. Donaggio's Methods for Early Degeneration.

Method I—
1. Fix in Müller's fluid or in 4 per cent potassium-bichromate solution. The tissue may remain in the fluid for any length of time.
2. Transfer directly, without washing, to alcohol. Dehydrate; imbed in celloidin; cut sections 20-30 microns. Place sections in distilled water for a few seconds.
3. Transfer to the following mixture for 10-20 minutes: To 20 per cent solution of ammoniated chloride of tin add an equal amount of 1 per cent aqueous hæmatoxylin. Allow to stand for five days. Keep in the dark, and in a cool place.
4. Wash rapidly in distilled water.
5. Differentiate in Pal's solution (oxalic acid 0.5 grm., potassium sulphite 0.5 grm., water 100 cc.) until the normal fibres are entirely decolorized.
6. Dehydrate; xylol; neutral balsam.

Degenerated fibres blue; normal, decolorized.

Method II—
1. Fix in Müller's fluid; imbed as in Method I.
2. Place sections in 0.5-1 per cent aqueous hæmatoxylin solution, 10-20 minutes.

3. Transfer directly to a saturated aqueous solution of neutral acetate of copper, 30 minutes. Renew copper solution once.
4. Decolorize as in Method I.
5. Wash rapidly in distilled water.
6. Dehydrate in graded alcohols; xylol; balsam.

Degenerated fibres black; normal fibres unstained, except for a narrow circle at periphery.

Method III—
1. Fix and imbed as in Method I.
2. Stain in 0.5-1 per cent aqueous hæmatoxylin solution, 10-20 minutes.
3. Transfer directly to 10-20 per cent solution of perchloride of iron. The section becomes black. After a few seconds they lose their color. If washed in water, they regain their color.
4. Without washing, differentiate in acid alcohol (0.75 cc. HCl in 100 cc. alcohol).
5. Dehydrate in absolute alcohol; xylol; balsam.

Degenerated fibres appear as small black streaks or circular areas.

C. Staining of Fat-granule Cells.

Fix in Flemming's or Marchi's mixtures; or in formol, staining with sudan III or scharlach R. The tissues may be examined also in the fresh condition.

D. Old Degenerations.

Use Weigert's myelin method to show absence of myelinated fibres. Van Gieson's method stains the, neroglia of degenerated areas a deep red; it is very useful combined with Weigert's myelin stain. Weigert's neuroglia stain may be used to demonstrate the relative parts played by neuroglia and connective-tissue in the formation of sclerotic patches. When Weigert's iron-hæmatoxylin is used with Van Gieson's the neuroglia remains unstained, while the connective-tissue stains red. With other hæmatoxylins the neuroglia cannot be sharply differentiated from connective-tissue when stained with Van Gieson's.

8. PERIPHERAL NERVES.

Use any of the above methods for the staining of myelin sheaths, ganglion cells, axis cylinders, etc. Van Gieson's is good for the demonstration of connective-tissue increase. For the demonstration of peripheral fibrils and nerve-endings consult textbooks on histology for Golgi methods, Ehrlich's vital methylene-blue method, and the modifications of May, Drasch, and others.

Platner's Method.

1. Harden in 25 per cent solution of liq. ferri sesquichlor., 1-5 days.
2. Wash in water, until the addition of KCNS to the water yields no reaction.

3. Place in 75 per cent alcohol containing an excess of di-nitro-resorcin, 2-30 days, according to the size of the piece of tissue.
4. Dehydrate in absolute alcohol.
5. Imbed; cut; dehydrate; clear; mount.

Axis cylinders, emerald green. A good method for the rapid demonstration of pathological processes connected with the peripheral nerves.

9. CHROMAFFINIC TISSUES.
Wiesel's Method.

1. Fix 1-4 days in 10 parts of a 5 per cent potassium bichromate solution, 20 parts of 10 per cent formol, 20 parts distilled water.
2. 1-2 days in 5 per cent potassium bichromate.
3. Wash thoroughly in running water, 24 hours; harden in graded alcohols; imbed in paraffin.
4. Stain sections in a 1 per cent aqueous toluidin-blue or water-blue solution.
5. 5 minutes in tap-water.
6. Stain 20 minutes in a 1 per cent watery safranin solution.
7. 96 per cent, and then absolute alcohol, until the blue color appears.
8. Xylol; balsam.

Chromaffinic cells green; other cells light blue, nuclei red.

X. SKIN.

Skin should be fixed in formol-Müller's or formol, and should not be left too long in alcohol or xylol. Imbed in celloidin preferably. For general use the ordinary stains suffice; for the study of pigment stain with alum or lithium-carmine. Use Weigert's elastic-tissue stain for the demonstration of elastic fibrils. The intercellular bridges may be demonstrated by Van Gieson's (remaining unstained), or by various special staining methods.

Herxheimer's Method for Epithelial Fibrillae.

1. Harden; imbed; cut.
2. Stain in a saturated watery solution of kresyl-echt-violett.
3. Dehydrate in absolute alcohol; clear in clove oil; balsam.

CHAPTER XXIX.
MICROSCOPIC EXAMINATIONS FOR MEDICO-LEGAL PURPOSES.

1. **BLOOD.** Fresh spots should be scraped off and examined in physiologic salt solution. Older spots are scraped off when possible, or if the spots are on clothing or other fabrics, a piece of the stained portion is cut out, and the scraping or piece of material is placed on a slide in a macerating fluid (30 per cent caustic potash; glycerin 3 parts and concentrated sulphuric acid 1 part; 15 per cent tartaric acid; equal parts alcohol and ether; or Pacini's fluid [mercuric chloride 1 grm., sodium chloride 2.0 grm., glycerin 100 cc., water 300 cc.]). Even in very old clots or stains some red cells may retain their characteristic form. The process of maceration should be observed directly under the microscope, as the macerating fluid gradually changes the cells after they become loosened. *Schmorl* advises the following method:—

Moisten a small piece of the fabric in water and stain with hæmatoxylin. Differentiate in acid alcohol, wash thoroughly in water, stain with 1/1000 watery eosin solution, wash in water (3-6 hours), place in alcohol, and then again in water. Tease with great care into fine threads on the slide, and examine the isolated fibres in a drop of glycerin. The red corpuscles are easily recognized; and the nuclei of the white cells or of the red cells of birds and amphibia stand out distinctly. Permanent mounts may be made by passing the specimen through alcohol, xylol, and mounting in balsam. A portion of the stained fabric may be imbedded in celloidin, sections cut, and stained with hæmatoxylin and eosin.

The **red cells** may be measured by the ocular micrometer. Those of man are somewhat larger than those of other mammals, but the difference in size is so slight that an absolute determination of the source of the blood is not possible from the consideration of size alone. Human corpuscles measure 0.0077 mm. in diameter; the nearest in size are the corpuscles of the dog, rabbit, hog, cow, horse, cat and sheep, in the order given, those of the sheep being smaller. The measurements of a large number of corpuscles must be taken if the question of size is to be considered. When red cells cannot be found the stains must be tested for the presence of **blood** pigment (*Teichmann's hæmin crystals*). A small piece of the scraping or stained fabric is placed upon a slide in glacial acetic acid; the fluid is expressed; and a small crystal of sodium chloride or sodium iodide is added to the fluid. Cover with cover-glass and heat gently until bubbles are given off, and continue carefully until the acetic acid has evaporated. The slower the evaporation the larger the crystals will be. Examine with a 1/6 inch or No. 7 objective. The hæmin crystals are brown or claret-colored, of the shape of rhombic plates single or superimposed. They are insoluble in water, alcohol and ether; dissolve slowly in ammonia, dilute sulphuric and nitric acids, and easily in caustic potash. The form of the crystal and the color determines the diagnosis of the presence of blood, but does not distinguish between human and animal blood. Old stains should be treated with acetic acid 12-24 hours before attempting to obtain the crystals. Contamination of the fabric with fat interferes with the reaction; the fat should be removed first with ether. If the suspected stain occurs on iron, steel, sand, clay or coal, the crystals usually cannot be obtained. Decomposition may also interfere with the reaction. In such cases a solution of the stain in a saturated solution of borax should be made and submitted to spectroscopic examination. The presence of blood-pigment on any substance can be demonstrated by means of the **spectroscope** or **microspectroscope**. Within recent years the **biologic** test for blood and albumins has been turned to medicolegal uses, in the differential diagnosis of human and animal blood or albumins. This test rests upon the principle that in the serum of an animal treated with human blood or albumin there are developed antibodies having a strong specific hæmolytic or precipitating action upon human blood or albumin.

2. **Semen.** Suspected seminal stains may be tested first by the **Florence sperm reaction.** A portion of the material is mixed on the slide with a drop of an iodine solution (1.65 iodine, 2.54 potassium iodide, 30 water). Cover and examine with low power. The formation of characteristic long rhombic, brown or violet crystals is evidence of the presence of semen. The reaction is hindered by decomposition. The **spermatozoa** may also be demonstrated in seminal stains by soaking the fabric, carefully flattened out, in a watch-glass containing dilute hydrochloric acid (1 drop to 40 cc. distilled water), for 5 minutes to 5 hours, according to the age of the stain. The fabric is then removed and gently rubbed on a slide; the smear is covered with a No. 1 cover-slip, and examined with the oil immersion or the highest dry objectives. The smear may be stained by adding

neutral red solution to the macerating fluid, or by drying the smear in the air, fixing in the flame, and staining with hæmatoxylin and eosin, neutral carmine or fuchsin. The staining and macerating solutions may be combined in one. The piece of fabric containing the suspected seminal stain is soaked in a mixture of methyl green 1 grm., hydrochloric acid 15 drops, distilled water 350 cc., for 1-6 hours. It is then removed with the forceps and smeared on the slide, examined in the moist state, or dried, fixed and mounted. The head is stained an intense green.

3. **Decidua and Foetal Tissues.** Clots, curettings and discharges may be examined in the fresh state by teasing; or the material may be fixed in formol, formol-Müller's or mercuric chloride. The characteristic structures of the decidual cells, chorionic villi and other fœtal tissues are easily recognized and the presence of any one of these determines the occurrence of pregnancy, abortion or child-birth.

4. **Hair.** The most important medicolegal question concerning hair is the differential diagnosis between animal and human. The following points must be considered:—

1. The cells of the outer layer (cuticle) of the hair are much larger in the majority of animals than in man, and are much more distinctly seen. The cuticle is much more dentate or serrate in the hair of animals than in that of man.

2. The cortical layer in human hair is much thicker than in animal hairs, as compared to the thickness of the medulla; in animal hair the medulla is thicker than the cortical layer.

3. The cellular structure of the medullary substance is indistinct in human hair; in animal hair it is very prominent. In human hair the medulla is often absent, especially in certain portions of the hair, while in animals it is rarely absent, and then only in sharply localized portions. The hair should always be examined throughout its entire length.

Hairs of the beard are usually thickest (0.14-0.15 mm. in diameter), then follow in order of size the pubic hairs of the female, the hairs of the eye-lids, male pubis, male head, and female head (0.06 mm. in diameter). There are, however, marked individual differences, and the hair of infants is much finer than that of older children and adults. The hairs of the new-born are pointed, as are also the hairs of adults that are protected from cutting, rubbing, maceration, etc. Cut hairs are at first blunt; later more rounded. Hairs that have been torn out usually show a bulbous end with the remains of the hair-follicle; fallen hairs have a closed, smooth, atrophic root. When the question arises as to the definite individual from whom certain hairs may have come a very careful comparison of the given hairs with those of the individual concerned must be carried out, as to color, size, thickness of different layers, shape and size of the transverse section, etc. Paraffin imbedding should be employed for this purpose.

CHAPTER XXX.
THE STUDY OF MOUNTED PREPARATIONS.

1. **Preparation.** Analyze the method of preparation of the specimen, noting methods of fixation, hardening, imbedding, injection, impregnation, staining, etc. Note the reaction of nucleus, protoplasm, red blood-cells and connective-tissue to the stain. Look for special staining reactions (hyalin, amyloid, mucin, etc.) and metachromasia.

2. **Histology.** Look for histologic landmarks by which the organ, or part of the body, from which the specimen is taken can be recognized. If such landmarks cannot be found, analyze the section, element by element, until its histologic features are fully noted and recognized. Answer the question, "From what part of the body does the tissue come?" Carry the differential diagnosis as far as possible, with regard to sex, age, side of the body or organ (for example, in the heart decide as to auricle or ventricle, left ventricle or right, etc.).

3. **Pathology.** Study next the deviations from the normal. Answer these questions: "Is the tissue normal?" "If not, in what respects does it differ from the normal?" Study pathologic conditions with the low power first, then use the high power for the finer details. Consider the histologic features of the organ (capsule, stroma, parenchyma, ducts, etc.) with respect to pathologic changes.

4. **Diagnosis.** After the pathologic changes have been fully studied, the diagnosis should be formulated. If the pathologic changes found can be correlated as factors in some specific conditions they should not be considered separately, but the specific condition itself would constitute the diagnosis. When the pathologic conditions have no definite relation to each other they should be classified separately. If a section of kidney shows cloudy swelling, congestion, œdema, small-celled infiltration, hæmorrhage and casts, these different conditions would all be included in the diagnosis of an acute parenchymatous degenerative nephritis. If the general picture corresponds to that of tuberculosis, syphilis, neoplasm, etc., the various associated changes need not be considered alone, but the broad and comprehensive diagnosis should be expressed in as concise terms as possible.

Written descriptions of microscopic appearances should be so full and clear that it is possible to make a diagnosis from the word-picture. A full and adequate analysis of the preparation set forth in concise and clear language is of more objective value than the bare diagnosis. Reproductions by means of drawings are also of great value in assisting the memory or in communicating the results of the observation to others. A technique sufficient for ordinary purposes may soon be obtained. Color work is usually easiest, since the majority of sections are stained in color. The camera lucida or Edinger's drawing apparatus may be of great service in the enlargement and placing of the various elements of the section; with these instruments but little practice is necessary to produce rapid and accurate representations. The close inspection of the preparation during the drawing often reveals features that previously had escaped attention. Many workers object to drawings on the ground of subjectivity, but the same criticism applies even more to word-descriptions. Especial attention must, however, be paid to this danger, both in the case of drawings and word-descriptions. In the case of scientific work the written description is best backed up by photographs, rather than by drawings. Microphotography has the very great advantage of being purely objective, although dishonest photographs are possible. There are, however, certain limitations to microphotography. Differential details are lost in sections; all parts of the section cannot be fairly represented; and focal and color limitations are great disadvantages. I believe, however, that for pure scientific work word-descriptions should be accompanied by objective microphotographs instead of drawings. The microphotographic outfit of Zeiss has already been recommended as the best. It is impossible to take up the subject of microphotographic technique in this book. The reader is referred to the chapter on "Microphotography" in Aschoff and Gaylord's Atlas, and to the works of Cresbie, Bagshaw, Kaiserling, Neuhauss, and others. (See article on *"Mikrophotographie"* in the *Enzyklopädie der mikroscopischen Tecknik.*)

INDEX.

A.

Abdomen:
  Inspection of..................... 45
  Section of........................ 140
Abdominal cavity, pathology of....... 102
Abdominal organs, pathology of....... 104
Abortion, death from................ 191
Acetic acid fuchsin.................. 220
Acetone 226, 237
Acetone-colophonium 278
Acetone-xylol 278
Acids:
  Acetic 220
  Chromic 228
  Fatty 268
  Mineral 220
  Osmic...............220, 230, 267, 299
  Picric 231, 258
  Poisoning with.................... 189
Acid fuchsin........................ 258
Acid stains......................... 253
Adrenals, examination of........145, 146
  Left 145, 155
  Right 146, 155
  Special pathology of.............. 155
African relapsing fever............... 284
Agar-formol 237
Age of newborn..................... 182
Alcohol 220, 227
Alcohol poisoning................... 189
Alkalies, poisoning with.............. 190
Alum carmine 256
Alum cochineal 283
Alum hæmatoxylin 254
Altmann's granules..............230, 265
Ammonium sulphide test............. 275
Amœba coli........................ 285
Amyloid, staining of................. 262
Aniline dyes 253
Aniline-xylol 270, 278
Animal parasites.................... 285
Anomalies 45
Antimony, poisoning with............ 190
Antrums, examination of............ 86
Aorta 120, 130
  Abdominal 158
Apathy's method.................... 300
Aronson-Philipp stain................ 292
Arsenic, poisoning with.............. 190
Artefacts 251
Asphyxia, death from................ 191
Atrophy 264
Atropine, poisoning with............. 190

Autopsy:
  General considerations............. 3
  Heller's method................... 30
  Importance of.................... 3
  Instruments 9
  Legal aspects of.................. 5
  Letulle's method for............... 30
  Medico-legal 187
  of newborn 177
  in animals 196
  Order of......................... 24
  Permit for....................... 8
  Preparation for................... 15
  Technique 20
  Time of.......................... 42
Axis-cylinders, staining.............. 299
Azur-blau 290

B.

Back, inspection of.................. 45
Bacteria:
  Acid fast........................ 280
  Actinomyces 278, 283
  Bacillus:
    Aerogenes capsulatus........278, 281
    of anthrax..................278, 280
    of bubonic plague...........279, 281
    of chancroid (Ducrez-Unna).279, 281
    Coli communis 279, 281
    Diphtheriæ 278, 281
    Dysenteriæ 279
    of epidemic conjunctivitis...279, 281
    of fowl cholera 279
    of Friedländer 282
    of glanders 279, 281
    of influenza 279, 281
    of Koch-Weeks 279, 281
    of leprosy 278, 280, 283
    of Lustgarten 280
    Mallei 279, 281
    of malignant œdema........279, 280
    of mouse septicæmia............ 278
    Paratyphoid 281
    Pestis 279, 281
    Pneumoniæ 279, 282
    Proteus 279
    Pyocyaneus 279, 281
    of rabbit septicæmia 279
    Rhinoscleroma 278, 282
    Smegma 280
    of swine erysipelas.............. 278
    of swine plague 279
    of tetanus 278, 281

INDEX.

	PAGE
Tuberculosis	278, 280, 282
of typhoid fever	279, 281
Cladothrix	283
Diplococcus pneumoniæ	278, 280
Gonococcus	279, 280
Gram-negative	278
Gram-positive	278
Leptothrix	283
Meningococcus	279, 280
Micrococcus:	
Catarrhalis	280
Melitensis	279
Tetragenus	278, 280
Nocardia	283
Oidium Albicans	278, 285
Spirilla and spirochaetes	283
Spirillum:	
of Asiatic cholera	279
Obermeieri	284
of recurrent fever	283
of Vincent's angina	284
Spirochæte:	
of African relapsing fever	284
of fowl-spirillosis	284
Pallida	279, 284
Refringens	284
Staphylococcus:	
Pyogenes albus	278, 280
Pyogenes aureus	278, 280
Pyogenes citreus	278, 280
Streptococcus pyogenes	278, 280
Vibrios:	
Staining of	283
of cholera	283
Balantidium coli	286
Basic stains	253
Basic aniline dyes	257
Beale's glycerin carmine	218
Béclard's center	181
Benda's method	268
Iron hæmatoxylin	273
Beneke's method	147
Best's glycogen methods	270
Bethe's method	300
Biebrich scarlet	293
Bielschowsky's method	299, 300
Bignami's method	286
Bile capillaries, demonstration of	297
Bile passages	151
Birch-Hirschfeld's method	263
Bismarck brown	257
Bladder, urinary	161, 163, 165, 169
Blastomycetes	285
Bleu Borrel	290
Blood:	
Biologic test for	306
Examination of	288
Fat in	293
Films	288
Fixing of	288
Medico-legal examination of	305

	PAGE
Parasites of	293
Sections	293
Size of red cells	305
Staining of	289
Blood content	39
Blood platelets	292
Blood vessels, peripheral	174, 176
Body, heat of	50
Böhmer's hæmatoxylin	254
Bone marrow:	
Examination of	173
Special pathology of	174
Staining of	293
Staining methods	294
Bones:	
Examination of	173
Special pathology of	174
Borax carmine	257
Bordeaux red	273
Brain:	
Basal vessels	89
Removal of	69
Section of	70
Section in skull	76
Section, Déjerine method	77
Section, Meynert method	77
Section, Pitres method	75
Section, Virchow method	70
Special pathology of	93
Bremer's reaction	292
Broad ligament	165, 172
Bronchi	118, 120, 128
Bunge's fluid	275
Burckhardt's fluid	231
Burns, death from	192
Buzzi's method	267

C.

Cadaver:	
Age of	42
Build of	44
External examination of	41
Facies of	44
Head of	44
Identification of	41, 187
Legal status of	5
Nationality of	42
Nutrition of	44
Occupation of	42
Orifices of	52
Palpation of	52
Percussion of	52
Restoration of	193
Sex of	41
Status of	42
Calcification	220, 264
Canada balsam	250
Carotids	134, 139
Carbol-kresyl-echt-violett	220, 263
Carbol-xylol	249
Carbon-monoxide poisoning	190

INDEX.

	PAGE
Carmine	256
Carmine, ammonia	258
Carmine and picric acid	260
Carnoy's fluid	231
Cartilage:	
Béclard's center	181
Costal	99, 105
Staining of	295
Cell granules	265
Cell inclusions	265
Cellodin	..234, 235, 239, 240, 243, 245, 247, 251
Cercomonas	286
Cerebellum:	
Examination of	92
Pathology of	92
Section of	74
Cerebrum:	
Examination of	90
Section of	70
Size	90
Weight	90
Cestodes	287
Chancroid, bacillus of	281
Chisel	12
Brunetti	15, 56
Curved	55
Esquirol	55
Straight	55
Tomahawk	55
Cholera, vibrio of	283
Cholesterin	266
Chorioid plexus	92
Chloral hydrate, poisoning with	190
Chloroform, poisoning with	190
Chromaffinic tissues	304
Chromic acid	228
Chromogen	300
Chromophilic cells	276
Claudius' method	223
Clearing	249
Clearing fluids	249
Cloudy swelling	266
Cocci, staining of	278, 279, 280
Coccidia	286
Cold, death from	192
Collagen, staining of	296
Colloid	266
Colophonium	250, 278
Color:	
of hair	48
of organs	35
Congo red	293
Connective tissue, staining of	295
Consistence	36
Copper, test for	276
Cord, spinal:	
Examination of	53, 61
Pathology of	61, 62
Removal of	57, 59
Size	61
Weight	61

	PAGE
Cornification	266
Courmont and Andre's method	276
Coverglass preparations	244
Cowper's gland	161
Cranium:	
Examination of	64
Examination of base	78, 93
Crushing	210
Crystal-violet	224
Cut surface	38

D.

Dahlia	271
Damar	250
Dark field	205, 284
Condenser	284
Death:	
Apparent	43
Icard's test for	43
Larcher's sign of	43
Magnus' sign of	44
Positive signs of	42
Ripault's test for	43
Tests for	43
Time of	42
Decalcification, methods of	232
Combined with fixation	232
Ebner's fluid	233
Haug's solution	233
Phloroglucin	233
Schaffer's	233
Sulphurous acid	232
Trichloracetic acid	232
Decidua, demonstration of	307
Deetjen's agar solution	292
Deformities	45
Dehydration	249
Déjerine method	77
Delafield's hæmatoxylin	255
Delépine's method	261
Diaphragm	98, 104, 148, 159
Differentiation	246, 247
Diffuse stains	258
Diffusion spots	51
Digestion	210, 217, 296
Diplococcus pneumoniæ	278, 280
Dissociation fluids	219
Donaggio's methods	302
Dorsal incision	60
Drawing	310
Duodenum	143, 150
Dura:	
Basal	93
of brain	88
of cord	60

E.

Ear	81, 82, 83, 94
Examination of	81, 82, 83, 94
Politzer method of examining	85
Microscopic examination of	297
Edinger drawing apparatus	310

	PAGE		PAGE
Ehrlich:		Formalin	229
Acid hæmatoxylin	255	Formol	229
Dahlia method	271	Formol-acetone	227
Triple stain	261, 292	Formol-alcohol	228
Ehrlich-Biondi-Heidenhain stain	273	Freezing and drying	229
Ejaculatory ducts	161	Heat	229
Elastic fibres:		Hermann's solution	230
Orcein stain for	296	Marchi's solution	230
Resorcin-fuchsin	296	Mercuric chloride solution	230
Staining of	296	Merkel's fluid	231
Weigert's method	296	Orth's fluid	228
Electricity, death from	192	Osmic acid	230
Eleidin	266, 267	Pianese's solution	230
Eosin	258, 259, 260	Picric acid solution	230
Epithelial fibres	304	Rabl's fluid	231
Ergot, poisoning with	190	Rawitz's fluid	231
Erlitzky's fluid	228	Rules for	226
Ether	220	Sublamine	230
Eustachian tube	83, 84, 85	Zenker's solution	230
Eyes	45, 94	Flemming's solution	230
Microscopic examinaton of	297	Flemming's solution and safranin	272
Pathology of	94	Fluids:	
		Burckhardt	231
		Carnoy	231
F.		Dissociation	219
Face	86	Ebner	233
Facies	44	Erlitzky's	228
Fat, in blood	293	Indifferent	219
Indophenol stain for	268	Maceration	219
Osmic acid stain for	267	Merkel	231
Scarlet R stain for	268	Müller's	228
Scharlach R stain for	268	Orth	228
Staining of	267	Pacini	305
Sudan III stain for	268	Physiologic	219
Fat-granule cells	303	Rabl	231
Fat tissue, staining of	297	Rawitz	231
Fatty acids	268	Fluorchrom	299
Fett Ponceau	220	Florence sperm reaction	300
Fibres, elastic	296	Fœtal tissues, demonstration of	307
Epithelial	304	Formalin	229
Sharpey's	295	Formol	229
Fibrin:		Formol-agar	237
Staining of	269	Formol-alcohol	228
Weigert's method of staining	269	Formol-gelatin	237
Fibroglia	296	Fowl-spirillosis	284
Mallory's stain for	296	Freezing	211
Filaria, staining of	287	Freezing and drying	229
Films, blood	288	Freezing microtome	211, 214, 216
Fisher's milk injection	218	Fresh material, examination of	208
Fixation	225, 288	Staining of	220, 243
Fixation and hardening	225	Treatment of	221
Acetone method	226	Fuchsin	257
Alcohol	227		
Altmann's solution	230	**G.**	
Burckhardt's fluid	231	Gaffky's method	281
Carnoy's fluid	231	Gall bladder	145, 155
Chromic acid and salts	228	Ganglia:	
Combined with decalcification	232	Cerebral	92
Determination of method	231	Spinal	60
Erlitzky's fluid	228	Sympathetic	148, 158
Flemming's solution	230	Ganglion cells, staining of	298
Flemming's chromacetic solution	231		

	PAGE
Gelatin preparations	223
Gentian violet	263, 279
Giemsa's method	291
Stain	284, 290, 291
Glycerin	219, 250
Glycerin-gelatin	250
Glycogen:	
Best's method for	270
in leucocytes	293
Staining of	270
Golgi's network	300
Gonococcus	279, 280
Gram-positive bacteria	278
Gram-negative bacteria	278
Gram-Weigert stain	269
Granules:	
Altmann's	230, 265
Basophile	290, 291, 292
Cell:	
Plasma	271, 272
Mast	271, 272
Eosinophile	290, 291, 292
Neutrophile	290, 291, 292
Nissl's	298
Green's method	263

H.

Hæmalum	255
Mayer's	255
Mayer's acid	255
Staining with	256
Hæmatoxylin	254
Alum	254
and acid fuchsin	259
and eosin	259
and orange G	259
and picric acid	259
Benda's iron	273
Böhmer's	254
Delafield's	255
Ehrlich's acid	255
Hansen's	255
Heidenhain's iron	273
Weigert's iron	255
Hæmolymphnodes	148, 158
Hæmosiderin	275
Hair	48
Medicolegal examination of	307
Hansen's hæmatoxylin	255
Hardening, methods of	225
Harke's method	85
Hasting's stain	290
Haug's solution	233
Head	44
Examination of	63
Inspection of	44
Heart:	
Left	125
Nauwerck's method of opening	114
Orifices and valves of	125

	PAGE
Prausnitz's method of opening	116
Right	124
Section of	107
Size and weight of	123
Special pathology of	126
Vessels of	125
Virchow's method of opening	113
Heat, death from	192
fixation by	229
Heidenhain's iron hæmatoxylin	273
Heller's method	30
Hermann's solution	230
Herxheimer's method	304
Hey saw	14, 85
Histologic features	39
Huber and Snow's plate method	245
Hyalin, staining of	271
Hydrocyanic acid, poisoning with	190
Hydropic degeneration	271
Hydroxides, potassium and sodium	220
Hypertrophy	271
Hypophysis	80, 92
Hypostasis	50

I.

Icard's test	43
Identification of cadaver	41, 187
Iliacs	158
Iliopsoas muscle	148, 159
Illuminating gas, poisoning with	190
Imbedding, methods of	234
Acetone	237
Celloidin	234, 235
Formol-agar	237
Formol-gelatin	237
Paraffin	234, 236
Pyridin	237
Incision, main	96
India ink method	284
Indophenol	268
Infanticide	191
Infiltration	234
Inflammation	271
Injection, methods of	217
Beale's glycerin carmine	218
Fisher's milk	218
Silbermann's	218
Thiersch's Berlin blue gelatin	218
Instruments, autopsy	9
Intestines	141, 150
Iodine-glycerin	220
Iodine, test for	272
Iodine green	263
Iodine test for amyloid	262
Iron:	
Ammonium sulphide test	275
Combined or masked	275
Potassium ferrocyanide test	275
Tests for	275

J.

	PAGE
Joints	174, 176
Jugulars	133, 139
Justus' test	272

K.

Kaiserling's method	222
Keratin	267
Keratohyalin	266, 267
Kidney:	
Left	145, 155
Removal of	145-147
Right	146, 155
v. Kölliker's method	295
v. Kossa's silver method	264
Kresyl-echt-violett	263, 273

L.

Laboratory, outfit	201
Utensils	207
Lævulose	250
Lake	253
Langhans' method	240
Larcher's sign	43
Larynx, section of	133
Pathology of	136
Lead, poisoning with	190
Test for	276
Legal aspects of autopsy	5
Leishman-Donovan bodies	286
Leishman's stain	290
v. Lenhossék's method	298
Leptothrix	283
Letulle's method	30
Leukocytes, staining of	291
Levaditi's method	284
Ligaments, broad	165, 172
Uterine	172
Lithium carmine	257
Liver, pathology of	153
Section of	144
Staining of	297
Location of organs	34
Luer's rhachiotome	14, 55
Lugol's solution	220
Lungs, section of	116
Pathology of	126, 127
Lustgarten's bacillus	280
Lymphatics	158
Uterine	172
Lymphnodes:	
Bronchial	118, 120, 129
Cervical	134, 138
Mesenteric	145, 155
Microscopic examination	293
Pelvic	165
Portal	145
Regional	174, 176
Retroperitoneal	148
Lymphocytes, staining of	292

M.

	PAGE
Maceration	210
Fluids	219
Macroscopic preparations	222
Magnus' sign	44
Malarial organisms	286, 291, 292
Mallory's method for actinomyces	283
for amœba	285
for fibroglia	296
for neuroglia	301
for reticulum	295
Mallory-Wright method:	
Serial sections	240
Tubercle-stain	282
Mall's digestion-method	296
Mamma	99, 105
Mann's method	287
Marchi's fluid	230
Method	302
Marking of plates	246
Mast cells, staining of	271
Material, examination of fresh	208
Treatment of	199
Mayer's acid-hæmalum	255
Hæmalum	255
Mediastinum, anterior	121
Medicolegal examination	305
Medulla	75, 92
Megastoma entericum	286
Melnikow-Raswedenkow	223
Meninges of cord	60, 61
Basal	89, 93
Inner	61, 89
Vessels of	88
Meningococcus	279, 280
Mercuric chloride fixation	230
Mercury, test for	276
Merkel's fluid	231
Mesenteric lymphnodes	145, 155
Mesentery	145, 155
Metachromasia	247, 254
Methods:	
Apathy's	300
Benda's	268
Best's	270
Bethe's	300
Bielschowsky's	299, 300
Bignami's	286
Birch-Hirschfeld's	263
Buzzi's	267
Claudius'	223
Courmont and Andre's	276
Delepine's	261
Donaggio's	302
Ehrlich's dahlia	271
Ehrlich's triple stain	261, 292
Fick's	267
Gaffky's	281
Giemsa's	284, 291
Golgi's	300
Green's	263

INDEX. 317

	PAGE
Herxheimer's	304
Huber and Snow's	245
India-ink	284
Jenner's	290
Kaiserling's	222
v. Kölliker's	295
v. Kossa's	264
Langhans'	240
v. Lenhossek's	298
Leveaditi's	284
Mallory's	240, 285, 295, 296, 301
Mallory and Wright's	240, 282
Mann's	287
Marchi's	302
Melnikow-Raswedenkow	222
Meynert's	77
Molasses plate	245
Morse's	263
Nikiforoff's	283
Nissl's	298
Noniewicz's	281
Pappenheim's	279, 292
Pianese's	265
Pick's	223
Platner's	303
Politzer's	85
Ramon j Cajal	300
Romanowsky	272, 286, 290
Schaffer's	233
Schmorl's	294
Schmorl-Giemsa	284
Schmorl-Obregia	240, 245
Silbermann's	218
Smith's	269
Strouse's	220
Trambusi's	293
Unna's chancroid	281
Collagen	296
Fungi	285
Mast cell	271
Van Gieson's	260
Warthin's plate	221, 245
Weigert's, elastic tissue	296
Fibrin	269
Gram	269, 278
Myelin sheath	299
Neuroglia	300
Westenhoeffer's	223
White's	261
Wiesel's	304
Williamson-Bielschowsky	299
Wolkowitsch's	282
Wood's	220
Wright's blood	284, 290
Ziehl-Neelsen	280
Zieler's	279
Methods of staining	246
Methyl blue	287
Methylene blue	257, 260, 289
Methyl green	257, 263
Methyl green-pyronin	279, 292

	PAGE
Methyl violet	262
Meynert's method	77
Micrococcus, catarrhalis	280
Melitensis	279
Tetragenus	278, 280
Micro-organisms, pathogenic	277
Microscope, accessories	201-205
Choice of	201
Polarization	205
Use of	203
Microspectroscope	205, 306
Microtome, choice of	206
Freezing	206
Knives	206, 211
Milk-injection	218
Mineral acids	220
Mitotic figures	272
Molasses method	221, 245
Mordant	253
Morse's method	263
Moulds, pathogenic	220, 285
Mounted preparations, drawing of	310
Photographing of	310
Study of	309
Mounting	243, 250, 251
Mouth	135
Muchæmatin	274
Mucin	273
Mucicarmin	274
Mucous membranes	49
Müller's fluid	228
Muscles	49, 102, 148, 159, 297
Myelin	274
Myelin-sheath staining	299
Myoglia	297

N.

Nails	49
Natural dyes	253
Neck	45
Neck organs, pathology of	135
Removal of	131
Section in situ	134
Necrosis	274
Negri bodies	286
Nematodes	287
Neoplasms	274
Nerve-degeneration	302, 303
Nerves, cranial	93
Inferior laryngeal	134, 139
Peripheral	174, 176, 303
Superior laryngeal	134, 139
Nervous tissue, staining of	298
Neurofibrillar structures	300
Neuroglia, staining of	300, 301
Newborn:	
Age of	182
Autopsy of	177, 182
Cause of death	185
Organs of	183
Size of	182

318 INDEX.

	PAGE
Nikiforoff's method	283
Nissl's granules	298
Method	298
Nitrobenzol, poisoning with	191
Nocardia	283
Nocht's stain	290
Noniewicz's method	281
Nose, pathology of	95, 136
Section of	85
Nuclear stains	246, 254
Nucleolus, staining of	258

O.

Occupation	42
Odor	37
Oedema	50
Oesophagus, pathology of	130, 136
Section of	120, 133
Oidium albicans	278, 285
Omentum	104
Opium, poisoning with	191
Orange G.	258, 259
Orbit, examination of	81
Orcein	279, 296
Organs, abdominal	104
of newborn	183
of special sense	174, 176
Thoracic	121
Orifices	52
Orr's osmic-acid method	299
Orth's fluid	228
Osmic acid	220, 230, 267
Ovary, pathology of	172
Section of	165

P.

Pacchionian bodies	88
Pacini's fluid	305
Palate	133, 135
Palpation	52
Pal's solution	302
Pancreas	144, 152
Panniculus	50, 102
Pappenheim's method	279, 292
Paraffin, imbedding in	234, 236
Mounting of sections	251
Ovens	207
Preparation of sections	244, 245, 246
Sections	241
Serial sections	242
Staining of sections	247
Parametrium	165
Parasites, animal	285
Parathyroids	134, 138
Parotid	86, 134, 138
Parovarium	165
Pathogenic, bacteria	277
Moulds	220, 285
Yeasts	285
Peduncles	92
Pelvis, examination of female	163

	PAGE
Examination of male	160
Penciling	216
Penis	163, 166
Percussion of cadaver	52
Pericardium	106, 122
Peripheral nerves	174, 176, 303
Peritoneum	148
Pharynx	133, 135
Phosphomolybdic acid	294
Phosphorus, poisoning with	190
Phosphotungstic acid	294
Pianese's method	265
Solution	230
Pick's method	223
Picric acid	231, 258, 259, 260
Picrocarmine	260
Pigment	274
Pineal gland	92
Pitre's method	75
Plasmodium malariæ	286, 291, 292
Plate method	245, 246
Platner's method	303
Plimmer's bodies	266
Poisoning:	
Acids	189
Alcohol	189
Alkalies	190
Antimony	190
Arsenic	190
Atropine	190
Carbon monoxide	190
Chloral hydrate	190
Chloroform	190
Ergot	190
Formalin	190
Hydrocyanic acid	190
Illuminating gas	190
Lead	190
Mercury	190
Morphine	191
Nitrobenzol	191
Opium	191
Phosphorus	191
Potassium chlorate	191
Potassium cyanide	190
Ptomaine	191
Strychnine	191
Suspected	188
Polarization microscope	205
Politzer's method	85
Polychrome methylene blue	264
Pons	92
Portal vein	145, 155
Potassium acetate	219, 250
Potassium ferrocyanide	275
Progressive staining	247
Prostate	161, 163, 168
Protocol	33
Pseudomucin	276
Purin bodies	276
Putrefaction	51

INDEX. 319

	PAGE
Pyridin	237
Pyronin	279, 292
Pyrosoma bigeminum	286

R.

Rabl's fluid	231
Rawitz's fluid	231
Reagents for fresh tissue	219
Rectum	161, 163, 165, 167, 169
Regeneration	276
Regressive staining	247
Repair	276
Resorcin-fuchsin	296
Reticulum	295, 296
Rhachiotome of Amussat	55
of Luer	14, 55
Rigor mortis	49
Ripault's test	43
Romanowsky method	272, 286, 290
Ross' electrical warmer	218
Russell's bodies	265

S.

Sarcosporidia	286
Scalp	87
Scalds, death from	192
Scars	46
Schmorl's bone methods	295
Schmorl-Obregia method	240, 245
Schmorl's method of examining blood	305
Scraping	209
Scrotum	167
Section cutting	210, 238
of celloidin blocks	239
of frozen tissue	239
of paraffin blocks	241
serial of celloidin	240
serial of paraffin	242
without imbedding	238
Sedimentation	209
Semen, tests for	306
Seminal vesicles	161, 163, 168
Sex	41
Shaking	216
Shape of organs	35
Sharpey's fibres	295
Silbermann's method	218
Silver, test for	276
Sinus, basal	93
Longitudinal	88
Size of organs	34
Skin	46
Staining of	304
Skull:	
Base of	78, 93
Pathology of	87
Periosteum of	87
Removal of cap	63
Smears	209
Soap, Venetian	298
Soaps, staining of	268

	PAGE
Sperm-reaction	306
Spermatozoa	306
Spinal cord	53, 57, 59, 61
Ganglia	60
Spirillum, Obermeieri	283, 284
of African relapsing fever	284
of fowls	284
of recurrent fever	283
of Vincent's angina	284
Staining of	283
Spirochæte:	
Pallida	284, 292
Refringens	284
Staining of	283
Spleen	140, 148, 293
Stage, mechanical	204
Warm	205, 218
Staining	246, 247, 253
General rules for	248
Huber and Snow's method	245
In bulk	247
Intravital	217
Methods	246, 247, 253
of bacteria in tissue	277
of blood	288
of celloidin sections	243, 247
of cover-glass preparations	244
of fresh tissue	220, 243, 247
of leukocytes	291
of paraffin sections	243, 247
of unimbedded tissue	243, 247
on slide	244
Plate method	245
Preparation for	243
Progressive	247
Regressive	247
Schmorl and Obregia method	245
Strouse's method	220
Supravital	217
Theories	253
Warthin's molasses method	245
Wood's method	220
Stains:	
Acid	253
Acid fuchsin	258
Alum carmine	256
Alum cochineal	283
Ammonia carmine	258
Aniline	253
Aniline blue	295
Aniline-gentian-violet	269, 282
Aronson-Philipp	292
Azur Blau	290
Basic	253
Basic aniline	257
Benda's	268
Benda's iron hæmatoxylin	273
Best's glycogen	270
Biebrich scarlet	293
Birch-Hirschfeld	263
Bismarck brown	257

	PAGE		PAGE
Bleu Borrel	290	Methylene blue	257, 260, 289
Borax carmine	257	Alkaline	257, 278
Bordeaux red	273	Morse's	263, 273
Carbol-fuchsin	280	Muchæmatin	274
Carbol-kresyl-echt-violett	220	Mucicarmin	274
Carbol-thionin	220, 286	Natural dyes	253
Carmine	256	Neutral red	217, 266
Carmine and picric acid	260	Nile blue	269
Combined	259	Nocht's	290
Congo red	267, 293	Nuclear	246, 254
Crystal violet	224	Orange G	258, 259
Dahlia	271	Orcein	279, 296
Delépine's	261	Pappenheim's	279, 292
Diffuse	246, 258	Phlosin-red	218
Eosin	258	Picric acid	258
Eosin and methylene blue	260	Picrocarmin	260
Ehrlich-Biondi-Heidenhain	273	Polychrome methylene blue.	264, 271, 276
Ehrlich's dahlia method	271	Pranter's	279
Ehrlich's triple	261, 292	Protoplasmic	246, 258
Erythrosin	253, 259, 261	Resorcin fuchsin	296
Fett Ponceau	220	Romanowsky's	272, 286, 290
Fuchsin	257	Rubin	259, 261
Gentian violet	263, 279	Safranin	272
Giemsa's	284, 290, 291	Scarlet R	220, 264, 268
Gram-Weigert	269	Scharlach R	220, 264, 268
Green's	263	Schmorl's, for bone	294
Hæmatoxylin	254	Schmorl-Giemsa	284
Alum	254	Selective	246
Böhmer's	254	Smith's	269
Delafield's	255	Specific	246
Ehrlich's acid	255	Sudan III	220, 264, 268
Hansen's	255	Thionin	220, 254, 264, 273
Weigert's iron	255	Thionin and phosphotungstic acid	294
Hæmatoxylin and acid fuchsin	259	Thionin and phosphomolybdic acid	294
Hæmatoxylin and eosin	259	Thionin-picric acid	294
Hæmatoxylin and orange G	259	Toluidin blue	253, 264
Hæmatoxylin and picric acid	259	Unna's mast cell	271
Hasting's	290	Unna's methylene blue	257, 271, 276
Heidenhain's iron	273	Unna's orcein	296
Indigo carmine	295	Van Gieson's	260
Indophenol	268	Vesuvin	253
Iodine green	220, 263, 265	Water blue	304
Jenner's	290	Weigert's elastic tissue	296
Kresyl-echt-violett	263, 271, 273	Weigert's fibrin	269
Leishman's	290	Weigert's neuroglia	297, 300
Lithium carmine	257	White's	261
Löffler's methylene blue	278	Wright's	284, 290
Magenta	286	Ziehl-Neelsen	280
Malachite green	265	Zieler's	279
Mallory's fibroglia	296		
Mallory's neuroglia	301	Staphylococcus	278, 280
Mallory's reticulum	295	Starvation, death from	192
Martius yellow	265	Status of cadaver	42
Mayer's acid hæmalum	255	Sternum	105
Mayer's hæmalum	255	Stomach	144, 151
Methyl blue	287	Streptococcus	278, 280
Methyl green	257, 263	Sublamine	230
Methyl green-pyronin	279, 292	Sublingual gland	134, 138
Methyl violet	262	Submaxillary gland	134, 138
Methylene azure	254	Sulphurous acid	232
		Supreme Court decisions	6, 7
		Surgical operation, material from	196

INDEX.

	PAGE
Surgical material, care of	198
Description of	197
Removal of	196
Surgical wounds	46
Sympathetic, abdominal	148, 158
Cervical	134, 139
Peripheral	174, 176

T.

Teasing	210
Technique, autopsy	20
Teeth, inspection of	49
Microscopic examination	295
Teichmann's crystals	301
Testicles	161, 162, 167
Tests, to determine death	43
Icard's	43
Ripault's	43
Tetanus bacillus	278, 281
Thiersch's Berlin-blue gelatin	218
Thionin	220, 254, 264, 294
Thoracic cavity	106, 121
Duct	120, 130, 134
Great vessels of	129
Vertebræ	120, 130
Thorax	45, 121
Thymus	106, 121, 184
Thyroid	134, 137
Time of death	42
Tissue, cultivation of	219
Tongue	133, 135
Tonsils	133, 135
Trachea	133, 136
Trambusi's method	293
Trauma, signs of	46
Trematodes	287
Treponema pallidum	284
Trichina	287
Trichloracetic acid	232
Trichomonas	286
Trichomycetes	283
Trypanosoma	286
Tubercle-bacillus	278, 280, 282
Tubes	165, 171
Typhoid-fever bacillus	279, 281

U.

Unimbedded tissue	243
Unna's alkaline methylene blue	257
Chancroid bacillus	281
Collagen stain	296
Glycerin-ether	271
Mast cell stain	271
Orcein stain	296
Polychrome methylene blue	271, 276
Stain for fungi	285
Ureters	158, 161
Urethra	161, 165, 168, 169

	PAGE
Uric acid	233, 276
Uterus	165, 170
Uvula	133, 135

V.

Vaccine bodies	287
Vagina	165, 169
Vagus	134, 139
Van Gieson's stain	260
Vena cava	158
Ventricles	72, 91
Venetian soap	298
Vermes	287
Vertebræ	60, 62, 139, 148, 159
Vessels, basal	89
Meningeal	88
Peripheral	174, 176
Uterine	172
Vesuvin	253
Vibrios	283
Vincent's angina	284
Violence, death from	192
Virchow method	70
Viscera, hollow	34, 40
Vulva	169

W.

Warthin's molasses method	245
Washing	248
Weigert's copper-fluorochrom	268
Elastic tissue stain	296
Fibrin stain	269
Gram method	269
Iron-hæmatoxylin	255
Myelin-sheath stain	299
Neuroglia	297, 300
Weight, of organs	34
Westenhoeffer's method	223
White's method	261
Wiesel's method	304
Williamson-Bielschowsky method	299
Wright's blood-stain	284, 290

X.

Xylol	249, 250
Acetone	278
Aniline	270, 278
Xylol-balsam	250
Xylol-damar	250

Y.

Yeasts, pathogenic	285

Z.

Zenker's solution	230
Ziehl-Neelsen method	280
Zieler's method	279

www.ingramcontent.com/pod-product-compliance
Lightning Source LLC
Chambersburg PA
CBHW051625170526
45167CB00001B/64